# RODALE'S HOME DESIGN SERIES™

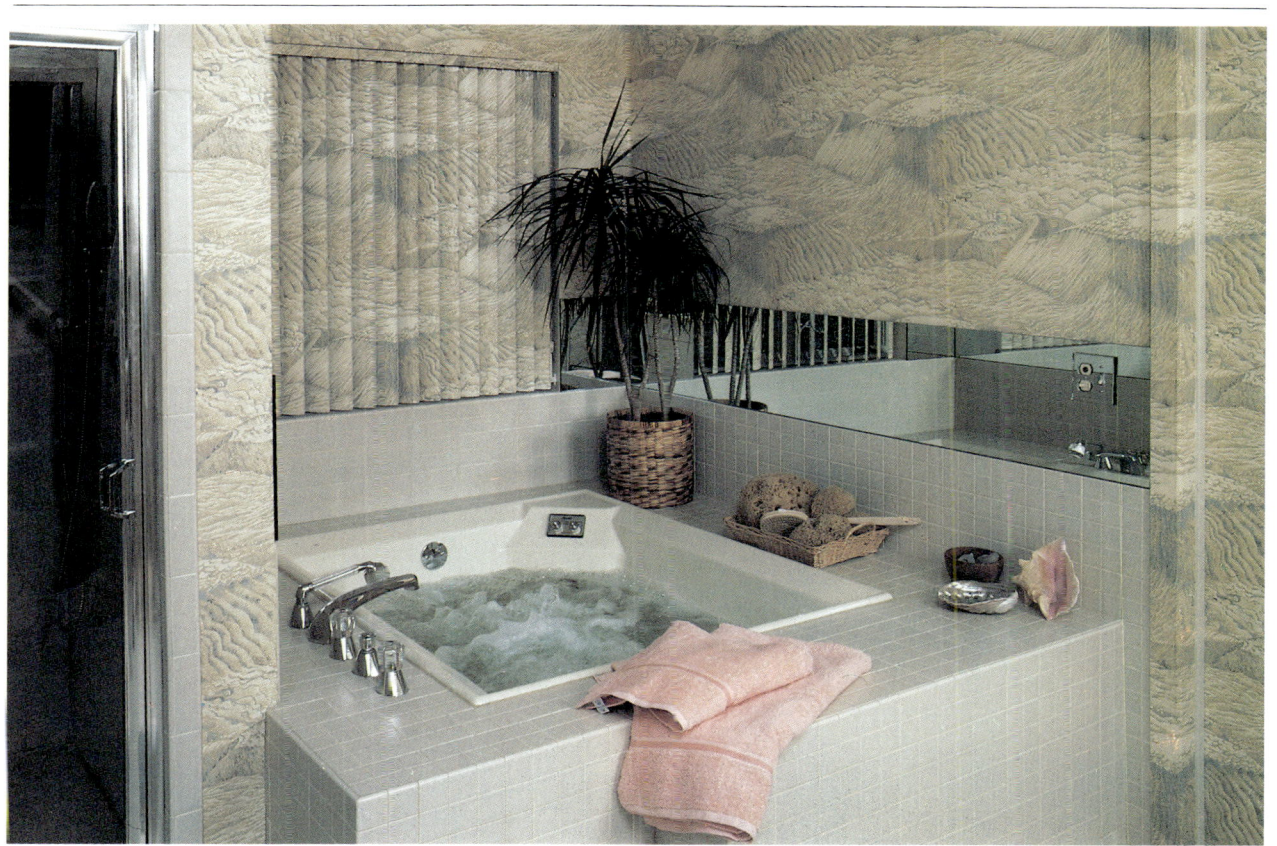

# BATHS

by the Editors of
*Rodale's Practical Homeowner*™ magazine

Rodale Press, Emmaus, Pennsylvania

Copyright 1987 © by Rodale Press, Inc.

All rights reserved. No part of this publication may be reproduced or transmitted in any form or by any means, electronic or mechanical, including photocopy, recording, or any information storage and retrieval system, without the written permission of the publisher.

Printed in the United States of America on recycled paper containing a high percentage of de-inked fiber.

Series Senior Editor: Ray Wolf
Series Editor: Margaret Lydic Balitas
Writers: Joe Carter, Catherine M. Cassidy, Ellen Cheever,
   Patrick J. Galvin, Michael Hamman, Suzanne Nelson,
   David Sellers, and Marguerite Smolen
Technical Reviewer: Fred Matlack
Editorial Assistance: Kerri Balliet and Bobbie Wanamaker
Copy Editor: Dolores Plikaitis

Director of Photography: T. L. Gettings
Series Photography Editor: Mitchell T. Mandel
Styling of Front Cover Photo: J. C. Vera

Art Director: Jerry O'Brien
Series Art Director and Book Designer: Karen A. Schell
Project Assistant: Denise Mirabello
Illustrator: John Carlance

**Library of Congress Cataloging in Publication Data**
Baths.

(Rodale's home design series)
Includes index.
1. Bathrooms—Design and construction. I. Rodale's practical homeowner. II. Series.
TH6485.B39   1987   643'.52   86-13007
ISBN   0-87857-639-8   hardcover
ISBN   0-87857-640-1   paperback

2 4 6 8 10 9 7 5 3 1   hardcover
2 4 6 8 10 9 7 5 3 1   paperback

Due to the variability of local conditions, materials, skills, site, and so forth, Rodale Press, Inc., and the authors assume no responsibility for any personal injury, property damage, or other loss of any sort suffered from the actions taken based on or inspired by information or advice presented in this book. Compliance with local codes and legal requirements is the responsibility of the reader.

# CONTENTS

ACKNOWLEDGMENTS — v

## DESIGN IDEAS
### NEW AND REMODELED BATHS — vi

#### A NEW VERSION OF THE BATH — 2
The philosophy of today's bath is quality space for quality time. Now a place for relaxing and enjoying life, the bath is a special world of elegance, spaciousness, and light.

#### THE WORKING PARTS — 20
What kind of fixtures (tubs, spas, whirlpools, toilets, bidets, sinks, showers) do you want in your new bath? New styles, colors, and materials offer stunning choices.

#### STORAGE IN THE BATH — 44
Everything in its place and a place for everything is the key to well-planned bathroom storage. Guidelines tell how to plan and "find" efficient storage space in the bath.

#### THE FINISHING TOUCHES — 60
Walls, floors, windows, lighting, and decorative accents have a profound effect on the look of a bath. Smart choices in the finishing touches complete a bath's decor.

## GALLERY
### A TOUR OF FINE BATHS — 78
Visit 30 of the best-designed baths in North America: master-suite baths, bodyrooms, family baths, spa rooms, children's baths, and powder rooms.

## WORKBOOK
### THE BASICS OF BATH DESIGN — 122

#### DESIGNING YOUR NEW BATH — 124
Learn design and construction tricks of the trade from professionals.

## HELPFUL ADDRESSES — 144

## CREDITS — 148

## INDEX — 152

# Acknowledgments

Margaret Lydic Balitas, series editor, gave this book form and nurtured its development from an idea into a book, and Catherine M. Cassidy wrote many parts of this book, including "A Tour of Fine Baths." Many thanks to the other writers who shared their expertise about the design and construction of bathrooms: Joe Carter, planning editor for *Rodale's Practical Homeowner* (formerly *Rodale's New Shelter*); Ellen Cheever, certified kitchen designer and member of the American Society of Interior Designers; Patrick J. Galvin, former editor and publisher of *Kitchen and Bath Business* and author of numerous books and articles; Michael Hamman, general contractor and writer; Suzanne Nelson, Rodale Press gardening editor; David Sellers, Rodale Press research engineer; and Marguerite Smolen, senior editor for *Rodale's Practical Homeowner*.

Fred Matlack, technical reviewer and manager of design at Rodale Press, read the manuscript to be sure that our information is accurate and up to date. Dolores Plikaitis, copy editor, ensured that we used correct English and that what we said made sense. Kerri Balliet diligently searched for photos to use in this book and checked numerous facts. Bobbie Wanamaker gave special research assistance.

The Rodale Press Photography Department is responsible for most of the lovely photographs in this book. Special thanks to Mitchell T. Mandel, series photography editor, who tirelessly scouted potential sites, who arranged for photo sessions, who reviewed hundreds of photographs, and who shot many of the photographs in this book.

Thanks, too, to photo stylists Lucretia Arpad, Kay Lichthardt, and J. C. Vera; and photo librarian Rose Reichl.

Many manufacturers lent photographs for use in this book. Larry C. Hatfield of American-Standard was always ready to answer technical questions.

Executive designer Karen A. Schell is responsible for this book's design and layout. Project assistant Denise Mirabello very capably assisted her and kept track of hundreds of details. Art director Jerry O'Brien was always available to offer suggestions. John Carlance's illustrations do much to show the basics of bathroom design.

Many people helped us locate the baths you see here, and we thank them. Special thanks to those who helped us locate the beautiful baths in "A Tour of Fine Baths": Lucretia Arpad, Carol Besler, Brion S. Jeannette, Heidi Kleinman, Mitchell T. Mandel, Karen Nelson, Anita Pearl, Dolores Plikaitis, Susan Smith, Alan Tariguchi, Vera Tweed, Susan Weaver, and Juanita Wall.

Without the gracious homeowners who welcomed us into their homes, "A Tour of Fine Baths" would not have been possible. Many thanks, too, to others who invited our photographers into their homes and willingly spoke to us about the design of their baths. The architects and designers mentioned in this book spent many hours discussing the fine points of design with us. And for this we are grateful.

So we have come full circle. Truly many people contributed to make this book one that we hope you will enjoy. And to all we give a heartfelt thanks.

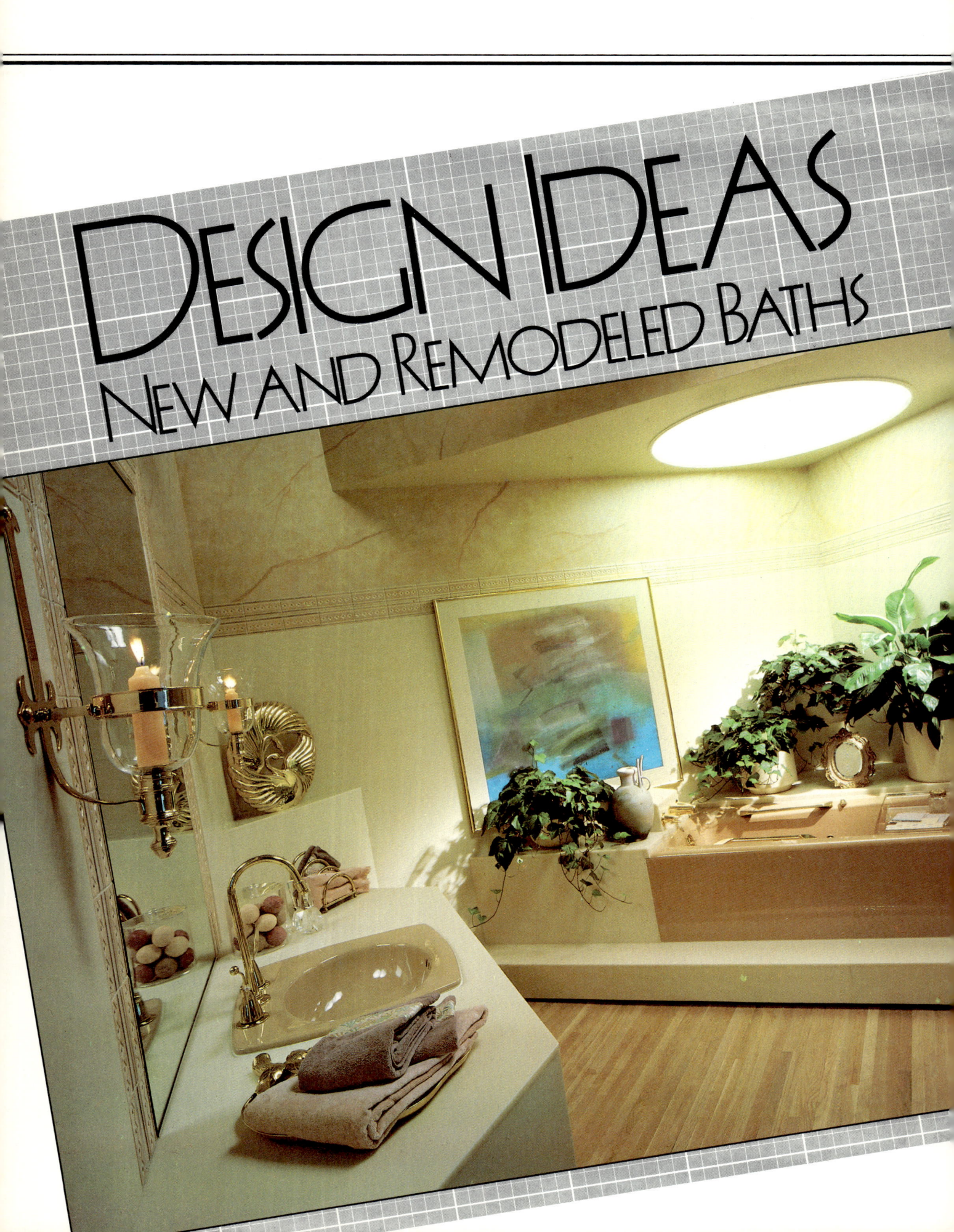

# Design Ideas
## New and Remodeled Baths

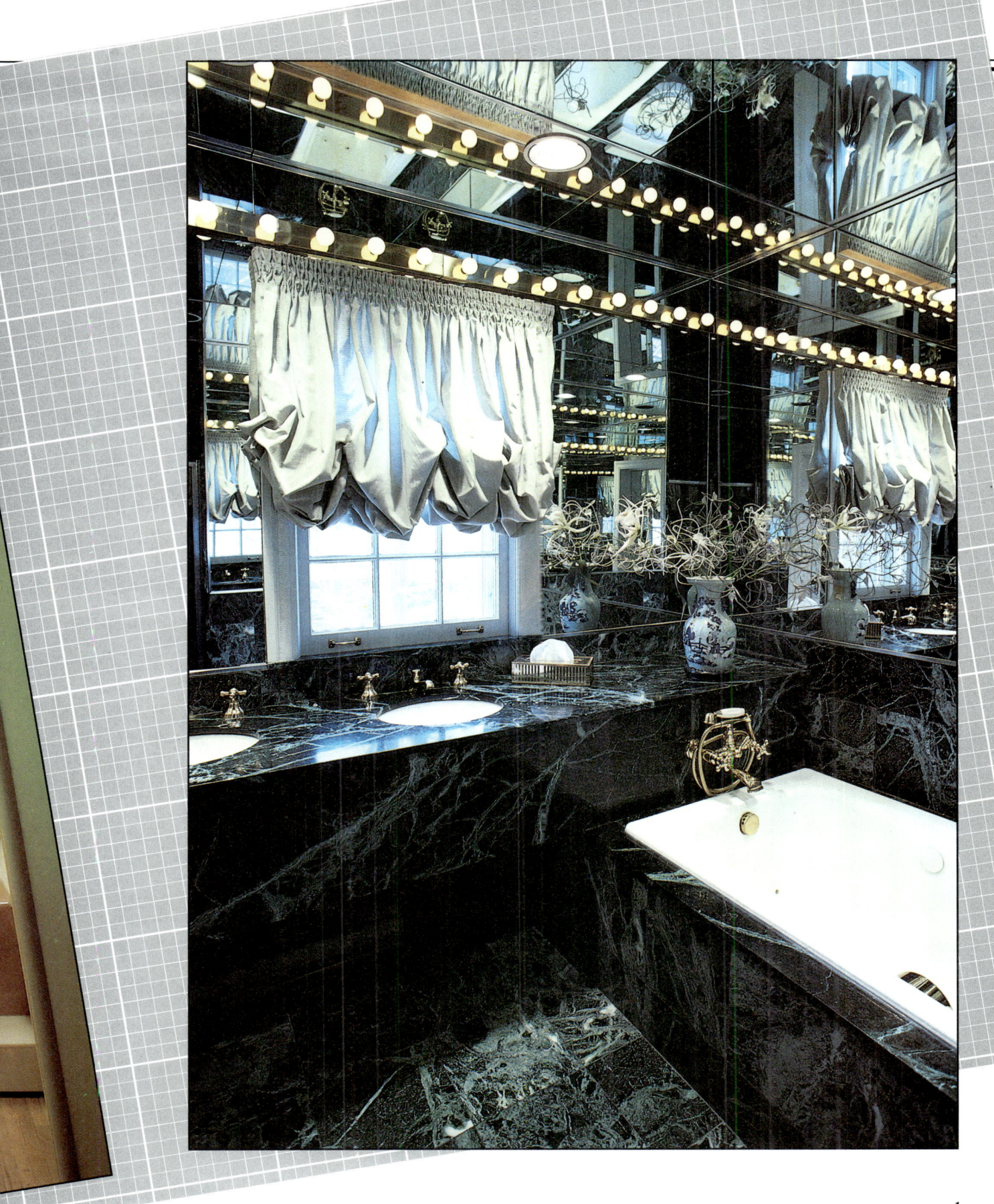

# A New Version of the Bath

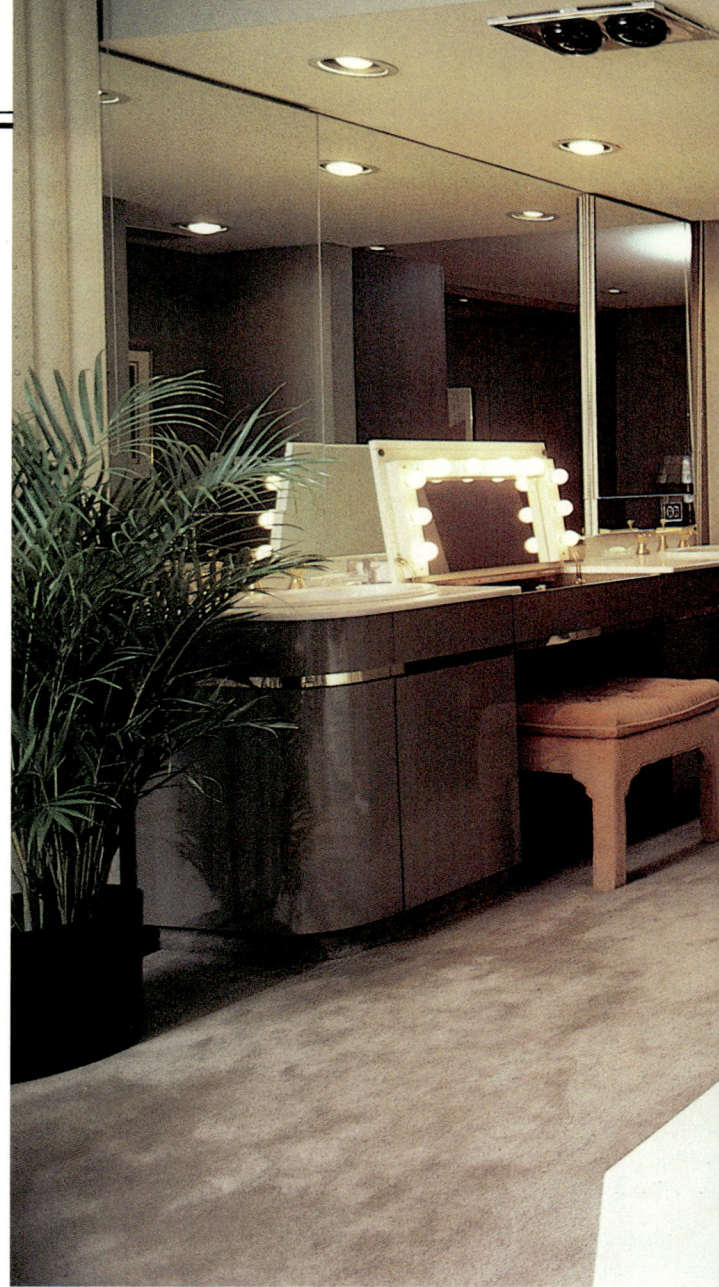

Think about a place in your home that provides total relaxation, a place that offers privacy, and that provides a very personal, pleasurable experience—a place in which you enjoy spending time. In today's home, you just might be talking about the bathroom.

If it sounds odd, it's because most of us are used to a startlingly different concept of the bathroom. Even as little as 10 or 15 years ago, the bathroom was not considered a room to be glorified. And with its unimaginative white fixtures, antiseptic features, and predictable design, it was hardly a place to pass time. Consequently, most of us have grown up with the notion that the bath is a room for necessary functions and little else.

But think about it: In how many places in your house can you *demand* complete privacy? Once you shut the bathroom door, you're free from the hustle and bustle outside. Barring interruptions, you can enjoy a few moments or hours of privacy, alone with your body, your thoughts, and your senses.

Western traditions and culture haven't made it easy for people to enjoy this private space. But times are changing, and the bathroom is finally being appreciated for the personal experience it affords. Today's bath concept is a reflection of that appreciation and a wonderful blend of the best of all bathing worlds.

It is no longer just a "necessary" space for perfunctory tasks. Like the Roman and Japanese baths of long ago, today's bath has again become a place to relax and rejuvenate the mind and body. It soothes and indulges the senses with color, light, and warmth, and it upholds bathing as an experience to be relished. Indeed, with its luxury appointments, the modern bathroom often bears far more resemblance to a Roman spa than to its lackluster American predecessors.

But unlike the communal baths of ancient times, today's baths are not designed for public experiences, but for private ones. Today's baths are for closing the door and hiding away, for lingering—for getting away from it all. They are places in which to wash away the cares of today's recklessly fast-paced world and to get in touch with body and spirit again. Today's baths are rooms to

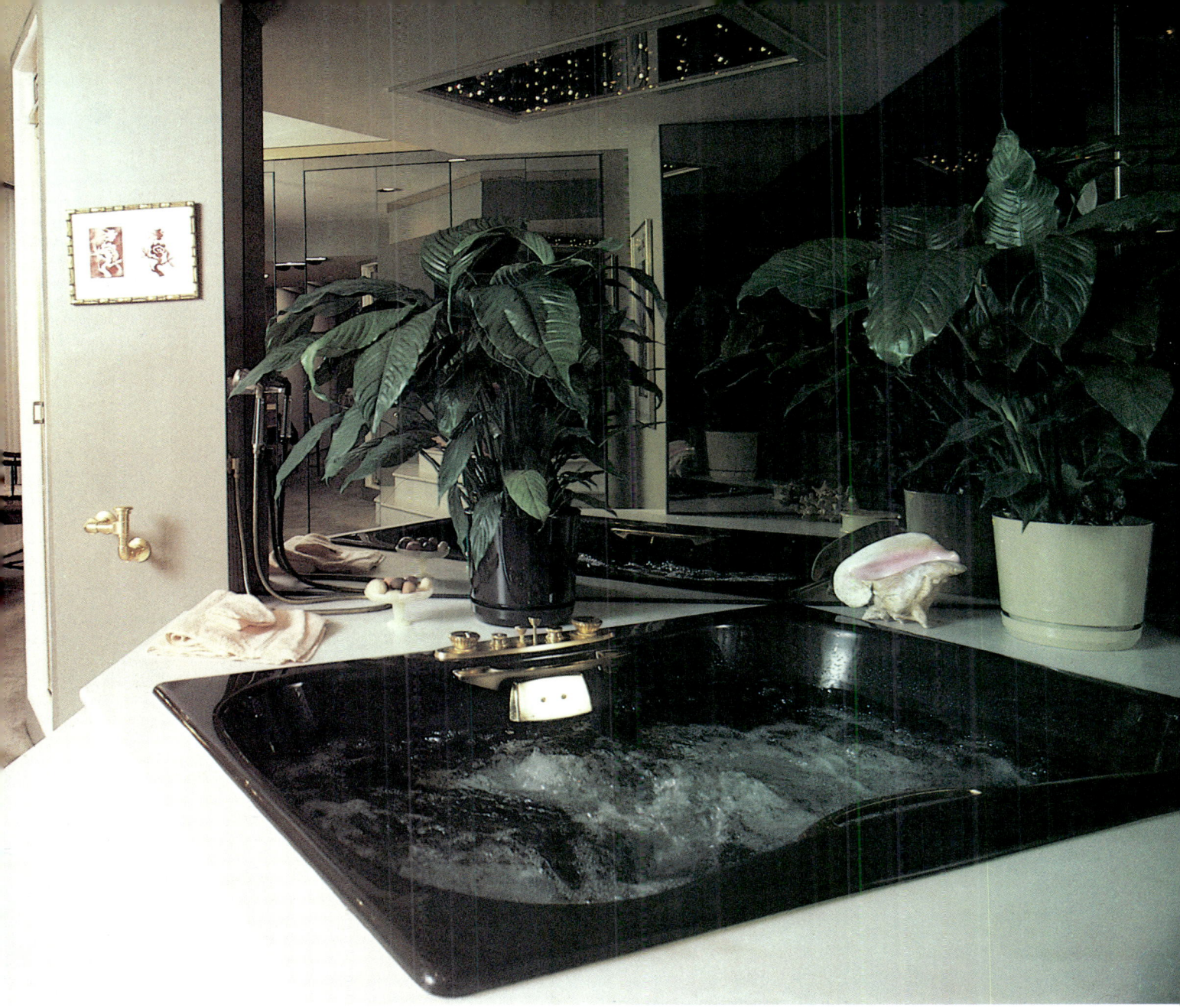

spend time in, and therefore rooms to love and embellish.

High design and luxury are watchwords among bath designers these days. But whether you're thinking about building a new bath, or renewing an outdated existing bath, the key word to remember when designing and decorating it is "personal." Your bath is your private, personal space in which to indulge your fancies and unwind. And this book will assist you in making the most of that space—whatever its size—by helping you create a bath that fulfills all your personal needs.

The ideal bath, however, is normally not what you'll find in the average home today. Because they were built 20, 30, or 40 years ago, many baths still have those dull white fixtures and traditional "bathroom style" wall and floor treatments. But these Spartan baths of yesteryear are no longer acceptable to modern homeowners, and they're going all out to make the bathroom a more pleasant place to spend time.

Some knock down walls and create brand new spaces for their baths. Others merely give existing bathrooms a face-lift by sprucing up walls and adding new fixtures and some well-chosen accessories. But while budgets and tastes may differ, the bathroom battle cry across the country is the same: out with the old and in with the new.

## What's New in Today's Bath?

Space, for one thing. The bathroom's size has virtually doubled in new home construction in the last 10 to 15 years, and remodelers are turning to closets and other cubbyholes to produce more space for bathroom redos. The more adventurous are transforming entire spare bedrooms into luxury bathing retreats. When space can't be bought—which is often the case—space-stretchers like mirrors and skylights are popular.

European bath design, with its sleek surfaces and high-contrast colors, has worked its way west and created bold new opportunities for bath designers. Clean lines and curves on cabinets, countertops, and tub surrounds, executed with smooth laminates (bench marks of the European-style bath), have become popular. The increasing use of bright primary colors, pedestal sinks, and bidets are other examples of the European influence.

Today's bath employs traditional materials in luxurious new ways. Rich-looking wood can be found not only in cabinetry but also on floors and walls. Marble graces tub surrounds and floors as well as countertops. Mirrors run from floor to ceiling, on several walls, and stained glass, glass block, and skylights add lighting interest. Ceramic tile, long a favorite in the bath because of its durability and easy maintenance, has taken on elegant new looks.

Fixtures today are as beautiful as they are functional. Manufacturers have commissioned top designers to produce sensuous-looking fixtures in the soft grays, blues, peaches, roses, and lavenders that are so popular with bathroom decorators nowadays. Faucets, hardware, and accessories, too, are designed both to work well and to look good.

Today's bathroom is a veritable playground for the imagination. You'll discover a wide variety of styles in the bath, each suited to a particular personal taste: Victorian romance, country charm, European high-tech, woodsy natural, marbleized elegance, contemporary luxury.

You'll also find a delightful array of items in bathrooms now that would never have been found there even 10 years ago: jetted whirlpool tubs, in-wall hair dryers, exercise equipment, plants (even patio gardens or greenhouses), furniture, fireplaces, artwork, wet bars, stereo equipment, television sets, telephones, and computers.

A luxurious bath doesn't have to be a resource waster, though. Today's homeowners are energy-conscious, and a number of new bathroom fixtures and devices reflect that consciousness. Tankless, point-of-use water heaters, water-saving toilets, radiant ceilings, and flow-restricting shower heads and sink faucets are among the energy-saving innovations found in today's baths.

And what's even more exciting than designing a beautiful new bath is that it all pays off. Studies show that people who are looking to buy a home place value on and will pay for a larger, better-appointed bathroom. Banks figuring to refinance your home recognize the value of an up-to-date bathroom. A remodeled, expanded bathroom will return 50 to 100 percent of its original cost when you resell the house; 40 to 130 percent when you go to a bank to refinance.

Quality space for quality time—that's the philosophy behind today's bathroom

Fine woods, custom ceramic tiles, and fixtures and accessories crafted in a wealth of luxurious materials make today's baths veritable showpieces.

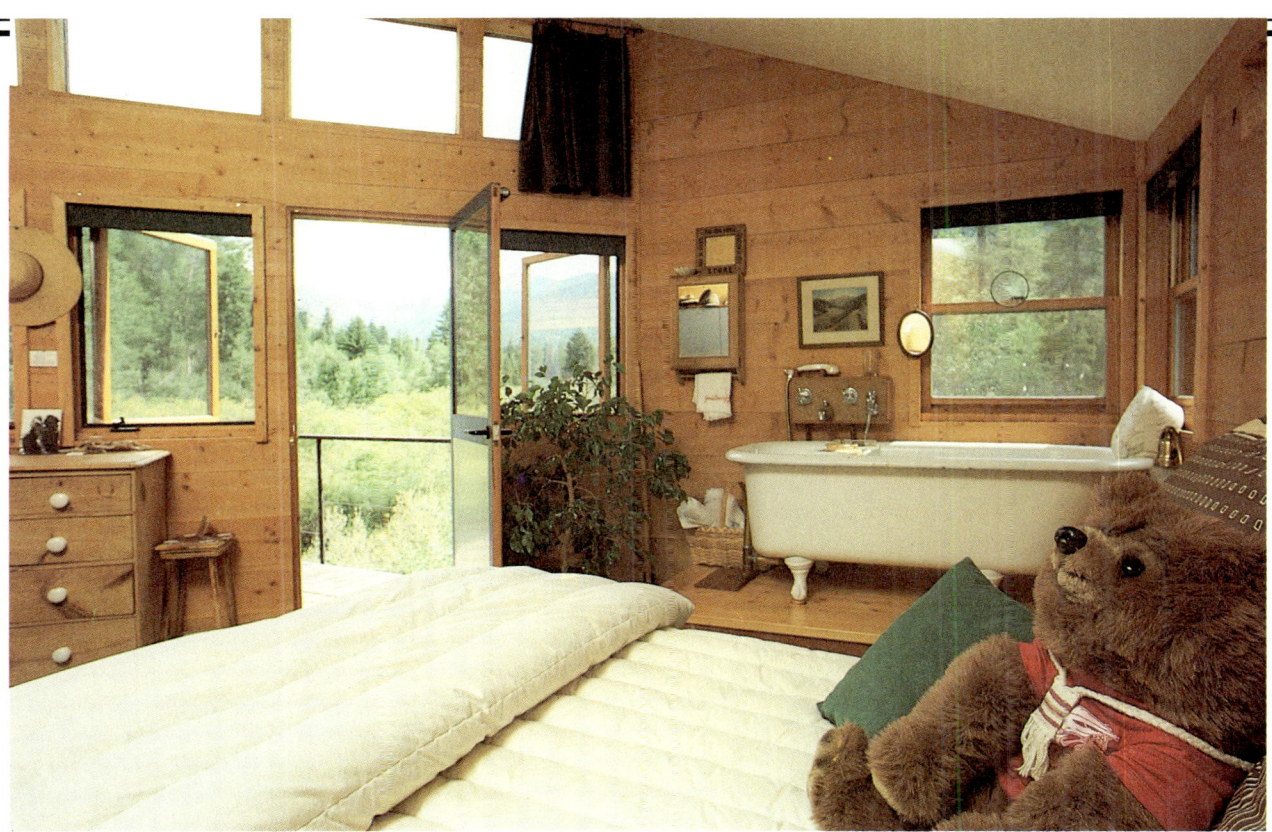

Combining bed and bath creates a sort of "cocoon" environment, a private space in which to unwind and relax.

designs. But all baths are not created equal, because they don't serve the same purpose. Let's look at some specific kinds of baths and some new ideas for each.

## The Master Bath: Luxury and Practicality

In no other bath have changes been more dramatic than in the master bath. As recently as 10 years ago, the master bathroom in most homes was nothing but a cubicle with a tiny shower stall, virtually no storage or counter space, and a cramped toilet area. Today's master baths are showpieces; designers like to refer to them as "master spas," a label that means luxury.

It is in the master bath that most homeowners are willing to splurge. These rooms are as big as space will allow, and often are integrated so well with the master bedroom that it's difficult to tell where the bedroom stops and the bath starts. Dressing areas are being moved out of the bedroom and into the bath.

The toilet is often partitioned off by itself in the master bath, making space for luxury items like steam rooms, saunas, and whirlpool tubs large enough for two. Many include "sunspaces," areas surrounded by windows to let in sunlight for sunbathing; some have doors that open out onto patios or verandas.

Media centers help to keep occupants in touch with the outside world while they're enjoying some private time. Accessories like heated towel bars; automatic soap, lotion, and shampoo dispensers; and scaled-down refrigerators make life in the master bath ever more pleasurable.

But while luxurious, today's master bath is also practical. It more than likely serves the needs of two people—who often both work—and so might include things like extra-large shower areas, double shower heads, double sinks, and spacious walk-in closets. A common trend in the master bathroom is to separate the shower and tub, which allows showering and bathing to take place at the same time.

## Bodyrooms:
### A Glorification of the Physique

The fitness boom that started 10 years ago has had a tremendous effect on today's bathrooms. As fitness became a way of life for more and more people, a whole new concept in baths appeared: bodyrooms (also called gym-baths). Designed for the serious fitness enthusiast desiring a private workout at home, the bodyroom is a unique celebration of human physical potential.

Bodyrooms, ideally, are complete personal fitness centers. They are spacious, to accommodate a wealth of amenities, and are designed with materials that, while luxurious, are easy to maintain. Wall-to-wall ceramic tile, rubber floors, and floor-to-ceiling mirrors are popular in this kind of bath.

While they usually contain standard bathware—sinks, toilet, and so forth—bodyrooms are also equipped with special extras. Stationary bicycles, treadmills, rowing machines, weight-lifting equipment, exercise mats, and other accessories offer a private workout. Computerized scales, heart rate and blood pressure monitors, and other electronic body analysis equipment keep the occupant apprised of his or her physical status.

Bodyrooms are places to cool down as well as warm up. A refreshing shower is

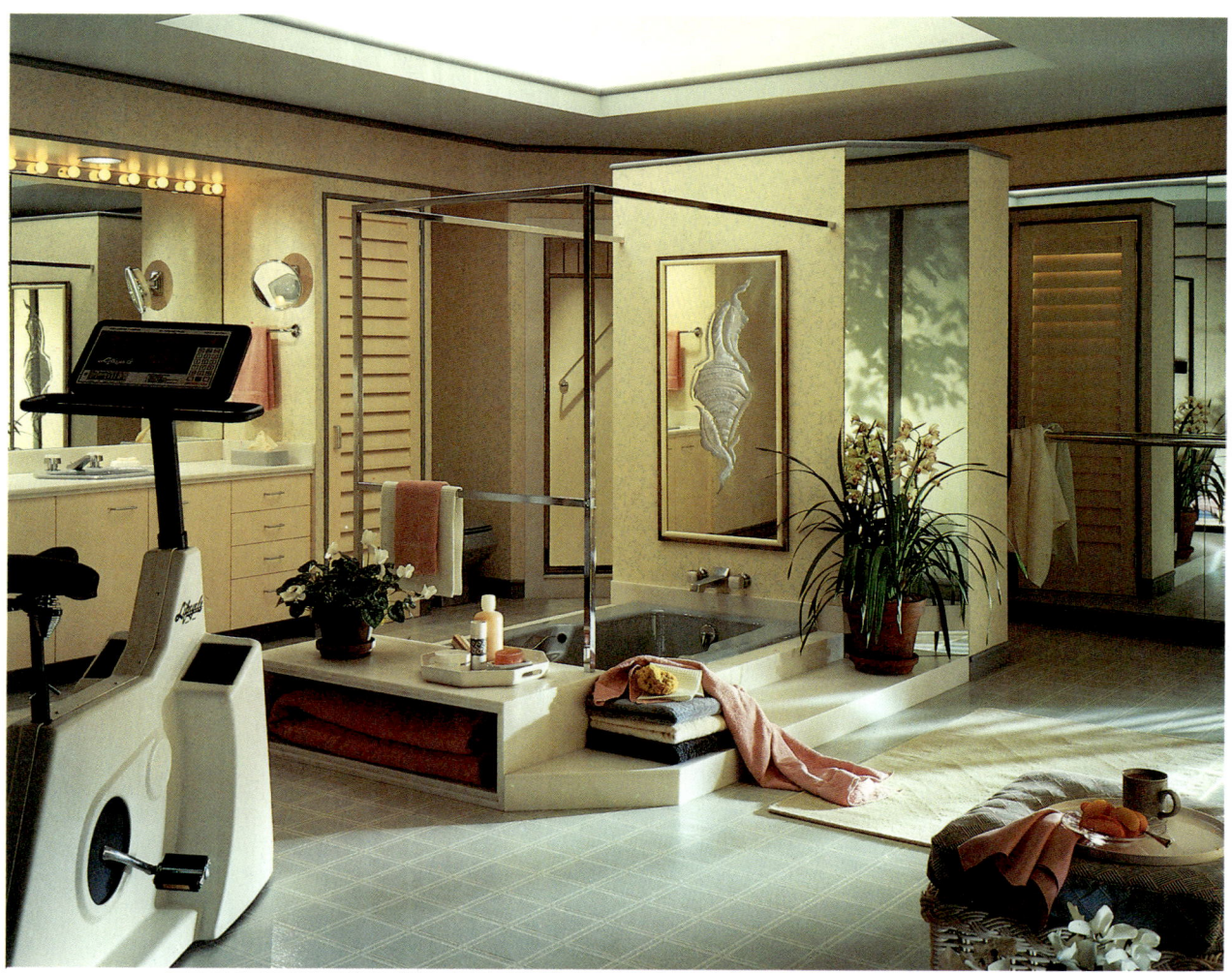

It's not unusual today to find exercise equipment right in the bath. "Bodyroom" baths are products of today's total fitness concept: fitness of both mind and body.

just steps away; after that, perhaps a sauna, or a relaxing soak in the whirlpool tub or spa while watching a videotape and sipping a cool drink. All of this is in an environment as soothing as it is stimulating. Many architects and designers believe that the bodyroom will become more and more popular in the years to come.

## The Family Bath: A Space for Everyone

While many homes have fabulous master-suite baths and exotic bodyrooms, almost all homes have at least one bath that must service a number of people daily. We can call this the family bath, or the standard bath. Again, the design emphasis nowadays is on comfort and convenience.

Today's family baths are being built and remodeled to handle high volume. The most popular means of accomplishing this is compartmentalization, or creating separate spaces for different components of the bath—for instance, partitioning off the toilet, or separating the shower and tub. (See "Making Room for the Bath" on page 15.)

Compartmentalizing keeps traffic in the bath moving smoothly; this can be especially important if a number of family members must use the bath at the same time (for example, to get ready for work or school in the morning). It's also helpful if the family bath must double as a guest bath.

Double sinks are desirable, as well as double mirrors and extra-long vanities with cabinets to store lots of items. A popular trend in very large households is to install small vanities with sinks in bedrooms, preferably on walls that back existing plumbing in a bathroom. That way, grooming can be done in the bedroom while others use the bath.

Laundry facilities are very often located conveniently close to family baths. Laundry chutes and two-way, two-door closets provide easy access to the washer and dryer. Some industrious people put laundry appliances right in the bathroom. (See "What about the Laundry?" on page 42.)

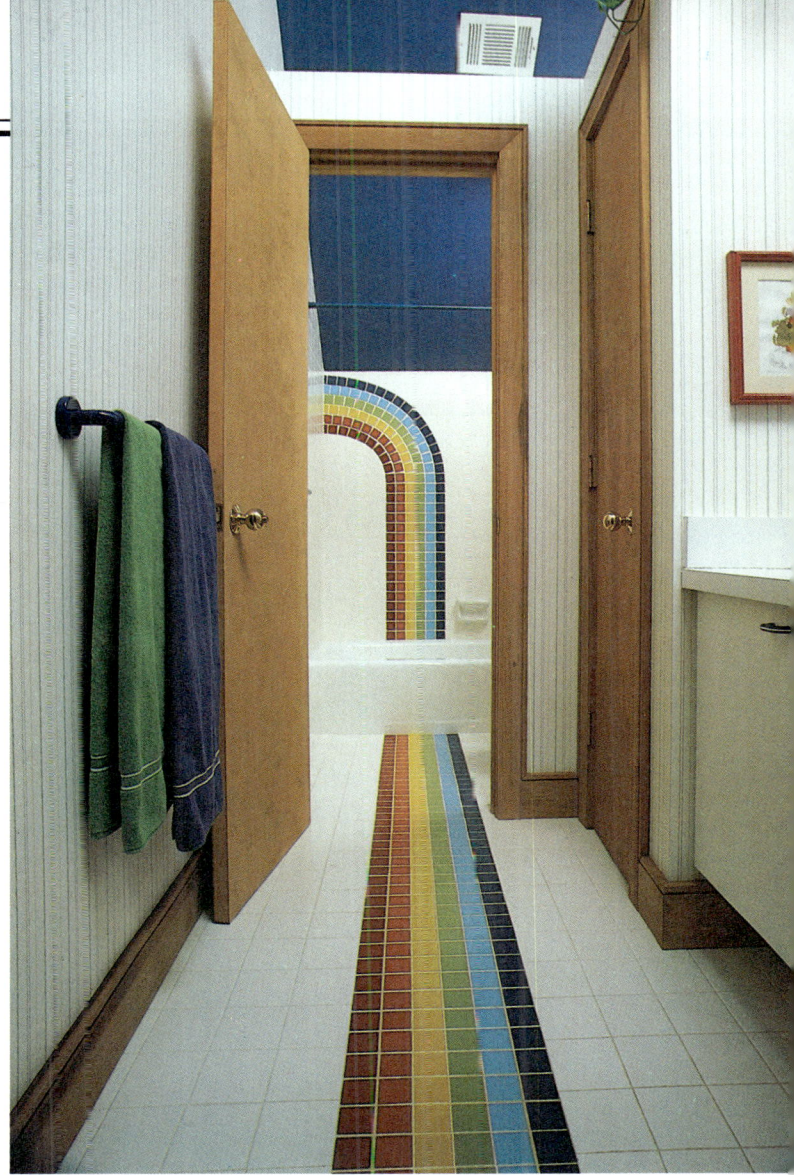

Bright colors help make this children's bath a pleasant place to play; durable materials hold maintenance to a minimum.

## Today's Small Baths

Some baths don't require a lot of space. Powder rooms or half baths—which most often contain a toilet and a sink, with perhaps a vanity and some storage space—are small, but benefit from luxury touches. Elegant materials, which might not fare well in a heavily trafficked bathroom, work nicely in a guest bath.

Children's bathrooms serve small people and therefore can be small spaces. But they should be happy spaces, too. Bright primary colors and cheerful designs make today's children's baths places to play as well as to bathe. Plastic toys, pretty mobiles, and pictures of favorite cartoon characters keep children interested in their surroundings.

Children's baths should be tough as well. Durable, high-gloss enamel is a standard choice for walls; it cleans up easily and can be changed if necessary. Low-maintenance vinyl wallpaper is another popular selection. Nonskid surfaces for floors and bathtub surrounds, and locking cabinet doors help prevent accidents.

Special accessories help both parents and children. Faucet spouts that adjust to different heights allow hair washing and hand washing in the same sink. Step stools that pull out of walls make it easier for children to brush teeth and comb hair; faucet handles with nonslip finishes are good for little fingers.

Other small baths are not glamorous but serve important functions. Basement or garage baths provide facilities for gardeners, weekend auto repairmen, woodworkers, and others involved in outdoor projects. Mudrooms, another ingenious idea from Europe, are places to shed soiled outer clothing and clean up before entering the house. Finished with durable, washable materials, these baths keep dirt out of the main baths in the house.

Homeowners with outdoor pools appreciate the utility of a small bath outdoors to service swimmers. These functional baths keep pool traffic out of the house. Most contain a toilet and small sink; some have a shower and dressing area.

## Specialty Baths

Bathing has become popular enough as a stress release and personal indulgence to spawn the creation of yet another genre of bath. "Water experience" rooms, as they have come to be known, are glorifications of the tub. Sometimes, that's all they contain—just a tub.

But what a tub! These are not your standard-size bathtubs, but four-, five-, and six-person hot tubs and spas with plenty of whirlpool jets. They might be made of fiberglass and finished with an elegant ceramic tile or redwood surround; or they could be completely custom-designed with tile.

The rooms that house these tubs are beautiful and functional. Often they are atriums or "sunspaces," rooms filled with lots of warm, natural light and many plants. Since they tend to be entertainment centers of a home, tub rooms are often finished with

*The rediscovery of the pleasures of bathing has spawned the creation of rooms designed solely for tub soaking.*

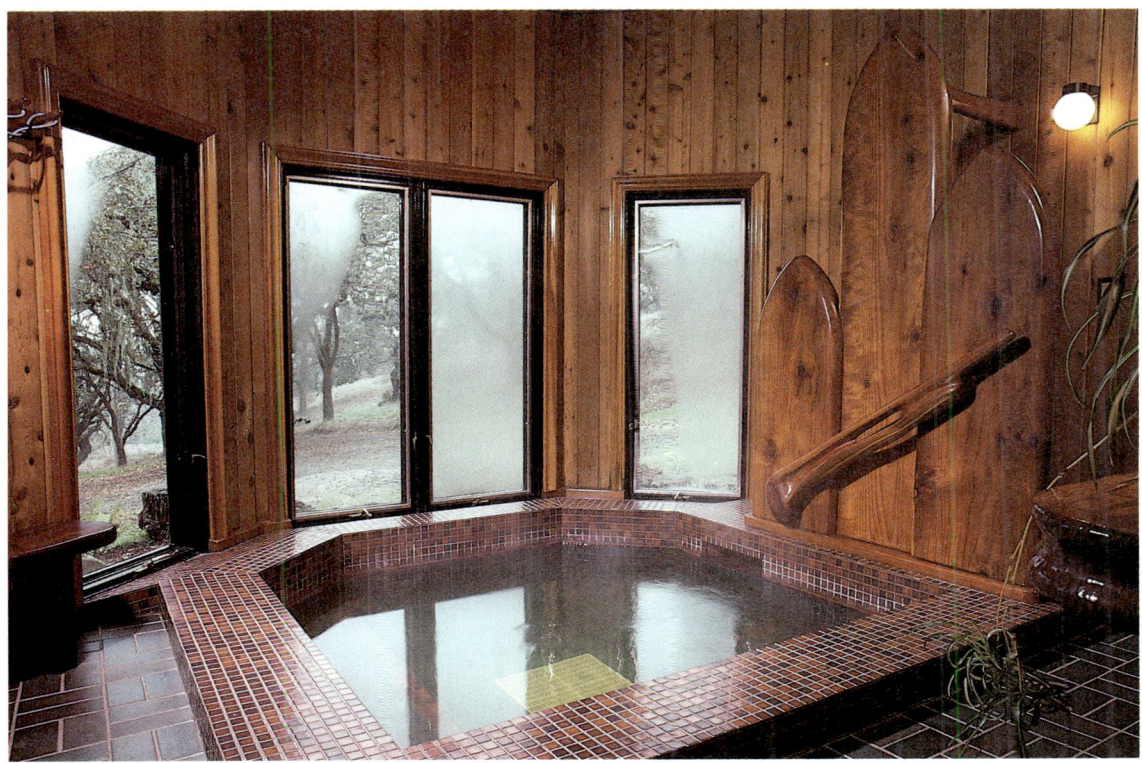

The walls of this spa room are cedar, an excellent choice for a room with lots of moisture. Three redwood monoliths of varying sizes stand guard and hide a toilet from view. Variegated blue penny and square red tile form the spa while handmade tile in shades from gray to teal cover the floor.

luxury treatments—fine wood, marble, plush carpeting, skylights, stereo equipment, wet bars, artwork, and other embellishments.

Those who live in areas with pleasant year-round climates might choose to do their "tubbing" outdoors. Hot tubs and spas in these areas are often located on decks overlooking pleasing countryside, or on garden patios. An outdoor tub room might be equipped with a roll-back roof and removable window covers for use in warm or cold weather.

## Baths for the Handicapped

The "handicapped" includes not only those with severe physical limitations but also the elderly and those with vision or hearing impairments. Baths designed for these people should help to improve the quality of their lives, not add more limitations —which bathrooms often do.

The key word in bath design for the handicapped nowadays is accessibility. An amazing number of manufacturers have responded to the needs of handicapped persons and have designed fixtures and other devices to make bathrooms more accessible to them.

Lowered lavatories with knee space accommodate wheelchairs better, while special electronically operated sinks that can be raised or lowered accommodate the needs of all family members. Elevated toilets, once found only in hospitals and other public facilities, are increasingly found in homes.

Hand-held showers are excellent for bathing the infirm, and barrier-free walk-in or "roll-in" showers are easily accessible to the wheelchair-confined. Grab bars, extra nonslip surfaces, and showers equipped with special benches further reduce injury risk. Such devices are great additions to *any* bath.

# Questions to Answer Before You Begin

It's obvious now that there are almost limitless possibilities for today's bathroom. But if yours, like most, is 5 by 7 feet and contains three basic fixtures and one or two fluorescent lights, you may wonder if there's hope. Don't despair. Great improvements are possible for even the smallest spaces. With good planning and awareness of the enormous range of fixtures, surface materials, and lighting options available today, you can design and remodel your existing bath to make a space that meets your family's needs.

Building a new bathroom or remodeling an old one is an expensive undertaking. Think of those initial expenses as an investment. Knowing what your bathroom needs are and how to design for those needs is the key to a high return on that investment, which is measured in increased value and, of course, better living. Before you begin designing your new bath (even the simplest 5-by-7-foot bath), you should gather information and answer some important questions.

### Who Will Use the Bathroom?

A bathroom may need to serve the entire family, one or more children, just the adults, or guests. The space should be carefully planned to suit the user.

If children use it, for example, determine what the schedule is: Do they use the bathroom individually, following a staggered schedule in the morning? Or do several

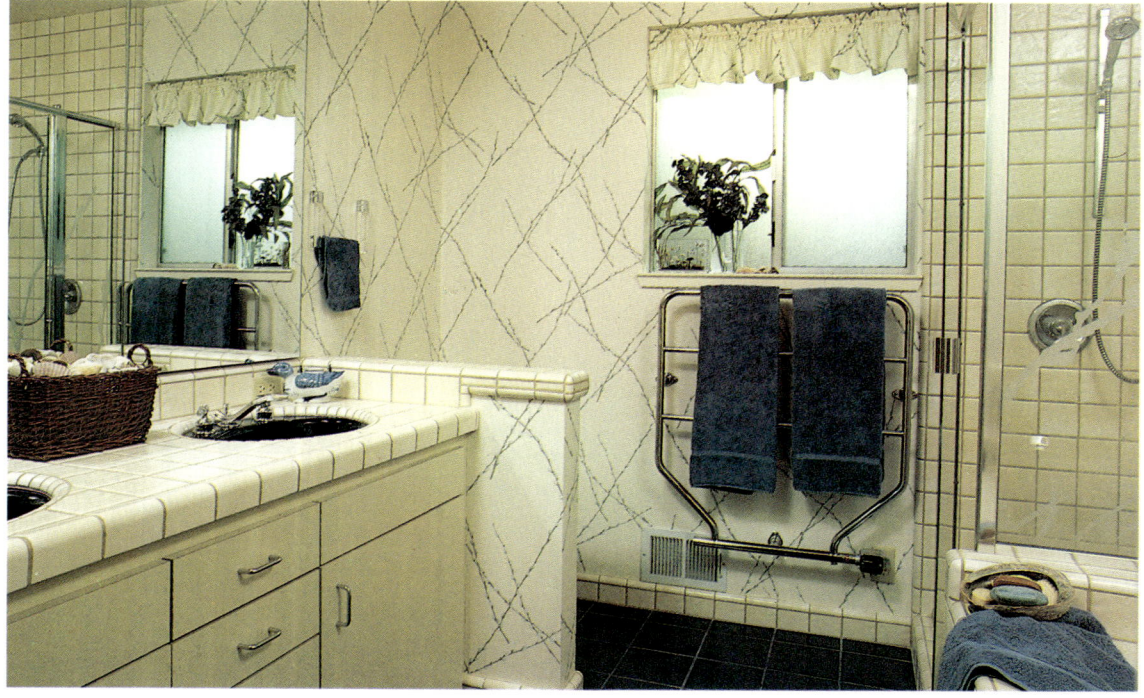

How many people will use your bath? The double sinks and extra roominess of this master bath make it practical for two people.

children use it at the same time as they get dressed each day? Does it seem as if a child is always in the bath? Could more people use the room if the toilet were in a separate compartment? If the bathtub or shower were also?

If a bathroom is your adult space, do you prefer privacy or company while grooming and dressing? Would you like the bathroom open to the bedroom? Open to closet space? If you'd prefer the bath brought out into the open, should the toilet be in a separate compartment?

### How Will the Bathroom Be Used?

Knowing your family's grooming patterns can help you decide how to use your space wisely. If, after morning showers, parents and kids retreat to their bedrooms to complete the grooming process, you probably don't need lots of storage and counter space for grooming in the bathroom itself. If family members prefer to stumble into the bathroom in the morning and not emerge until they are ready for the day in perfect order, another plan is called for. It might make mornings easier to give more of the bathroom's space over to large counter and mirror areas as well as storage for toiletries.

Don't automatically say, "I can't have any of this—there is simply no room!" You're going to be surprised at all the places you can find space. Manufacturers are making it easier to have these extras, too.

### What Equipment Do You Store in the Bathroom?

Designing the storage system in a bathroom is a major part of any plan. Equipment should be stored in its center of use and be clearly visible and easily accessible. To help you decide just what sort of storage will be right for you, make a list of all the supplies—hair dryers to soap, lotion to towels, even books and magazines—that you want to store in the bathroom, and who uses them. These answers will help you block out areas of storage and begin to designate cabinet areas.

### How Would You Like the Room to Look?

You will want to create a space as handsome as it is functional. Should the new

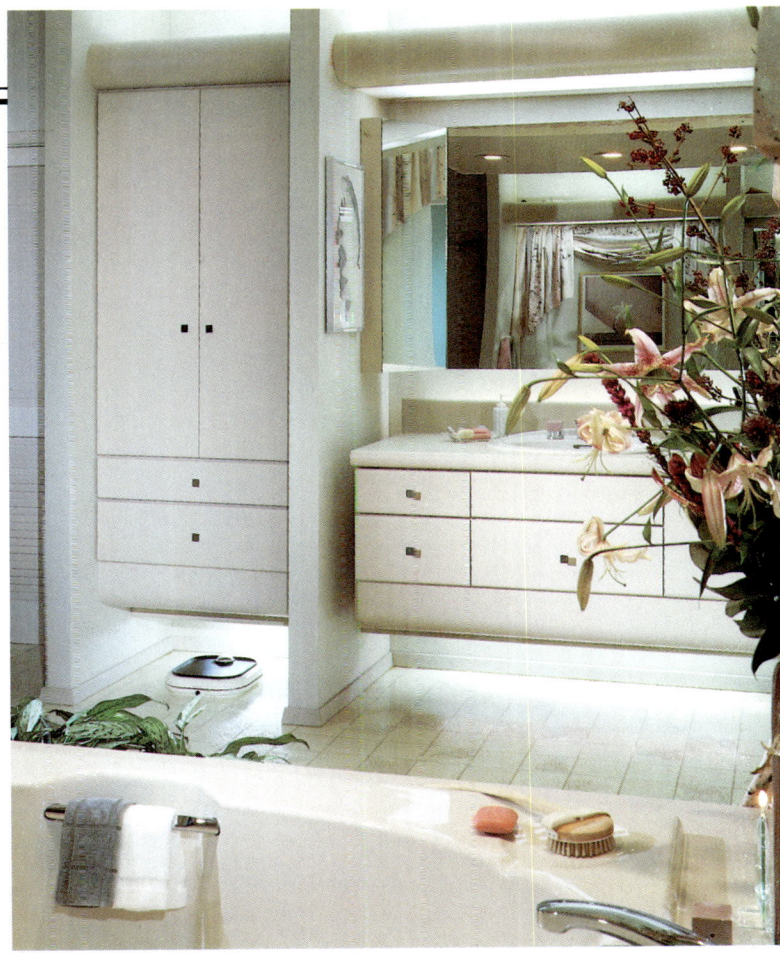

How much storage space will you need? Whether it's a little or a lot, cabinetry should meet your specific needs.

bathroom be restful and understated or colorful and stimulating? Should it be formal or as warm as Grandma's house on a wintry day? Whatever your dream, you must identify it before you can create it.

### What Construction Constraints Exist?

Where is the bathroom located in the dwelling? The physical space must be carefully measured. Draw a plan of the bathroom and surrounding rooms to scale, and on it indicate the present fixtures, windows, doors, and floor and wall coverings. Note if each is to stay in the new bathroom or go out with the old. (For more assistance, see "Workbook: The Basics of Bath Design" on page 122.) Open cupboards and go into the basement or utility rooms to mark the locations of the water-supply lines and the outgoing drain-waste-vent system. (For more details, see "Making the Right Connections" on page 130.)

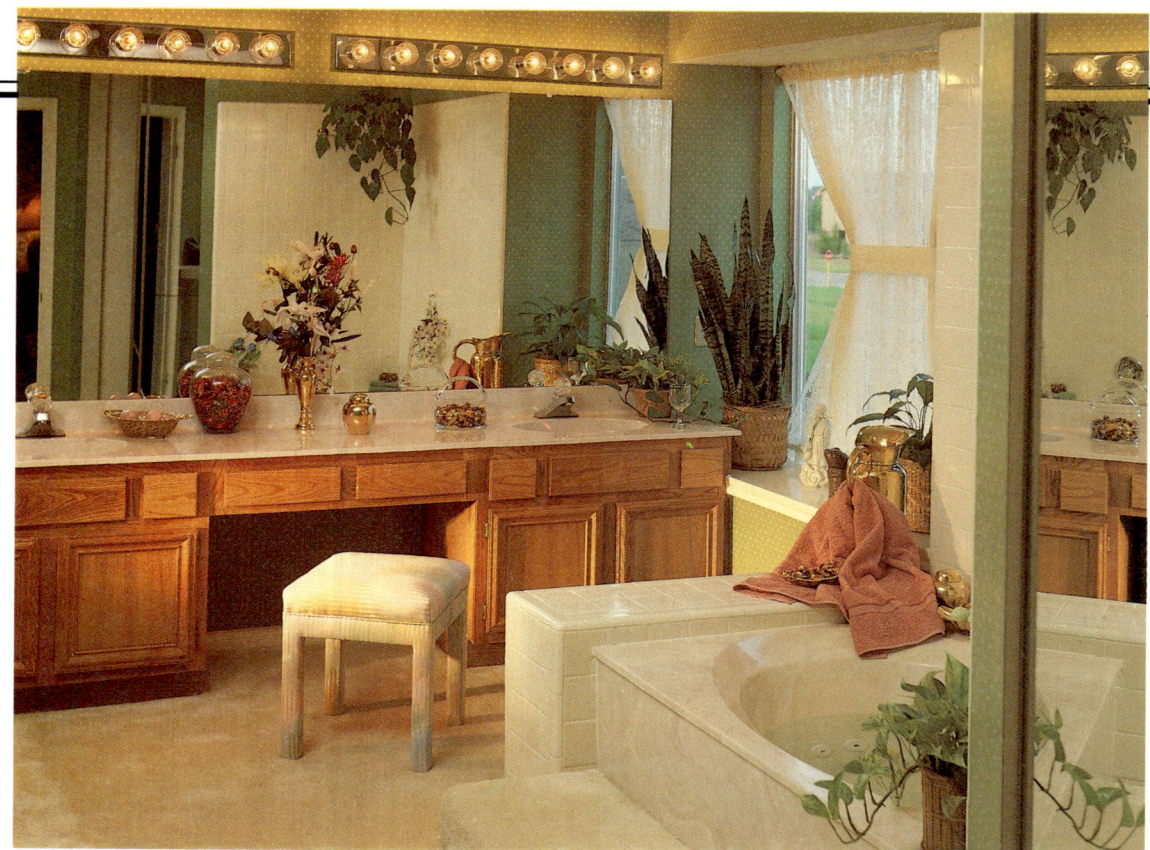

What kinds of fixtures and accessories do you want in your bath? Tastefully chosen fixtures set the perfect tone for the whole room.

### What Plumbing Fixtures Would You Like in the New Bathroom?

Once you've examined the old fixtures, make a list of *ideal* fixtures for your new bathroom; indicate whether they'll be new or recycled from the existing bath. If the bath will be a place for reenergizing after a long day, for example, consider installing a sauna, steam room, or whirlpool tub. Think of fixtures and accoutrements that would enhance the space—lighting fixtures, special window treatments, mirrors, and so forth.

Your answers to these questions will enable you to complete the first stage of the planning process: identifying the scope of the project and setting the budget. Your answers may reveal, for example, that the existing fixtures and their placement are fine and that storage space is adequate, but that the general condition of the room—inappropriate colors and patterns, bad lighting, and aged, hard-to-clean surfaces—make for a not-too-enjoyable room.

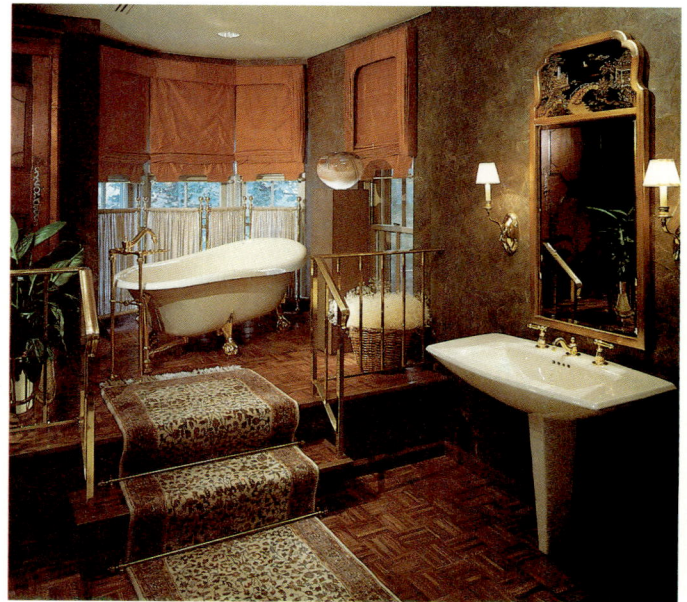

How do you want your bath to look? There are almost limitless possibilities from which to choose; use your imagination to create your own special bath retreat.

## Renew

To make an adequate bathroom more pleasant, the least costly approach is a facelift. It involves simply freshening up the surfaces and possibly replacing the vanity area (leaving the tub and toilet where they are).

Material and labor costs are generally each about half of the total budget. Prices can range from $1,000 to $6,000 for a professionally planned and installed project. This option—the least expensive—also has the lowest return when you go to resell or refinance.

## Replace

If your answers to the questions on pages 10 to 12 indicate that the fixtures are in dire need of replacement, the storage space is far from adequate, and there isn't enough counter space around the sink or there aren't enough sinks, a major change will be required. Strip the room to the bare walls, and leave all major plumbing and electrical systems in the original positions. Replace all fixtures, cabinets, and surfaces.

When standard equipment is used, materials will account for about 40 percent of the cost, and labor for about 60 percent. You should anticipate an investment of $4,000 to $10,000 for this project, if it's to be planned and installed professionally.

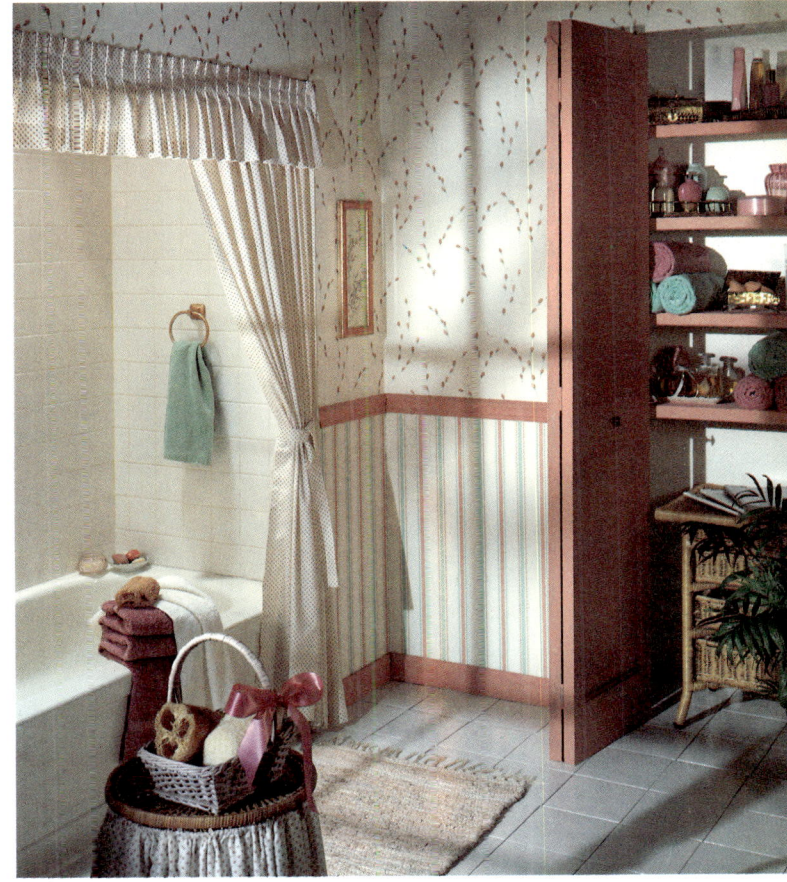

**Renew:** Resurfacing countertops or walls is a low-cost way to liven up any bathroom. The use of wallpaper with green and peach pussy willows and stripes enhances the clean, white look of this bath.

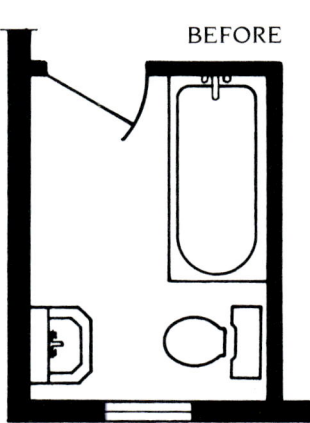
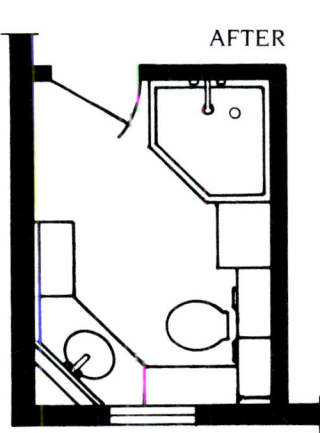
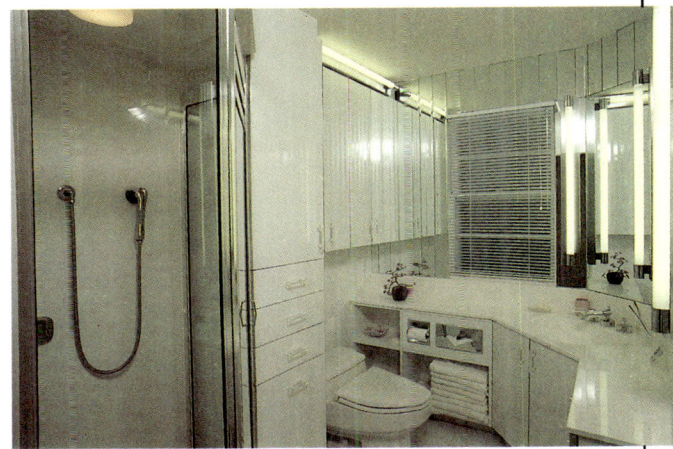

**Replace:** New bathroom fixtures and surfaces modernize and add value. Here one material, one color, and simple lines add up to make a small bathroom seem much larger. Moving the fixtures around a bit and utilizing corner space also helped designer Robert Gelormino to fit in three times the storage space the bath once had. Now the room serves as a full bathroom as well as a linen closet.

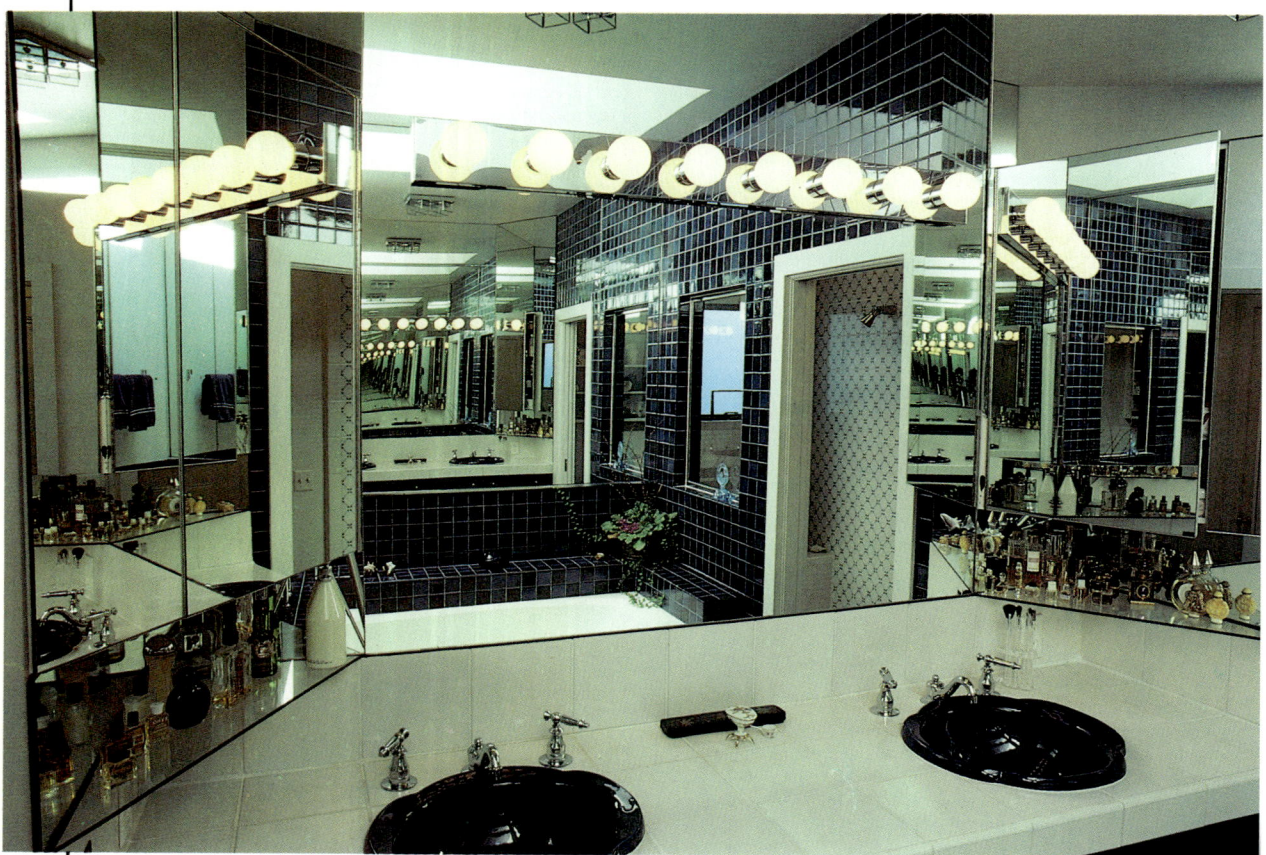

**Redesign:** Adding space and rearranging bathroom fixtures make living easier and give the best return on your remodeling investment. Here, the bath adjacent to the master bedroom used to be in a narrow hallway. Architect Fred Karren borrowed closet and bedroom space to bring the bath into the master-bedroom suite. Karren likes to compartmentalize the various bathroom functions as much as possible; sacrificing a little extra space pays off in easier living. Every remodeled bathroom should suit its owners' life-style. In this bath two sinks allow the couple to get ready for work at the same time; lots of mirrors make the space seem larger and help to spread the light around. The shower and toilet are in private compartments; increased privacy means more accessibility.

## Redesign

If your answers to the questions on pages 10 to 12 indicate that the space just doesn't suit your life-style, the room really needs to be completely rearranged or even expanded.

Redesigning a bathroom is the most elaborate type of project. Strip the room to the bare walls; construction and plumbing and electrical work will have to be done to create the new design. Labor costs for these changes will account for approximately three-quarters of the overall investment.

All fixtures, cabinets, and surfaces will have to be replaced. Expect an average investment of $8,000 to $20,000 for a professionally planned and installed project. This option gives the highest returns when you go to sell or refinance. Only adding a second or third bath has a higher investment value.

If these costs seem out of reach, remember: These estimates are based on entirely professional labor. You can keep costs low by doing some of the work your-

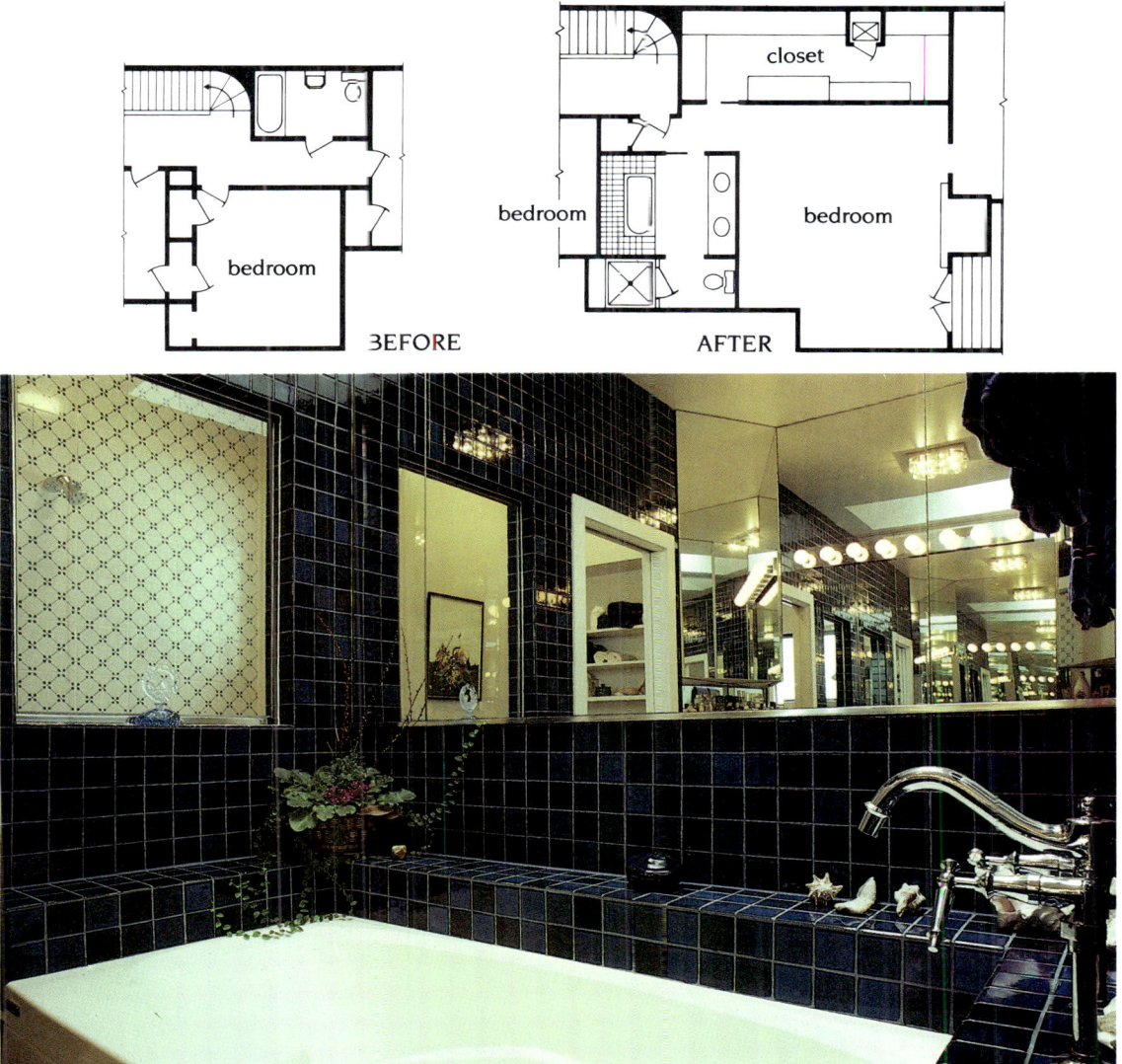

The bathtub gets extra special treatment. Building the tub into a platform creates space around the tub and ties it to the rest of the bathroom. A skylight above the tub bathes the area in natural light and enlarges the space. A window between the shower compartment and bath adds to the spaciousness.

self. If you are a skilled do-it-yourselfer, consider doing the wiring and plumbing yourself. Or take on the painting, wallpapering, and trim work. If you're less skilled, you can still save money by handling the demolition, cleanup, and hauling.

Also, remember that fixtures and wall coverings in standard colors and sizes are less expensive than unusual, designer, or custom-made products. See "Fixture Sizes and Clearances" on pages 124-25 for the dimensions of standard fixtures.

Carefully surveying your family's wants and dreams, taking a close look at the construction of your home, and being familiar with the space required for the various fixtures is the first step in a successful plan. It is, however, only a beginning!

## Making Room for the Bath

The next step is to find space for your bath. Sometimes a simple rearrangement of fixtures and storage will create all the space you need within the room's existing perimeter. Other situations may call for additional space. In most cases, more bathroom space can be carved out of a home's existing floor plan—without the expense of a room addition. All it takes is some creative rearranging.

Your first task is to determine the main problem with your home's existing bathroom situation. Rarely can every inconvenience be remedied, so try to identify a single, realistic remodeling goal. Writing out your priorities as the plan develops will help you make the trade-offs that are always part of a renovation project.

Take, for example, a home with a children's bath that suits the youngsters fine, but is a continual source of embarrassment when friends drop by. In this case, a powder room (reserved for guests) should be the top priority.

If, to take another example, the family bath is a center of traffic tie-ups and tension in the mornings, the goal should be to break up the existing space into compartments—or divide it into two smaller baths—so that more than one person at a time can get ready for the day.

Or perhaps the adults in the household are fed up with sharing a bathroom with the kids. It may be time to add a master bath—or to expand the old one into the minispa of your dreams.

### Finding the Space

If redesigning a bathroom will involve expanding the space, you may wonder where you're going to find the extra square footage. If at all possible, try to stay away from actually adding on to your home to make the bathroom bigger. Unless the bathroom will be part of a major family-room or bedroom project, it is just too expensive to "bump out" the bathroom.

An easier way to increase the size of the bathroom is to steal floor space from other areas, either by creating space in other rooms for typical bathroom activities, or actually engulfing square footage into the bathroom. For example, a vanity with a lavatory could be placed in your bedroom. (Locating it against the bathroom plumbing wall will minimize expenses.) Side-wall medicine cabinets, a duplex outlet, and good lighting will increase storage and create a total grooming center.

Take a look at how the square footage in adjacent rooms is being used. Often, it makes sense to make the master bedroom smaller and the bath larger.

Look at closets that are close to or adjacent to the bathroom. Could such closets be made smaller or eliminated and the space incorporated into the bathroom? Could the closet access area be a part of the bathroom, enlarging space and allowing dressing functions to be joined with those of grooming and bathing? Is there an entryway or other transitional space close by that could be incorporated into the bathroom?

Often separate bathrooms are built back to back. To gain space, try combining the two baths into one larger bath. By using compartments to separate the tub and toilet from the vanity area, two people can still use the new larger space without sacrificing privacy.

Two bathrooms can also sometimes share a single fixture. One tub, shower, or toilet may serve two separate vanity areas. The vanity sections can open into two bedrooms or into one hall and one bedroom. This is a great way to provide the feeling of two bathrooms, gain space for more vanity area, yet conserve on total floor space used for bathrooms.

**Powder Rooms.** If a guest bath is what you need, you can keep it simple; powder rooms normally require only a toilet and lavatory. Very little storage is necessary: just a decorative towel bar and an attractive soap dish. An efficient, quiet ventilation system and good lighting are also key elements. And since the surface areas involved are tiny, elegant coverings for floors, walls, and ceilings may be an affordable luxury.

Powder rooms can fit into very small spaces—as little as 36 by 72 inches, or 48 by 54 inches. The smallest space we recommend for a toilet is a yard wide, with a minimum of 24 inches in front of the bowl. (See "Fixture Sizes and Clearances" on pages 124-25.)

The lavatory can be either a small pedestal fixture or a sink on top of a cabinet. Most bathroom vanities are 21 inches deep and 24 inches wide, although they are also available in 18-by-24-inch sizes. The extra 3 inches of floor space gained by using the smaller fixture sometimes make all the difference.

Space for such a tiny bath can be carved out of an existing floor plan in several ways. Could the powder room go under a stairway? Maybe the entryway coat closet could be reassigned or a bedroom closet shortened to make way for the guest bath. Or consider replacing a side-by-side washer-dryer combination with a stacked unit, thereby freeing space for a half bath adjacent to the utility room. (Vertical laundry units are no longer downsized, stripped-down models; at least two major manufacturers—Maytag and Speed Queen—have recently introduced full-size, stacked appliances.)

When considering any of these possibilities, make sure that the entrance to the powder room is shielded from areas where guests are apt to assemble. Comings and goings to the "privy" shouldn't be in full view of the dinner party.

*Family Baths.* If your family is plagued by morning gridlock in the bathroom, keep in mind that having a toilet, lavatory, and tub in one room means that a single occupant monopolizes all three fixtures. As a solution, you could divide the existing family bath into two separate rooms. But it's doubtful you'll find space enough for two full baths. You'll need to determine which fixture is most in demand.

If the lavatory is the most sought-after spot, you could create an additional grooming center outside the main bath. A child's bedroom or a sectioned-off part of a bedroom closet is a good potential site. Another possibility is to make the utility-room sink do double duty as a spot for morning and bedtime routines, as well as for the usual laundry chores. All any sink needs in order to become a grooming station is a drawer or two, a recessed medicine cabinet with a mirror, at least one duplex electrical outlet, and good lighting.

It's equally possible that the toilet or shower is responsible for the traffic jam. In that case, consider borrowing some space from an adjacent bedroom or closet for an additional toilet and shower. If you arrange the space so that both pairs of fixtures are accessible from a common lavatory area, you will have created the feeling of two bathrooms in the floor space of one and a half.

To make the most of the available floor space, consider exchanging a 60-by-32-inch tub for a 48-by-32-inch stall shower. The shower will be safer and more pleasant to use than a tub/shower combination, and it frees 12 precious inches to be used in other ways. Narrow vanity cabinets (18 inches deep rather than 21 inches) can add 3 inches to the walkway space. Also, avoid swinging doors in the bathroom entrance. Pocket doors, which slide into the wall are great space savers.

*Master Baths.* Adding a new master bath—or expanding an existing one—means that something has to get smaller. Can you eliminate a linen closet? Can you relocate your clothes closet? Can you transfer clothing storage from a closet to some additional furniture pieces, such as an armoire or a chest of drawers?

Another option is to make the bedroom itself smaller so that an adjoining hall bath can be widened. Then squeeze a new bathroom behind the existing reshaped facility. (See "Masterful Minibath" on page 127.)

Be creative in your search for space. Often you can find it in areas of your home that you might never have considered. If children have grown up and left the home, consider turning a spare bedroom into a large master bath. (Keep in mind that some real estate experts think that decreasing the number of bedrooms from three to two diminishes the resale value of a home, whereas from four to three is all right.) Or convert the attic into a luxury retreat.

A good way to fit a big tub into a small space is to select a fixture that is shorter but deeper. The Kohler Company, for example, offers a tub called "The Greek," which is only 48 inches long. Its 22-inch depth and 32-inch width, however, make it comfortable for most average-size adults.

Space may be at such a premium that none of these options offers enough space for that big, luxurious bathtub you've been hankering after. You may need a small room addition. If the roof overhang outside your bedroom is at least 24 inches long, perhaps you can "bump out" the wall enough to create an inviting bathing retreat.

But the chances are good that you'll find the needed inches for more (and more functional) bathroom space within the boundaries of your current home. Make a scale drawing of your floor plan, and cut out some templates of basic fixtures and furniture. Then ask yourself, "What if?"

## Inexpensive Ways to Spruce Up Your Old Bath

If a tight budget is dictating your redo plans, take heart in the fact that you don't have to spend a fortune to wake up a worn-out bath. In many cases, an eye for detail, a little elbow grease, and ingenuity can take you farther than you probably imagined.

*Cut a lot of the expense right from the start by planning to redo yourself.* Hiring designers, builders, plumbers, and electricians can get costly—and that doesn't even include the price of new fixtures, wall and floor coverings, and accessories. For ideas, consult home building and remodeling magazines, bath product catalogs, and brochures; visit showrooms and department stores, and ask lots of questions.

*Consider color first.* Color can pull a room together like no other design element. Sometimes just changing the color of the walls can breathe life into an oppressive bathroom. Painting is your least expensive redecorating option.

Experiment with color. One nice shade —on walls and repeated on towels and other accessories—can tie the whole bath together visually. Or play with several different shades of the same color, or two or three completely different colors. Walls could be white, while shower surround, towel bars, and window curtains are cornflower blue. A wallpaper with both colors makes a nice accent.

Pastels and neutrals are pretty, but don't be afraid of primaries. Used in the right amounts, they can really brighten a boring bath. Don't forget floors and ceilings when planning color for the bath, and remember that dark colors decrease space while light colors expand it.

*Patterns and textures can also create visual excitement in your bath without eating a hole through your wallet.* Rough-hewn wood is reasonably priced and contrasts wonderfully with smooth, lustrous fixtures. Covering walls and ceilings with fabric (treated to resist moisture) or wallpaper is another inexpensive treatment that adds pattern and texture. Painted ceramic tiles can be used to create patterns on walls, shower surrounds, and countertops. Repeat patterns on window curtains, towels, throw rugs, and wall hangings.

*Consider lighting and space.* Sometimes a different kind of light can make all the difference in the world. If you have fluorescent fixtures, try the new warm-toned tubes; they emit a light that is much more representative of natural light. Employing reflective surfaces—like shiny laminates, chromes, or porcelains—increases the intensity of light in the bath. Unusual fixtures like track lights, glass hurricane lamps, or theatrical light bulb strips add more interest.

Don't forget windows when evaluating your lighting options. Instead of curtains, consider using mini- or microblinds, which come in an attractive array of colors. Stained glass is another dramatic alternative to conventional window treatments.

If you cannot add space to your bath, create the illusion of more space. Mirroring walls, ceilings, and cabinets is an excellent way to do this. Clear glass shower enclosures also make baths look bigger by opening up to view a normally closed-off area of the room. Skylights, too, can visually enlarge and enhance your bath. You can create a skylight effect by covering a lighted ceiling with translucent paneling. This disperses light more evenly and creates the illusion of daylight.

You can also create the illusion of more *storage* space in a minuscule bathroom. Several-tiered hanging baskets hold towels and other accessories, and a plant as well. Cube-shaped shelves (which can add color

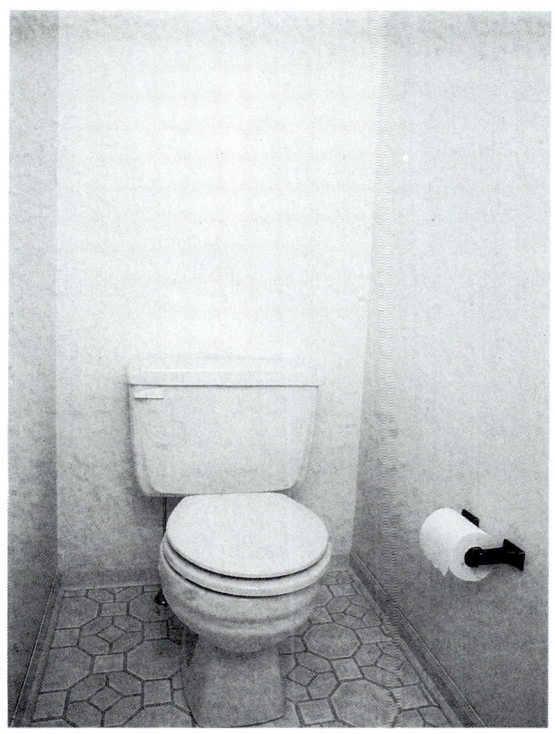

You don't have to spend a fortune to brighten a boring bath. A little paint and a little ingenuity gave the plain-Jane half bath (above) a new lease on life (right).

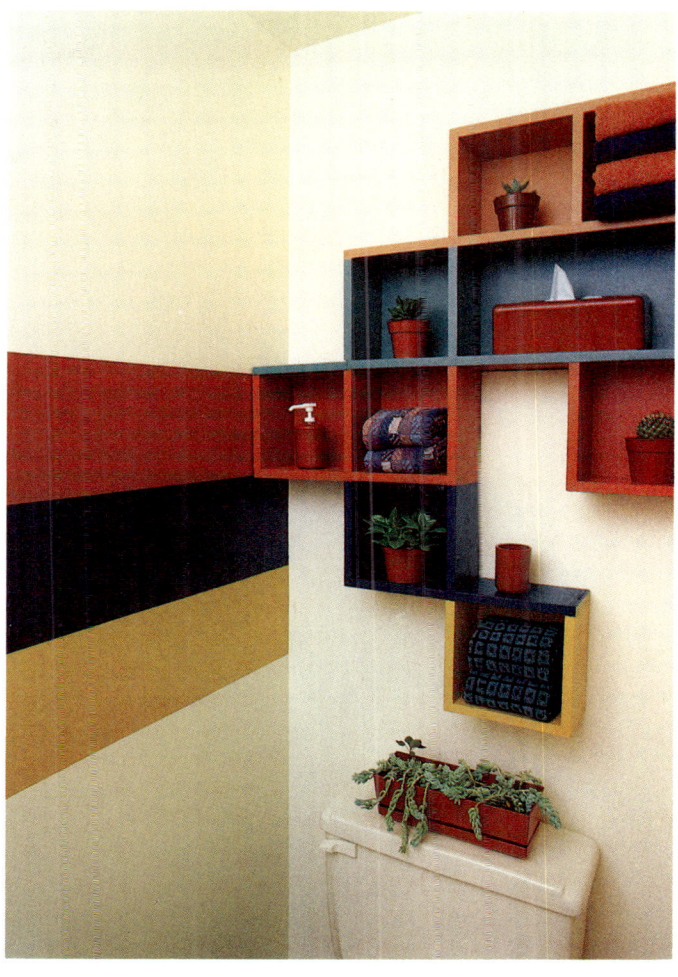

as well as storage space) can be stacked on top of one another or spread out in an interesting pattern on the wall.

You can create recessed storage alcoves by bumping out small portions of the wall between studs. If you don't disturb plumbing or bearing walls, this doesn't have to be too expensive, and it's a wonderful way to show off pretty towels.

*Consider replacing outdated fixtures.* It could be that the fixtures wore out their welcome 20 years ago. If so, consider replacing them. Manufacturers have upgraded fixtures tremendously even in the last five years, and they're available in many different sizes, styles, and colors.

If new fixtures are out of the question, use some of that ingenuity and "disguise" the old ones. A new vanity and countertop can do wonders for an old sink; or "dress" it up with a fabric skirt that matches curtains or wallpaper. Retiling a surround can downplay a homely tub, while a new seat and a towel shelf positioned above it give a less-than-attractive toilet a face-lift.

*Ultimately, attention to detail is what will convince others you've spent thousands of dollars on a renovation.* Things like faucets, towel bars, vanity drawer and door handles, shower curtain rods, trim around windows and mirrors, and bathroom toilet-paper holders are small items, but in a 5-by-7-foot room, those little things become important vehicles for your decorating theme. Special touches like artwork and wall hangings, treasured pieces of furniture, antiques, glass objects, hanging plants, and other interesting curios will help make your bath a more pleasant and relaxing place.

# The Working Parts

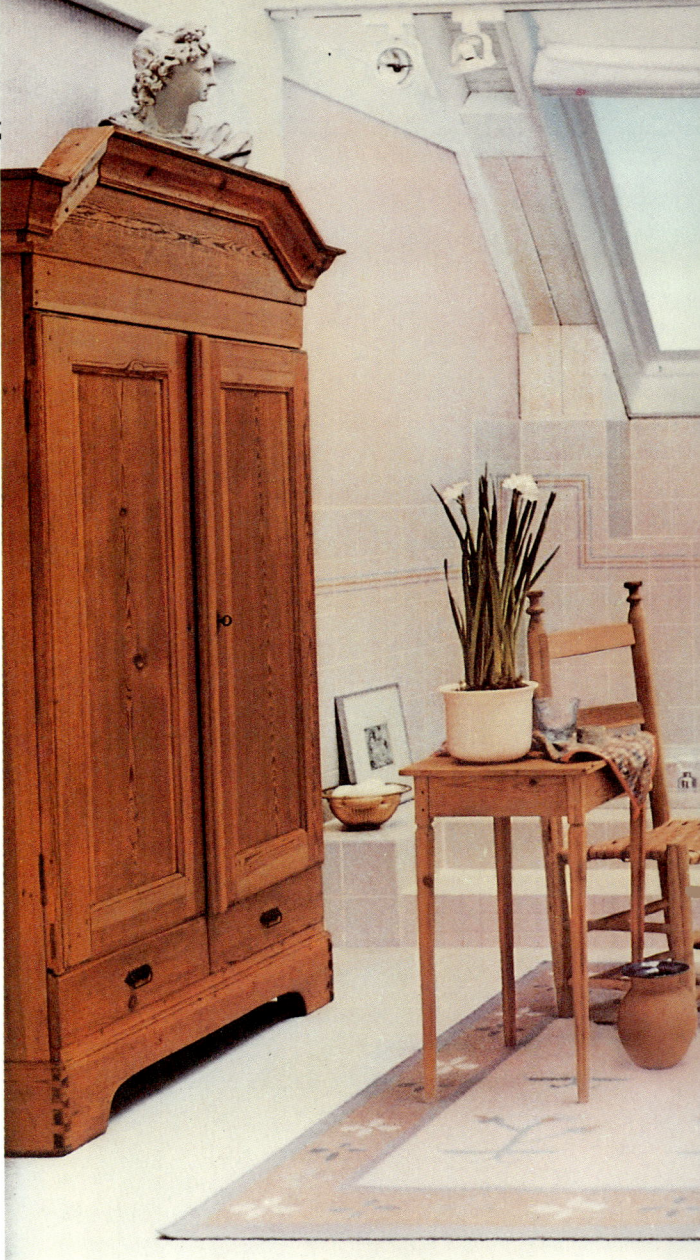

Choosing bathroom fixtures used to be easy—the plumber's joke was that you could get anything you wanted as long as it was white porcelain. But we want more out of our bathrooms now, and bathroom fixtures in new combinations of beautiful colors and innovative materials have emerged to fill those needs. You now have literally hundreds of choices with a range of prices to match.

Consider these fixtures—tub, shower, toilet, and sink (lavatory)—as major design elements in your bath. Remember that, while you are replacing them now, you probably won't want to do so again. So plan your design carefully to meet your needs and your personal tastes. Examine your current bathroom. Determine where traffic is the heaviest and which facilities get the most use; this will help you to decide where to place new fixtures. Moving the toilet to its own partitioned area, for example, might free up more room in the bath for storage space. Or perhaps double sinks would solve the problem of "rush-hour" bathroom crowding.

Look into the advantages and disadvantages of different fixture materials. Will a fiberglass tub suit your needs best, or does the durability of enameled cast iron sound more attractive?

Explore the various color schemes available. Plain white toilets and tubs are still around—and still in demand—but fixtures can also be found in a stunning array of bright primaries, pretty pastels, and blended hues.

No matter what color or material you select for your new tub, toilet, or sink, however, consider these points before you buy:

• Damage is more noticeable on dark-colored fixtures than on light-colored ones. A scratch will be more apparent on a chocolate brown basin than on a white one.
• Never use abrasive cleaners on *any* bathroom fixture—they destroy a fixture's luster, pit its surface, and simply make it harder to clean as the years go by.
• Don't expect colors of different materials or from different manufacturers to match. Even in white, vitreous-china toilets, fiberglass tubs, and Corian vanity tops are all different shades. If you're very particular about this, purchase a full line of fixtures from the same manufacturer.

Some innovative companies do collaborate to offer fixtures, wall coverings,

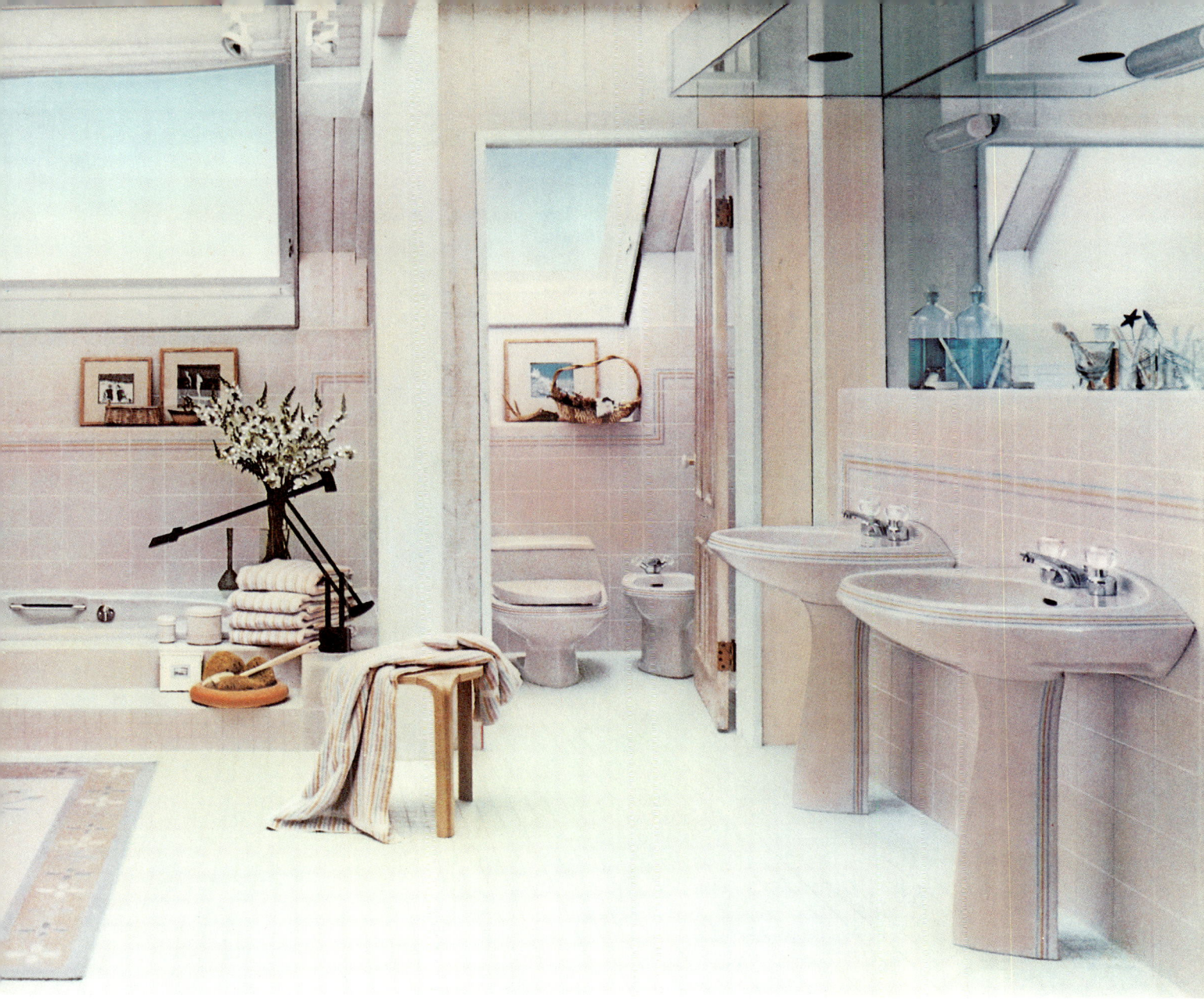

and countertops in matching and coordinated colors. The Whisper Colors and Patterns by American-Standard and American Olean Tile Company, and the Cerámica Companions of tile and fixtures by Eljer Plumbingware and American Olean are two such team efforts. The Kohler Color Coordinates program is a way to match Kohler fixtures with those of seven manufacturers. Matching products include: laminates, cabinets, tile, towels, wall and floor coverings, and paint. For a complete listing of manufacturers, see "Helpful Addresses."

Plan on spending as much as you can afford for fixtures. Generally speaking, sinks, tubs, and toilets are priced according to the quality of design and workmanship; the more expensive models last longer, work better, and are more attractive.

If you're working with a limited budget, replace the fixtures in your bathroom before starting any other major renovations. You'd be surprised at just how much a new toilet, sink, or bathtub can do to spruce up a dreary old bath. Walls, floor coverings, and countertops can be upgraded at a later date.

If the sky's the limit, be prepared for sensory overload in the fixtures department. The bath as a restful and luxurious room is the credo of fixture manufacturers today. Now top-of-the-line products bear virtually no resemblance to their counterparts of 30 years ago. Even toilets are designed for comfort rather than utility.

## An Efficient Flush

Today's toilets look different and work differently from their counterparts of 30 years ago. New low-profile, one-piece toilets are sleek and stylish. Modern toilets have elongated bowls that are far more comfortable than old-style round bowls and are much easier to clean as well. One-piece, wall-hung units (no part of the fixture touches the floor) make floor cleanup even more of a breeze, though they do require special drainage systems and therefore are more expensive than conventional floor-standing models.

You can find a toilet to fit any niche. Some are designed for very odd spaces: Several manufacturers offer a model with a triangular tank that fits cozily into a 2-by-2-foot corner—great for tiny half baths. Tanks come in a number of sizes and shapes—tall and rectangular, short and squat, even rounded—making it easier for you to choose one that meets your particular design needs. Many of the newer models have "invisible" tanks that sit almost flush with the seat and lid.

Seats are also available in a variety of contours, so that you can "customize" toilets for children or adults. Most standard models have seats that are 14 inches off the ground, but there are toilets with higher, 18-inch seats, which are helpful if a handicapped or elderly person will be using the bathroom. When looking for a seat, make sure it has corrosion-resistant hinges; some hinges allow easy removal of the seat for quick cleanup.

Then there's the flush. There are two basic flushing actions to choose from: reverse trap and siphon jet. Another, the washdown, can be found in older bathrooms, but most municipal codes will no longer accept this type of flush mechanism in toilets for new or remodeled rooms. It's very noisy and uses water inefficiently. And because very little of the bowl surface is covered with water, it stains easily and is difficult to keep clean.

Both the reverse trap and the siphon jet flush mechanisms use siphon action to whisk away waste, but the reverse-trap models are less expensive. A water jet located at the inlet to the trapway or outlet channel

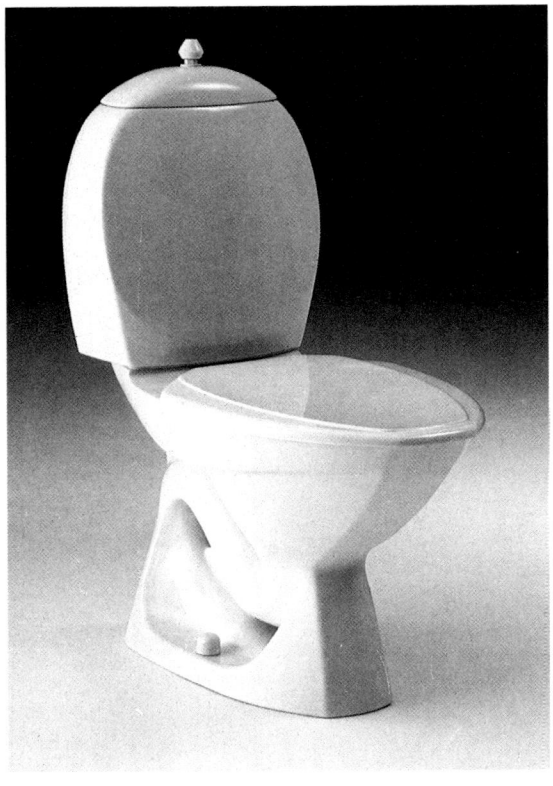

A low-flush toilet, like the Ifö Cascade, can save you thousands of gallons of water per year.

promotes the siphon action of the reverse trap. The trapway itself has a 1½-inch diameter. Because of the water jet, a reverse trap is noisier than the siphon jet, and the relatively small trapway makes reverse-trap models more prone to clogging.

An updated version of the siphon jet is the "siphon action" mechanism. This type of flush action can be found in newer, one-piece toilets; it is almost silent as it operates, and it leaves no dry surfaces in the bowl. As you might expect, it is also the most expensive. Many of today's new water-saving toilets use this flush mechanism.

Today, most standard toilets are engineered to save water, using only 3½ gallons per flush compared to the 5- to 7-gallon flushes of older models. Water-saving toilets are more expensive than the old standards, but the long-term benefits of a water-saving toilet more than justify the initial expense. An average family can save 20,000 gallons or more of water a year (reducing water and sewer maintenance costs) by switching to one of the new standard models.

Some innovative toilets operate on an even more frugal flush. Colton Wartsila's ultra-low-flush Ifö Cascade unit requires only 1 gallon. Mansfield Plumbing Products also markets several water-saving toilets, including the Quantum, which flushes on just 5.9 quarts of water. The Superinse by the Thetford Corporation uses just 1 gallon of water. (See "Helpful Addresses.") Before you install any kind of water-saving model, make sure it meets the building codes in your area. Also, be certain that your existing plumbing water-supply system has adequate pressure. The water pressure is a critical element in most water-saver toilet designs. Without at least 30 pounds of pressure per square inch, the toilet will not provide a complete washout with each flush.

Most toilets today are made of vitreous or low-porosity glazed china, which is easy to clean and resists stains and acids. No matter what material you are shopping for, make sure the toilet surfaces, both inside and out, are free from pits, ripples, or burrs. The tank lid should sit level and tight, and the toilet base should be flat so that the fixture will sit level on the floor.

Figure on paying anywhere from $40 to $700 for a new toilet. Two-piece, floor-standing models are the least expensive. The sleeker and more modern the design, the more you can expect to pay. Super water savers are on the high end of the price range. One-piece, wall-hung units cost the most.

### Urinals: Are They Feasible in the Home?

You might not care for one in your luxury master-suite bath, but under certain circumstances, urinals can be very practical choices for home baths. Basement bathrooms near work areas, pool-side baths, and highly trafficked baths are prime locations for urinals. Most models designed for home use are highly efficient water users, consuming just a quart or two of water per flush.

And they don't have to be unsightly. While many urinals in commercial buildings have unsightly pipes and hardware, some fixture manufacturers, like Mansfield, offer sleek, modern designs that all but hide water-supply lines. You won't find them in many decorator colors, however; most are white vitreous china.

## Bidets

A bit of mystique surrounds the bidet, primarily because most Americans don't really know what it is or how to use it. A popular fixture in European baths, the bidet

### No-Flush Toilets: Are They for You?

The ultimate water-conserving toilet is one that doesn't flush at all. A composting toilet is, in essence, a big box that stores wastes and turns them into humus—odorless fertilizer you can use in your yard.

In theory, composting toilets are a great idea. But in reality, they're plainly not for everyone. Part of the problem is cultural—let's face it, not everyone is comfortable with a toilet that doesn't flush.

On top of that, your local plumbing codes may not allow composting toilets, although many codes have been rewritten to permit them. And there is the cost—keep in mind that your initial investment will probably top $750.

Despite those disadvantages, many homeowners have found flushless toilets to be quite suitable for their homes. Even with its high purchase price, a composting toilet can save you money with every flush you don't make. The average family can save about 40 percent of its annual water bill. Several companies manufacture them (you may have heard of Clivus Multrum), and most look very similar to regular flushing toilets. Another advantage of composting toilets is that they are ideal for remote vacation homes.

If you do decide to get a composter, be aware that it will require more owner involvement than a regular toilet. Your best bet is to visit someone who has one before you buy one. A little first-hand experience will let you know whether you're ready for one.

was first conceived and used in Europe as a means of improving personal hygiene for both men and women. The user sits astride the fixture facing the faucets at the back, which control the temperature of a gentle spray that cleanses the genital area.

Bidets require a 3-by-3-foot space next to a wall and are usually placed alongside the toilet. Normally a spray, mounted in the bottom of the bowl or attached to the faucet, is used by the bather. Most bidets are also equipped with a stopper to retain the water for foot-soaking or sitz-bathing.

You won't find these fixtures in many older homes in this country. For years, bidet manufacturers concentrated their marketing efforts in Europe. But with the growing number of American homeowners creating total body relaxation areas and sleek, European-style baths, bathware giants like Kohler, Eljer, and American-Standard are beginning to introduce color-matched, toilet-bidet sets here and to advertise the bidet as a necessary luxury.

And it is a luxury. Because bidets need both hot- and cold-water connections and a separate drainage system, plumbing involves opening walls and flooring, and it can get quite expensive. But if you're willing to foot the extra expense, the bidet is a marvelous personal pampering item for a luxury or master-suite bath.

## Sinks

As unglamorous as it might sound, the bathroom sink offers hundreds of design possibilities. Lavatories come in a myriad of sizes, shapes, colors, prices, and materials; whichever you choose will make a definite design statement in your new bath. But before you start thinking about exotic, museum-caliber washbasins, you should determine which basic style will best suit your needs. There are three styles of sinks: wall-hung, freestanding pedestal, and vanity-top.

Wall-hung sinks can be an undesirable option. They provide no storage or counter space, and pipes are exposed under the sink. If your storage space will be concentrated elsewhere, however, a wall-hung model can add a unique design element to your bathroom. Stainless-steel, laboratory-style sinks, for instance, might lend a sleek, elemental look to the bath. And other new models incorporate the plumbing right into the sink's design, making it appear attractive and contemporary. Wall-hung units also require the least amount of space and are nice for small baths and half baths. Specially designed, three-corner, wall-hung sinks fit cozily into corners.

Freestanding pedestal sinks are a more graceful space-saving solution. The pedestal hides the pipes and drain, and its sleek design gives the bath a continental air. These types of sinks normally have very large, flaired bowls with extended ledge room for soap dishes, toothbrush holders, and so forth. However, pedestal sinks provide no storage or counter space, although you can custom-build a countertop around one.

Vanity-top sinks are popular because they offer storage space and come in a wide variety of styles. They are also ideal when two sink basins are needed in a bathroom. These types of sinks are available either molded into the counter (the entire unit sits on top of the cabinetry) or separate and ready to drop into a countertop.

### Separate Sinks

You can choose from three styles of separate sinks. A flush-mounted sink requires a metal ring to hold it in the countertop. Surface-mounted models eliminate the metal ring; the sink overlaps the mounting hole in the countertop. Under-the-counter units are secured by metal fasteners underneath the counter.

Separate sinks are made of four basic materials—enameled, formed steel; fiberglass; cast iron; and vitreous china. Formed-steel sinks with glazed-enamel surfaces are the least expensive. These sinks are available in a limited number of colors. They're lightweight and easy to clean but are also very easy to chip. If anything heavy is dropped on the sink, the formed steel expands upon impact, then quickly contracts, but the enamel finish doesn't. Instead, it cracks or flakes off.

Fiberglass sinks are in the middle of

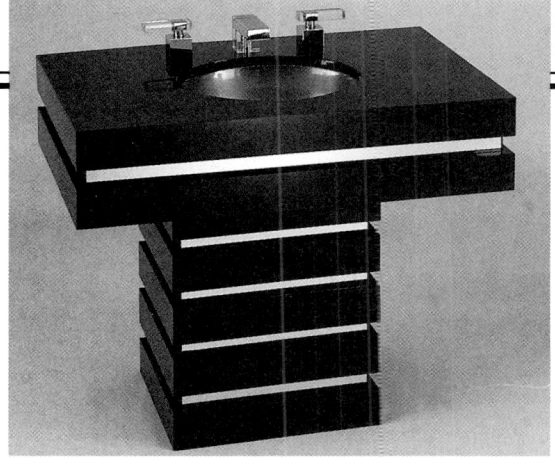

The Haviland Vanity by Paul Associates is made of acrylic with contrasting acrylic bands. The basin shown here is vitreous china coated with a bright silver finish.

the price range. They're available in an enormous selection of colors and shapes and come with either an acrylic or polyester gel coating. A great debate rages over which finish is better for home use. Acrylic is the stronger of the two—it's more resistant to scratching, abrasion, chemical damage, and fading from the sun. But acrylic is more expensive and more difficult to repair than polyester gel coating, which is strong enough to stand up to normal household use.

Cast-iron sinks are the most expensive ready-made variety and also the most durable. The enamel finish on cast iron is several layers thick and baked on at high temperatures. The coating is thicker than that on formed-steel sinks, and the cast iron itself is stiffer, so the enamel coating is much less prone to chipping and cracking.

Vitreous china has long been revered for its durability in other bathroom fixtures and has recently been put to use for sinks. It's chip-resistant, holds heat well, and is easy to clean. And because of its smooth texture, a vitreous-china sink pairs well with a countertop of ceramic tile. Eljer recognized this and collaborated with American Olean to introduce the Cerámica Companions, color-coordinated tiles and vitreous-china sinks.

For those who'd like to lend an extra touch of opulence to the lavatory, there are several unusual and quite expensive washbasins from which to choose. The line of decorator basins from Sherle Wagner International, which are richly designed with precious metals and lavish hand-painted porcelains, can add style to the bath. Villeroy & Boch has the "Lift" sink that moves up or down with finger pressure from about 18 to 35 inches high. This is great for children or for washing feet. You can also find basins of hammered copper; hand-thrown, glazed pottery; even giant seashells! Just be sure that the material you choose is appropriate for its intended purpose; a bright brass washbasin is certainly lovely, but not practical for a heavily trafficked family bath.

### Integral Countertop Sinks

Molded one-piece, or integral, vanity-top sinks are normally made of cultured marble, cultured onyx, Corian made by E. I. Du Pont de Nemours & Company, or 2000X made by the Formica Corporation. Cultured marble sinks are the least expensive and are actually cast polyester. Plan on paying about $110 for a 25-by-22-inch integral countertop sink. The polyester resin forms are filled with crushed marble, calcium carbonate, hydrated aluminum, or glass bubbles to give the sink color and texture.

Although manufactured by similar methods, cultured onyx is less opaque than cultured marble. Cultured onyx looks and feels much more like polished stone. It costs more than cultured marble, too—figure $225 for a 25-by-22-inch cultured onyx sink top.

Both cultured products come in a wide variety of colors and styles, usually finished with a polyester gel coating. They're easy to maintain, but cultured marble and onyx can scratch and stain. If chips or cracks occur, you can't repair them. When shopping for cultured marble or onyx, look for evidence of certification by the Cultured Marble Institute.

You can also buy one-piece counters and sinks made of Corian or 2000X, which are similar products that are marvelous for surfaces that take a beating. Because these man-made marble materials are the same color throughout, you can rub or sand out surface damage. Corian and 2000X resist stains, scratches, chipping, and cracking and won't burn. These materials are extremely easy to maintain and are similarly priced.

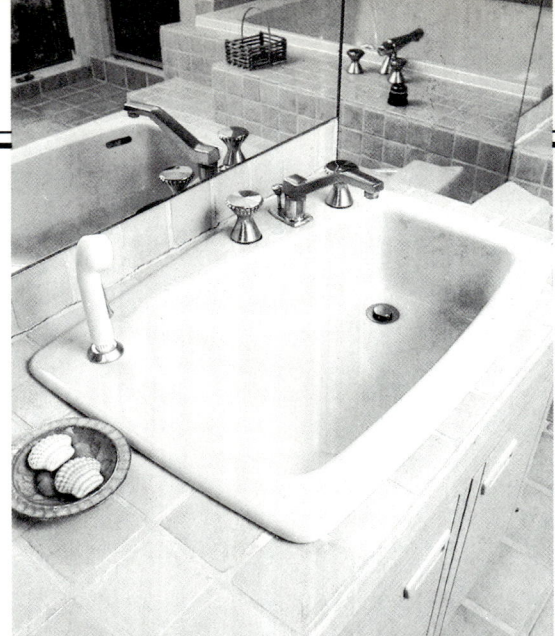

An extra-large sink basin by Kohler is versatile. It can also be used for infant bathing and hair washing.

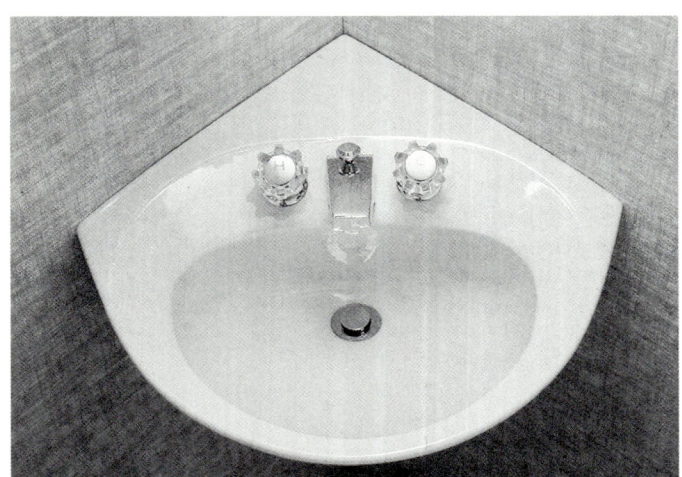

Corner sinks like this one from Eljer fit nicely into tight spaces in small baths.

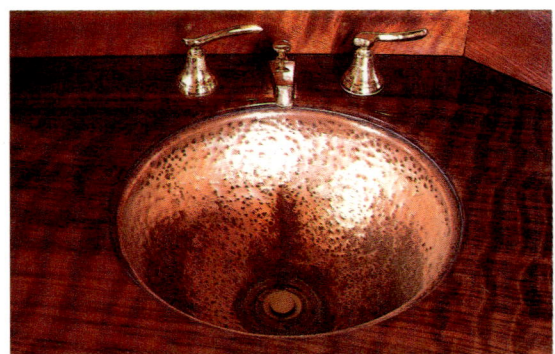

This hammered copper basin gives just the right luxury touch to a redwood burl countertop.

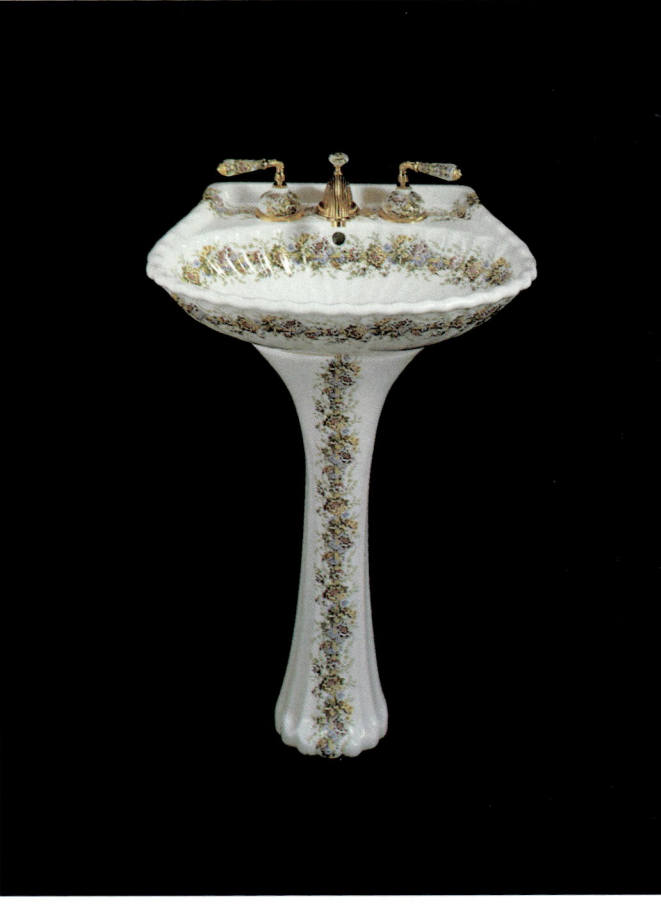

Many fixtures, like this hand-painted pedestal sink from Phylrich, are veritable works of art.

The futuristic look in fixtures that is so popular in Europe, such as this model from Hastings Tile & Il Bagno Collection, has now worked its way west.

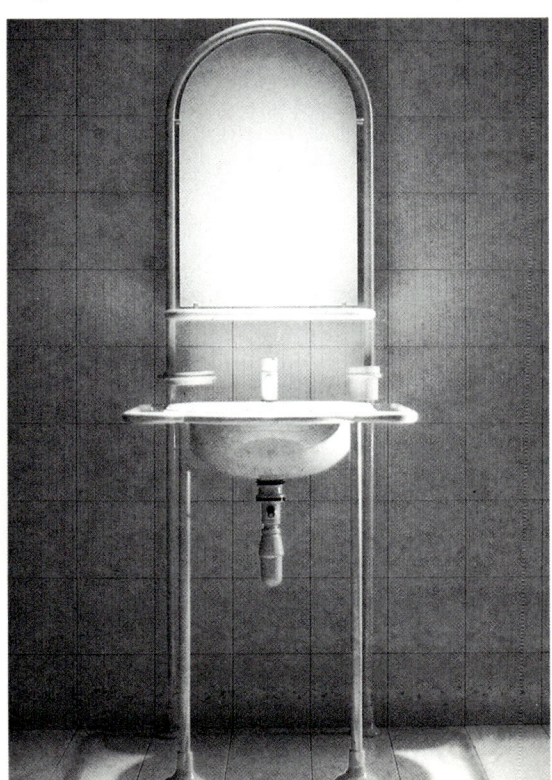

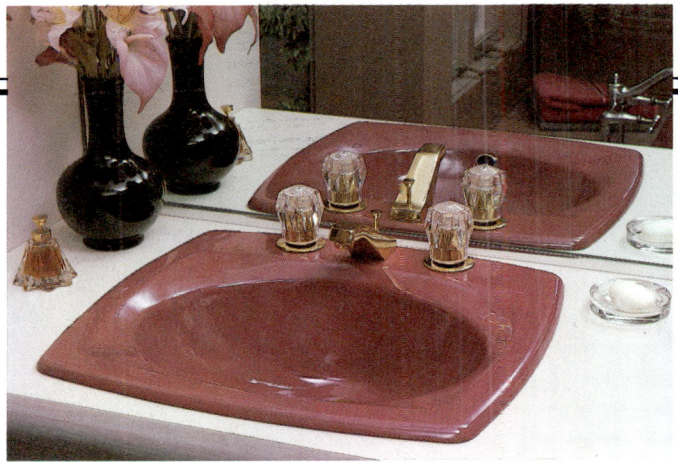

Sinks come in a wide variety of colors as well as styles. This is Kohler's raspberry puree.

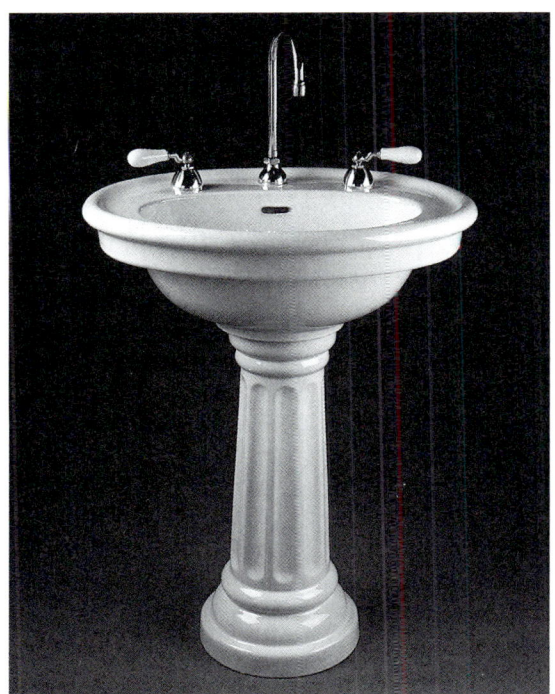

Amazingly authentic-looking reproductions from Sunrise Specialty Company offer nostalgic charm with modern plumbing efficiency.

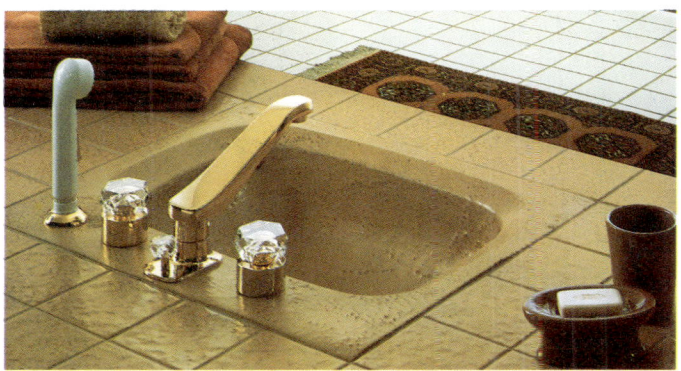

The Cerámica Companions sink by Eljer pairs up nicely with made-to-match tile by American Olean.

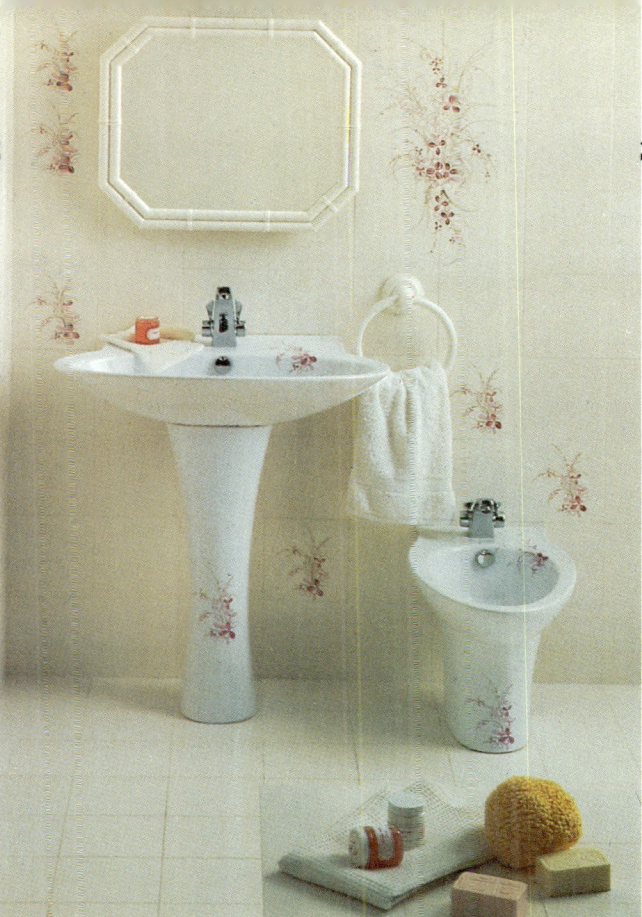

Many fixtures, like these from Porcher's hand-painted collection, can be color-coordinated.

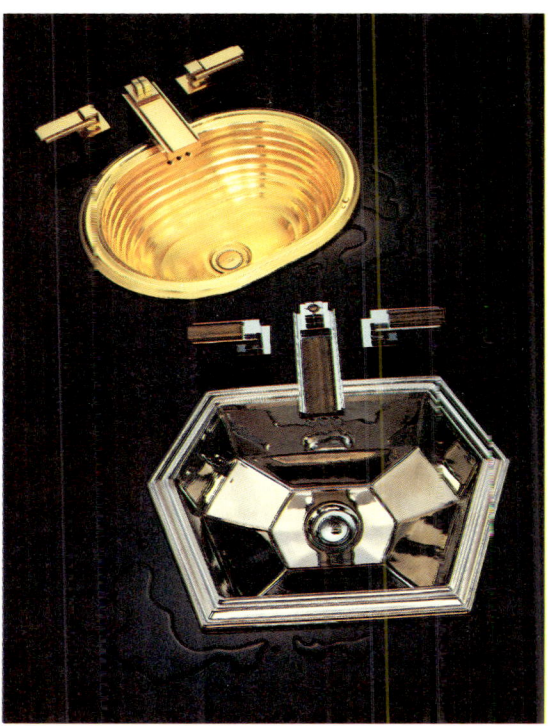

Basins of precious metals, like these gold and platinum sinks from Sherle Wagner, require special care.

## The Basic Bathtub

Bathtubs have gotten a face-lift in the last several years. Traditionalists can still soak in a standard 5-foot, rectangular model, but the more adventurous bathers have many more choices: round tubs; square tubs; modular tub/shower units; old-fashioned-style, claw-foot tubs; sunken tubs; oversize tubs; undersize tubs—even Japanese-style soaking tubs!

This should not discourage you from considering a standard model. Despite the popularity of luxury models, manufacturers report that 5-foot tubs still account for 85 to 90 percent of tub sales.

Today's basic bathtub doesn't have to be utilitarian. Manufacturers have upgraded both the design and the materials used in standard rectangular tubs, as well as equipping them with attractive side moldings, grab bars, nonskid textures, and built-in lumbar supports and contours for more comfortable soaking.

Some standard models feature drains located at the opposite end from the faucets, allowing for easier cleaning; others accommodate special dispensers for soap and shampoo. Standard tubs come in a wide variety of colors to match other bath fixtures and are readily available at plumbing or building-supply stores.

If you're in the market for a standard bathtub that's a bit more customized, you have a few alternatives from which to select. Rectangular tubs vary in length to meet differing space requirements. If your bathroom is small or primarily used by children, consider a 4-foot model; an extra-large bather might be more comfortable in a tub that is 6 feet long.

Square tubs fit nicely into corners and give the bathroom a special appearance. They may be small or large and often feature small seats in the corners. They require a great deal of water, however, and are difficult for small children or elderly persons to get in and out of. You can find oval tubs, round tubs—even octagonal tubs—that fit into standard-size bath areas.

Bathtubs come in the same basic materials as drop-in sinks (formed steel, fiberglass, and cast iron) and have the same basic properties. The least expensive tubs start at $100; you can pay up to $2,000 and more for top-of-the-line models.

Formed-steel bathtubs are the least expensive. Like the sinks of similar material, they're lightweight and easy to clean but are not chip-resistant. Because of the thinness of the steel, formed-steel tubs can also be very noisy. These tubs are available in a limited number of colors.

Fiberglass tubs, regardless of whether they have an acrylic or polyester gel coating, tend to be noisy because of their thinness; they also scratch easily and so require special care. But they come in a wide variety of decorator colors and shapes and so are an attractive choice. When shopping for a fiberglass tub, look for consistent thickness along the edges of the tub and a smooth surface free of cracks or creases. Better tubs are reinforced along the bottom.

Cast-iron tubs are the most expensive and also the most durable. Cast iron is also thicker than other bathtub materials, so it holds heat well. (It is possible to insulate the underside of a tub, which will also keep the water warmer.) Because cast-iron tubs are much heavier than those made of other materials, installing one could require extra work. You might, for example, have to reinforce the bathroom floor joists. When shopping for cast iron, look for a tub with a surface free of ripples or indentations. A thick enamel coating is an indication of a well-made tub.

## Beyond the Basic Bathtub

Sure, the old Saturday-night soak is still around, but with today's hectic pace, many people want more from their tubs than mere immersion. They want total relaxation. And makers of bathroom products have obliged with a number of unique alternatives to ordinary baths.

With the emergence of the bath as an enjoyable place to relax and spend time, oversize tubs are becoming more and more popular. They are much wider than the standard 30- to 34-inch-wide tub and are deeper as well; two adults can easily enjoy a sensuous, neck-deep soak. Available in a dazzling array of colors and almost as many shapes and textures, the oversize tub turns the bath into a focal point in a room. It's a perfect setting for after-dinner conversation and cordials—guests will relish "soaking" parties.

If you plan to include an oversize tub in your bath design, be sure to consider its extra weight and water requirements. You will need substantial support framing and possibly a back-up water heater. And don't embarrass yourself: Make sure you can get the tub into your house through existing doorways.

Sunken tubs add even more luxury to the bath. Almost any size bathtub can work as a sunken tub, including the standard 5-foot model. Again, you'll need to do some checking before you begin installation. A sunken tub needs adequate ground support, so make sure there is enough room underneath the floor to hold one. Second-floor sunken tubs may require special framing supports. Also, in a renovation the plumbing drain system may not allow such an installation. Keep in mind, too, that sunken tubs are hard to clean.

The Soft Bathtub Company has taken the fiberglass tub one step further, with—what else?—the *soft* tub. These comfortable tubs are lined with a 1-inch layer of plastic foam, which is covered with a tough, flexible surface that resists scratches and punctures. Noise in the tub is reduced considerably, and the soak is easier to settle into. The standard 5-foot size retails for about $1,200.

## Platforms

A major disadvantage of oversize and sunken tubs is the potential hazard they create, especially in households with small children or elderly residents. Oversize tubs can be very difficult to navigate. And sunken tubs, which are flush with the floor, pose the possibility of someone taking an unplanned step and hurting themselves. One way to alleviate this problem and at the same time create a luxurious bathing space is to "sink" the tub into a raised platform.

A platform can add to the attractiveness of your bath by creating a special space

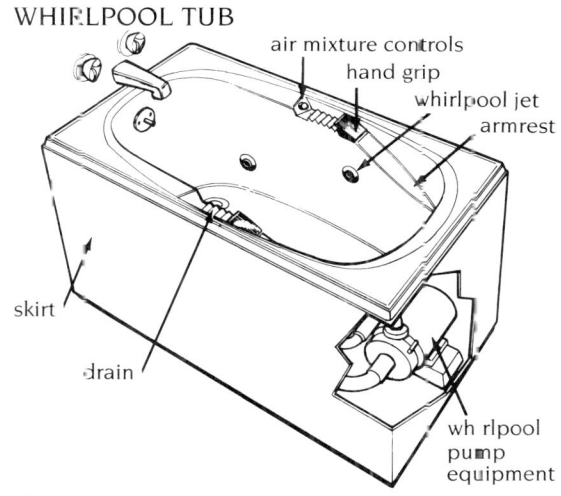

WHIRLPOOL TUB
air mixture controls
hand grip
whirlpool jet
armrest
skirt
drain
whirlpool pump equipment

for your special tub and will double as a plant holder or towel shelf. You can use a number of different waterproof materials for the platform surround, including ceramic tile, laminate, Corian, 2000X, treated wood, or stone.

Your platform will require a considerable amount of space, however; if you are remodeling, installing one might mean expanding the size of your existing bathroom. You could "borrow" needed space from a linen closet or part of a spare bedroom. Or you might consider bumping out a wall to create a sunspace type of enclosure for the bathtub area.

Platforms need to be well-built, since they will be supporting weights that can reach in excess of 1,300 pounds (that's two people in a 6-foot, 700-pound tub filled with 50 gallons of water). Floor joists underneath the tub may have to be strengthened. If you will be doing the work yourself, make sure you check with a contractor, plumber, or other building professional to make sure the platform will provide adequate support for the tub.

## Whirlpool Tubs, Hot Tubs, and Spas

Whirlpool tubs have all the trappings of a regular bathtub, and you can still take an ordinary bath in one. But there is an important difference. A whirlpool tub comes with jets that, when turned on, create a strong bubbling or swirling current in the tub. Whirlpools are both relaxing and therapeutic.

CLASSIC HOT TUB

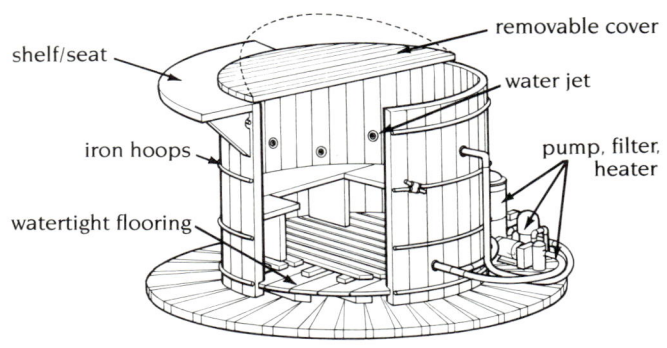

SPA

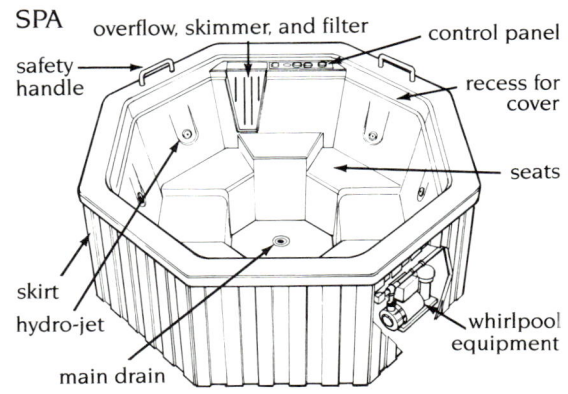

They are available in a variety of sizes: Some are little bigger than an average shower stall; others fit standard tub enclosures; still others are big enough to hold three or four people. They come in just as many shapes: square, oval, round, triangular, and rectangular.

Some whirlpool tubs have only three jets; most have four, while others come equipped with as many as eight. The price of the unit varies with the number of jets. A standard 60-by-32-inch whirlpool tub may cost only $1,100, but with eight jets, the same tub can cost $3,000. And there are other extras. Underwater illumination systems, for example, run an extra $500; designer faucets can cost you a few hundred dollars more.

If you'd like the soothing, swirling action of a whirlpool but can't afford the price of a built-in whirlpool tub, a portable whirlpool can allow you to enjoy a bubbly soak in your existing tub. It costs about $250. Be sure that such a device is UL-approved (Underwriters Laboratories).

Hot tubs are self-supporting wood tubs, 4 to 10 feet wide and about 4 feet deep. They are usually made of oak, redwood, mahogany, cypress, cedar, or teakwood, held together with metal bands. When the tub is filled with water, the wood swells and makes a watertight seal. Japanese soaking tubs are fashioned similarly but are deeper and are often designed for only one or two persons. Water spas are like hot tubs, except that they're made of fiberglass, tile, or concrete and measure 5 to 6 feet wide and about 3 feet deep.

Like swimming pools, spas and hot tubs are kept filled with water and must be filtered, drained, and cleaned periodically. Maintenance costs vary greatly depending on numerous factors: the size, the amount of use, whether the spa or tub is indoors or outdoors, the climate, and so forth. Spas and hot tubs come equipped with either electric or gas water heaters, pumps, and filters. They cost between $3,000 and $5,000. Both hot tubs and spas can be fitted with special covers to keep the water cleaner and to prevent accidents from occurring

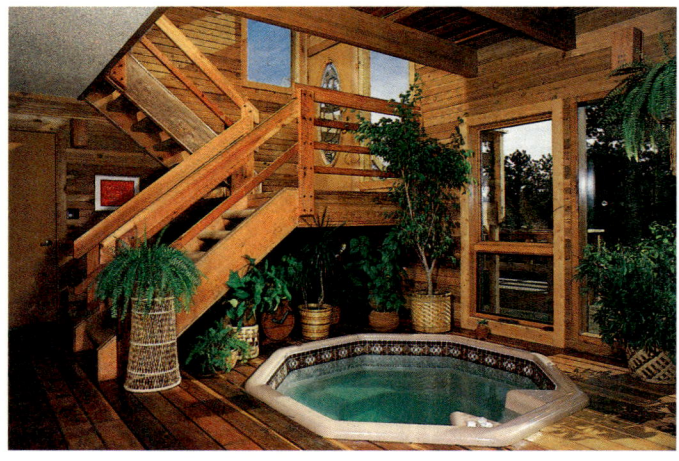

If you're going to locate a spa indoors, remember that adequate ventilation is a must.

when the tub or spa is not in use. Some of the newer models sport special "party tables" on which you can play a board game or cards or rest a cool drink.

One new type of spa, the portable spa, is becoming increasingly popular. Because it has self-contained plumbing and is relatively lightweight, it can be installed just about anywhere—and you can take it with you when you move. It's not as deep as a permanent spa, but it's less expensive, costing just over $3,000.

You can buy whirlpool tubs and spas that are made from enameled cast iron, but most of the ones sold today are made of fiberglass, which offers far more variety of color and style. If you're in the market for a fiberglass spa, get one that has an acrylic rather than a polyester gel coating finish. Acrylic is more resistant to ultraviolet and infrared light and chemicals. Check to make sure the edges of the tub are the same thickness all the way around and that there are no cracks on the rim or the lining. Molded units should be reinforced at the steps, across the bottom, and around all outlets.

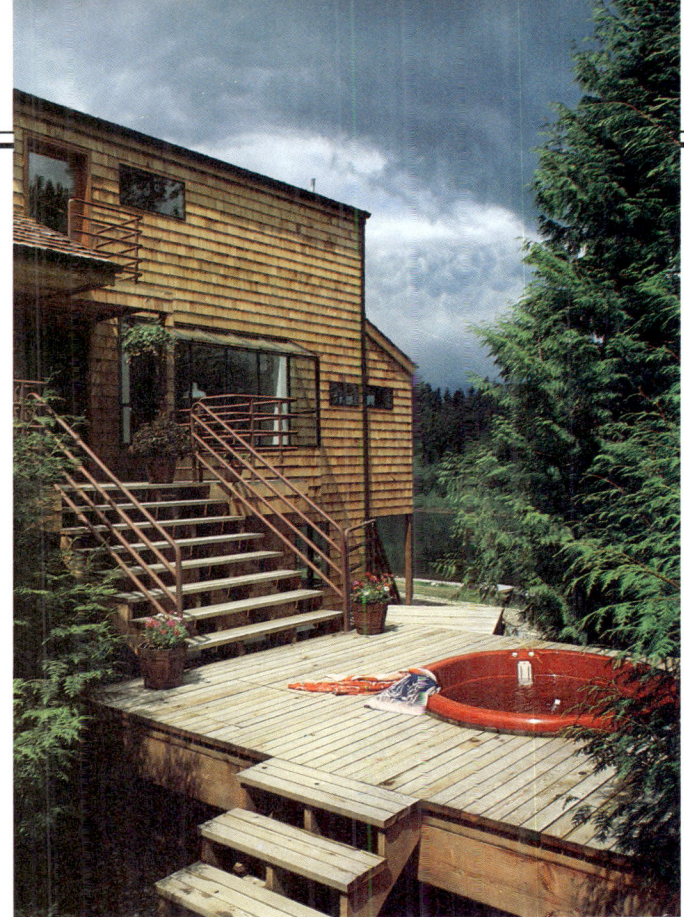

Outdoor spas are wonderful—as long as they are maintained properly. Timed filtering devices can make maintenance much easier.

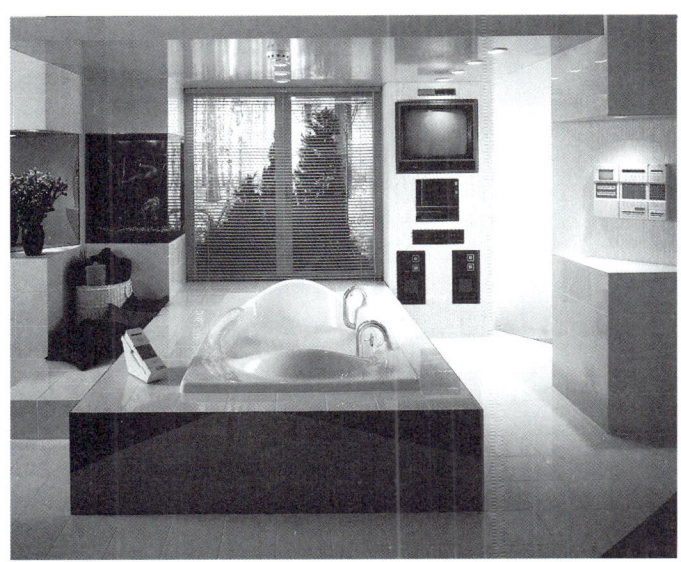

American-Standard's Sensorium whirlpool is equipped with Ambiance, a special computer that ensures a luxurious bathing experience.

## The Ultimate Soak

There are whirlpools and then there are *whirlpools*. The BathWomb by Water Jet Corporation, for example, is an anatomically contoured tub that sports a water-safe electronic panel that controls a nine-jet whirlpool, a stereo, a Touch-Tone phone speaker system, a digital clock, a pillow and body massage, and a facial mister. Available in 55 colors, the BathWomb offers sybaritic soaking for a price. (It retails for about $11,000.)

Kohler's Environment Masterbath which retails for over $19,000, is another total bathing experience. It's a built-in, enclosed tub unit that offers a variety of "environments": a heat-lamp "sun"; junglelike steam; dry, desert sauna heat—even cool rain and warm breezes—in addition to the whirlpool bath and shower.

American-Standard's Sensorium whirlpool is another bath for the self-indulgent. A special computer (it's called Ambiance) built in to the tub allows bathers to set the proper mood for a regal soak. The $25,000 system controls room lights, door locks, telephone, stereo, and, of course, the hydromassage in the spacious whirlpool itself. The only thing it won't do is pour drinks for you.

## Questions to Answer before You Buy a Spa

Before you financially commit yourself to a spa or hot tub, be sure you have the answers to these questions:

*Is it in your budget?* The overall cost of a spa includes much more than a fiberglass shell and a heating unit. Installation is normally not included in the base price of a spa. In-ground spas require foam insulation, and modifications to the plumbing and power source may be necessary. And don't forget the inevitable increase in your monthly heating bill.

*Is the intended location of the spa a practical one for the household?* An indoor spa must be easily accessible, but you won't want spa traffic tracking through your formal dining room. A spa is a luxurious addition to a bathroom, but keep in mind that people will want to use the bathroom for other reasons. And while it's tempting, remember that you can't use soaps or oils in the water while you soak; they will clog the filter.

An outdoor spa should be private and close to the house—you won't want to skip through several feet of snow to soak in the wintertime. Try to keep your tub out of direct sunlight, which promotes algae growth. Wind currents, too, are important to monitor; too much breeze can make it difficult to maintain the water temperature at its recommended level.

*Is it a practical location for the installer?* The farther your outdoor tub is from the house, the farther it is from heat and water sources, and therefore the more costly installation will be. Indoor installations are even trickier. Floor joists have to be strengthened, fans must be installed to vent humidity outside the house, and all surfaces in the spa area should be moisture-resistant. And, of course, you'll have to have some way to get the spa (they are one-piece, fiberglass units) into your house!

*Who will maintain the spa?* You won't be happy if there is bacteria growing in your spa. So make sure that *someone* has the time to clean it properly. If your household is too busy to follow a maintenance schedule, consider investing in automatic feeders, ozonators, and timed measuring devices.

*Is the spa area safe?* Indoors or out, the spa should be well-supervised; if you have young children, plan for a locking door at the entrance to the area. The floor surrounding the spa should be covered with a nonslip surface. Everyone who has a spa or who is considering installing one should read *The Sensible Way to Enjoy Your Spa or Hot Tub: An Essential Safety Guide*, available for $1.75 from the National Spa & Pool Institute. (See "Helpful Addresses.")

## Shower Stalls

As much as the bath has become a personal pampering parlor, it can't adequately serve a busy household without the utility of a shower. But in today's bath, the shower is as aesthetically pleasing as it is functional. You can be as original as your imagination and your budget allow.

The most economical way to include a shower is to install a shower head on the wall above an existing bathtub, or to add a movable spray head on a flexible cable. (See "Tub and Shower Faucets" on page 37 for more information.) A popular trend is to separate the shower from the bathtub, to isolate the tub as the essence of your bathroom design. This requires the installation of a separate shower stall.

Two-piece, all-fiberglass units are the least expensive kind of shower stalls. The pan on a two-piece unit sits on the floor and houses the drain opening; the sides cover the wall and accept the shower head, doors, or curtain. Or you can buy just the pan, then customize the walls and floor with tile or cultured marble.

Going custom all the way with tile or other materials floor to ceiling is the most expensive option, but it does produce striking results. If you do plan to use tile on the floor of your shower, make sure it's skid-resistant—even in water. And pay attention to waterproofing the joints; water seepage can cause major damage.

Although the minimum size of a shower stall is 32 inches square, 36 inches square is generally much more comfortable. The best shape is rectangular—36 by 42 inches or 36 by 54 inches. That leaves room to fit in a built-in bench or seat for safety and comfort. The starting price for a two-piece fiberglass shower stall is about $400.

If your bath does not allow space to separate the shower and tub, consider a one-piece fiberglass model. Factory-made tub/shower combinations are easy to install (provided you have some way of getting them into your house) and are available in a spectrum of brilliant colors. Some, like the Bath Wraps line by Plaskolite, have built-in seats, soap dishes, washcloth holders, and special nooks for hair-care products, back brushes, and bathing oils.

Because there are no joints or grout lines, the smooth, contoured surfaces of these units are easy to care for, although they do scratch easily (use a nonabrasive cleaner). If you are planning to include a one-piece unit in your bath, make sure you install it before the walls are finished; otherwise you won't be able to get it into your bathroom.

Unless you specially design a shower large enough to function without it, you will need some kind of enclosure for any shower style you choose. A curtain is the least expensive but the most difficult to keep clean. Another option is the door. Most are made of durable, corrosion-resistant materials and have screens of shatterproof glass or Plexiglas. You can choose from a single, swing-away door or a sliding or accordion-style door (good for a shower/tub combination).

A two-sided or angled model converts a corner of your bathroom into a shower;

## Living with a Shower Curtain

A shower curtain doesn't have to be an ugly, mildewy piece of plastic. In fact, it doesn't have to be plastic at all. You can use just about any fabric you wish for the outer curtain and pair it with a separate piece of vinyl that will protect it from splashes.

Let your curtain continue the design statement of your bath. Coordinate it with your towels and other bath linens, and accessorize it with a gleaming brass, chrome, or brightly colored acrylic curtain rod. You'll be looking at the curtain both inside and outside the shower, so make it attractive from all angles.

To combat the mildew and grime that often build up on a shower curtain, air it out as completely as possible after each use. Wiping it down is even more effective, if you can get into the habit. Make sure the shower area is well-ventilated with windows or exhaust fans.

Mildew often builds up despite faithful cleanup efforts. Fortunately, most curtain materials are machine-washable. Just launder the curtain with mild soap and cool water; throw in a few old towels to aid in the scrubbing action. Or keep several inexpensive inner liners on hand to use with the decorative outer portion. When one mildews, toss it out and replace it with another one.

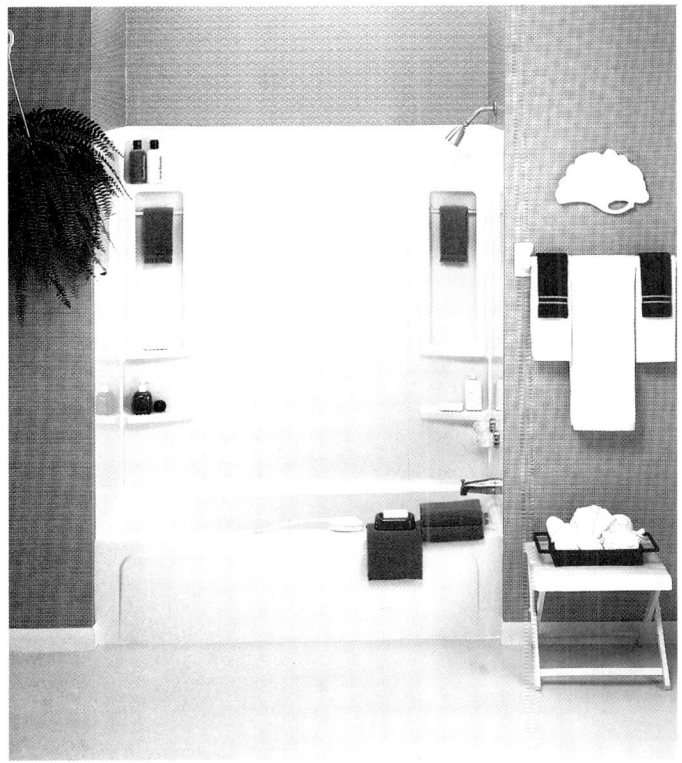

All-in-one systems like this provide a tub, a shower, and nooks and crannies for bathing needs.

this is especially nice if your shower walls will be covered with waterproof laminate or tile, since it precludes the need for an additional stall. Showerlux Canada and Alumax/Magnolia Division, among others, make rounded enclosures that serve the same purpose and add a touch of elegance.

Shower enclosures should be well-built. Doors should open and close efficiently and glide smoothly and quietly. Most major manufacturers make enclosures with rounded corners, which decrease the chance of injury. For ease of cleanup, Huppe has introduced a sliding door that sits flush with the tub rim or shower base—the groove-free surface eliminates the buildup of grime.

Yet another enclosure option is the "shower room" concept, which eliminates doors and curtains completely. The Shower Shell by Swan Corporation is just that—a shell-shaped enclosure that serves as an open but private and protected shower room.

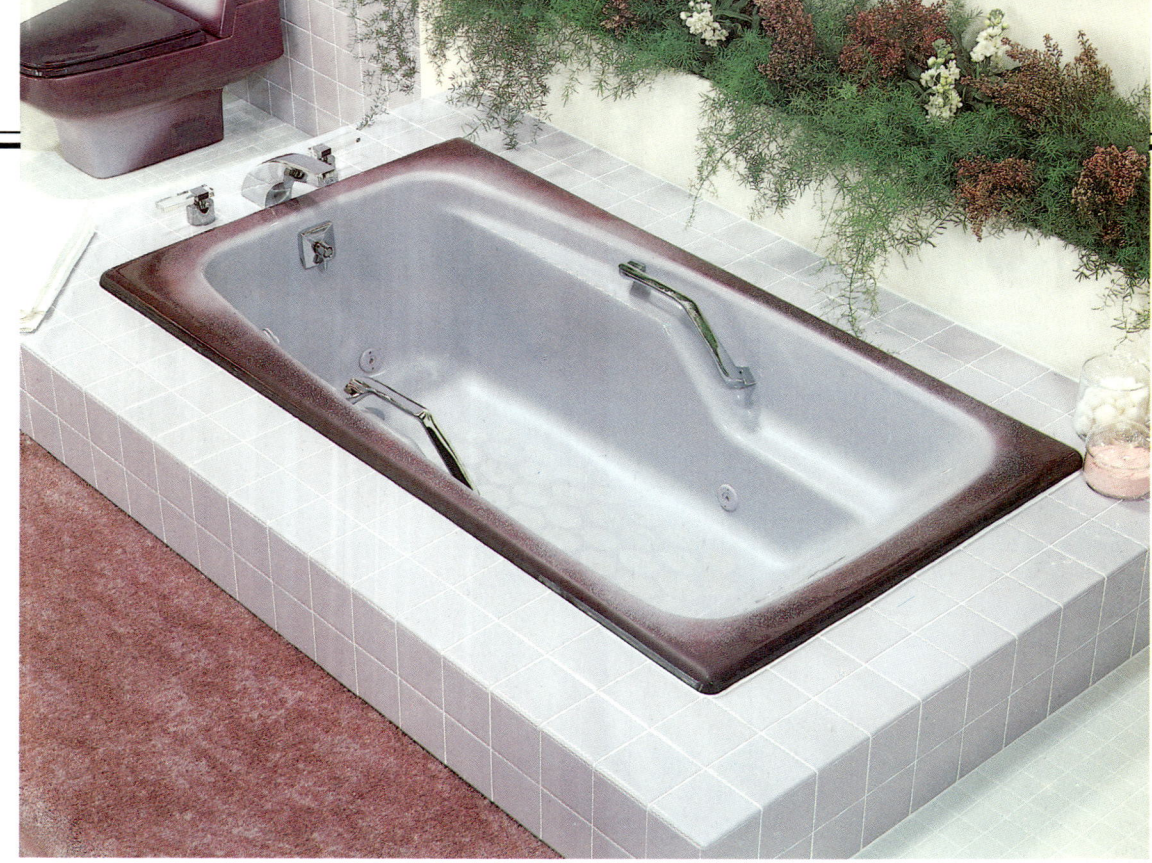

Lavender and dark purple, blended together in Eljer's Blended Hues, make this tub a masterpiece.

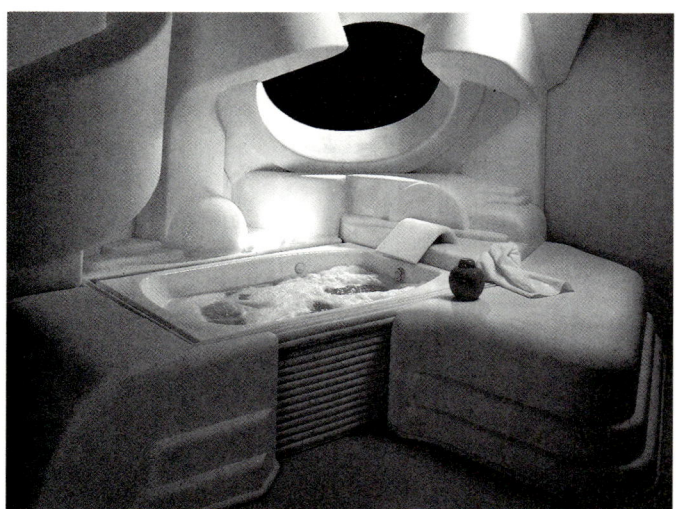

Soft-surface tubs keep water warm as well as offer a more comfortable soak.

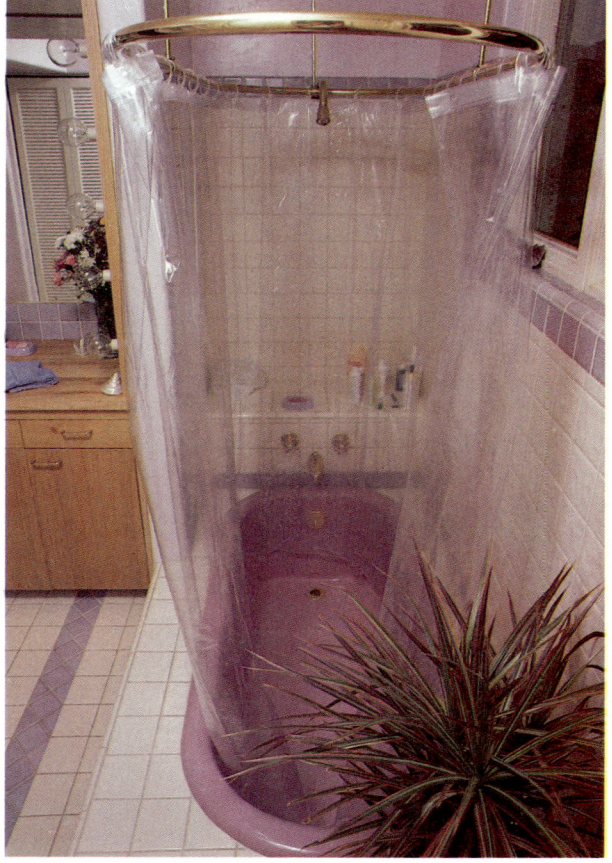

A brass converter rod can turn an old-fashioned tub into a unique shower system.

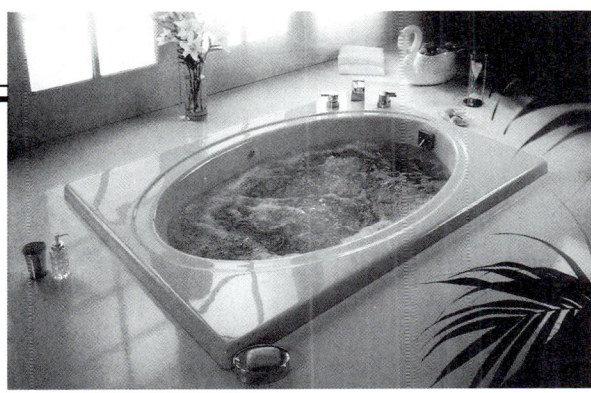

Oversize whirlpool tubs can be set into platforms or installed in a sunken area, like this one, directly into the floor.

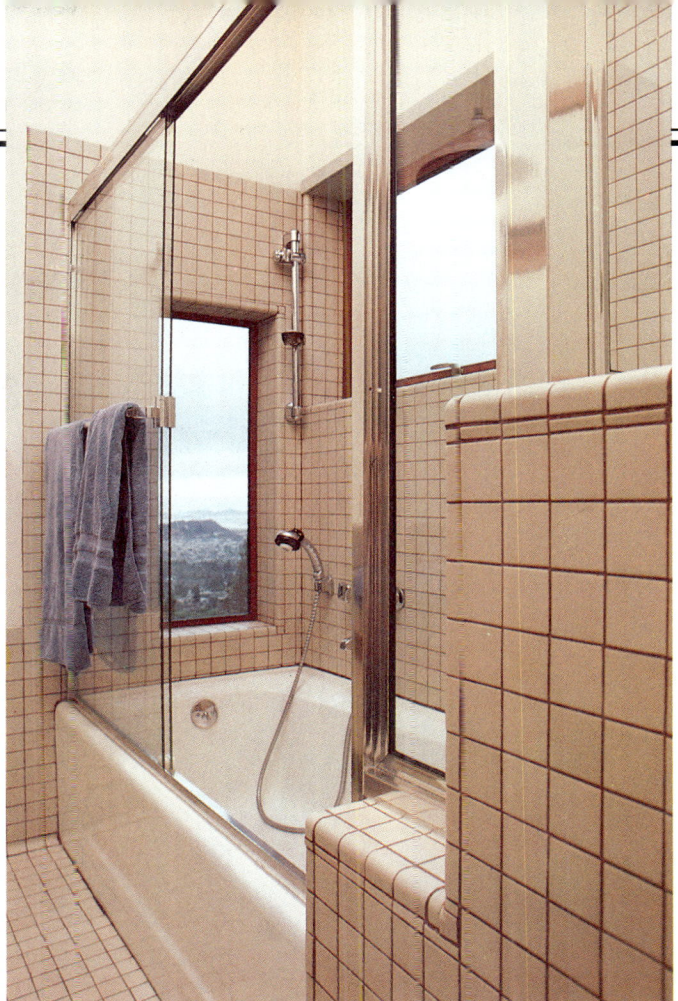

Dark red grout gives this tile shower surround a unique look.

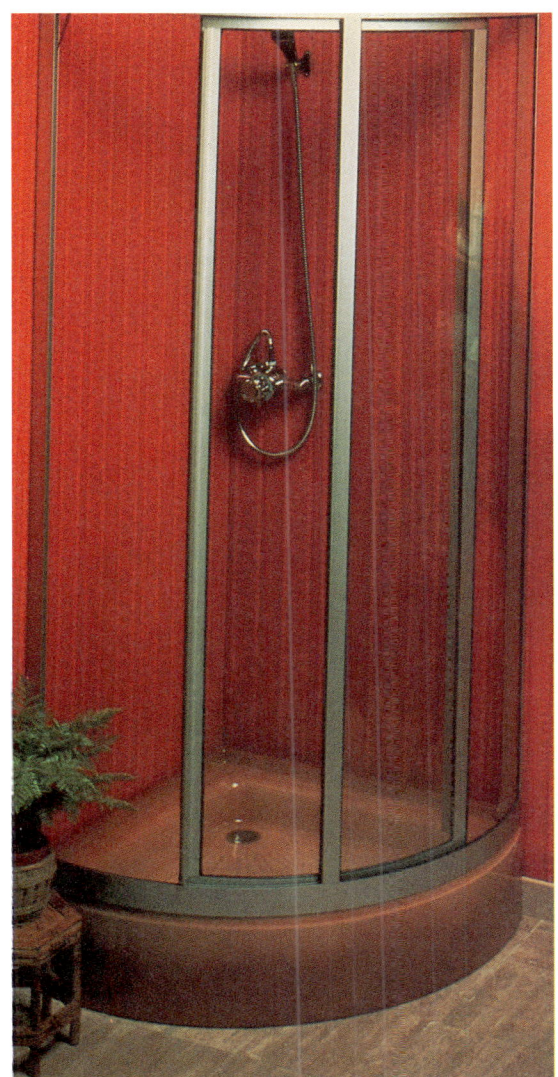

Corner showers can make it possible to install a shower in even the smallest bath.

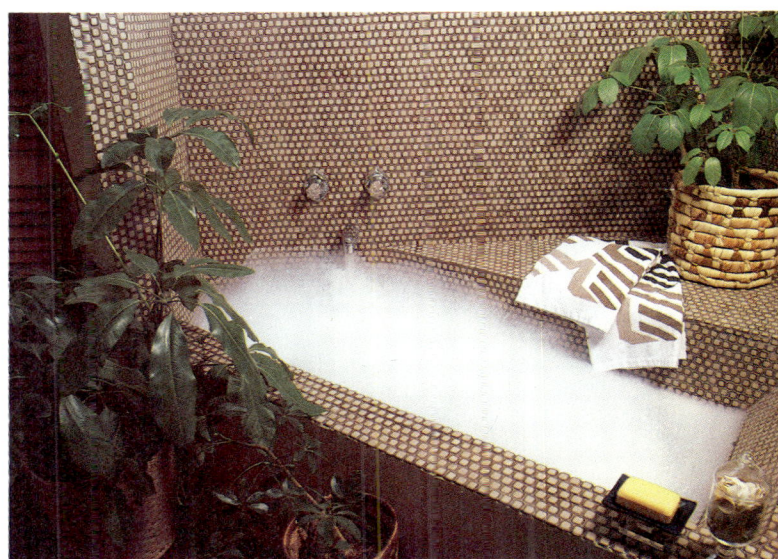

You can use ceramic tile to custom-design a tub in any shape you desire.

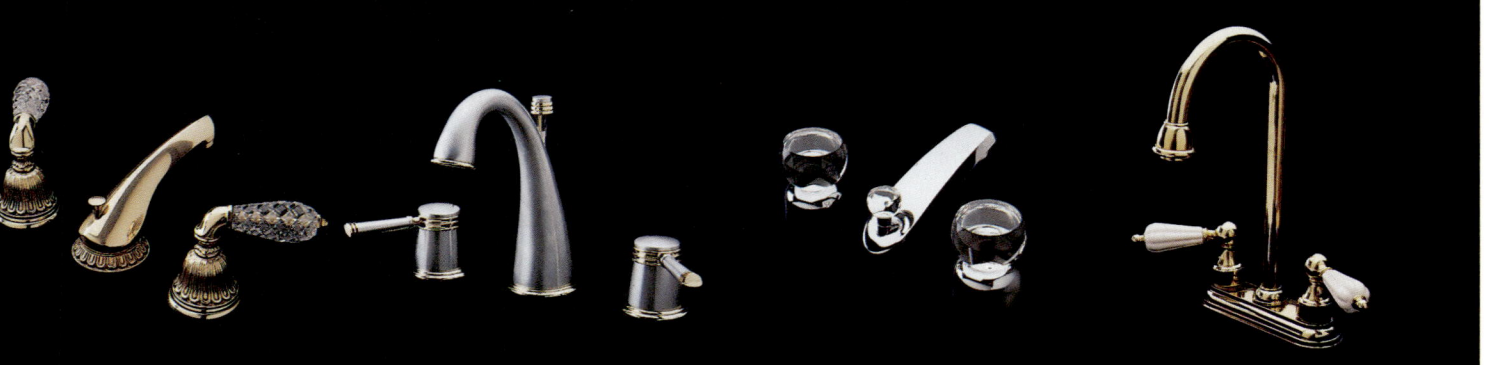

**Jewels of the Bath:** Faucets are available in just about any style and material you can imagine. From left to right: Moen Widespread from Moen Group/Stanadyne, polished brass with cut crystal handles; Dual-Finish Lever Handles (76 series) from Artistic Brass, satin chrome and polished brass; Ellisse from American-Standard, chrome with clear acrylic handles; and La Coquille Petite suite from the Broadway Collection, polished brass with porcelain handles.

## Faucets: Plain and Fancy

Looking at bathroom faucet displays these days is like browsing past a showcase of fine jewels. Alluring new designs, crafted in a wealth of fine materials, make the simple act of turning on hot water a rich experience. Some faucet sets are quite ornate, with lavish fittings of gold and brass complemented by cut-crystal, porcelain, or onyx handles. The new European designs, with their sleek, modern lines, impart a high-tech look to your bath. American-Standard makes a faucet with a digital readout on the handle to indicate water temperature. Although there are literally hundreds of faucet sets on the market, your answers to the following questions will help narrow your choices.

*Who will be the primary users of the bathroom?* Faucets for a children's bathroom should be easy to use, with durable finishes and nonslip handles. A sink used for hair washing in the master bath might benefit from a graceful, gooseneck faucet spout that can be moved out of the way when it's not needed. Moen makes a gooseneck faucet that can be raised for washing hair and then lowered when not in use. In a luxury bath, you can give your imagination free rein. Just make practical faucet choices for the type of bath you are creating.

*Are you more concerned with the mechanical design of a faucet or with its aesthetic appeal?* Professional bathroom designers generally agree that the more ornate the faucet, the less attention the manufacturer is likely to have paid to its fittings. But durability *can* be quite stylish; manufacturers like American-Standard, Delta Faucet Company, Grohe America, Kohler Company, and Moen Group, among others, make some quality faucets that are as elegant as they are efficient.

*Will you be happy with a chrome finish on a faucet, or are you interested in something fancier?* Most fittings today are constructed from brass (it resists corrosion well) and are coated with some type of finish. From a maintenance standpoint, chrome is your best bet. Gold is a soft finish and requires gentle care and delicate use. Uncoated brass will tarnish, and the lacquer or epoxy topcoats used to protect brass from tarnishing must be carefully maintained so that the finish is not scrubbed off. However, if you are willing to maintain them, these finishes can help you make an important design statement in your bath.

*Is it important to you that all of the faucets and accessories in the bathroom match?* Many manufacturers do not offer a complete line of sink, tub, and shower faucet sets. Even fewer product lines include towel bars and toilet-paper holders. Although various finishes can complement each other quite nicely, if you've got your heart set on a perfect match, consider only full-line manufacturers.

Bathroom-sink faucets come in two sizes: a 4-inch-wide set with one or two

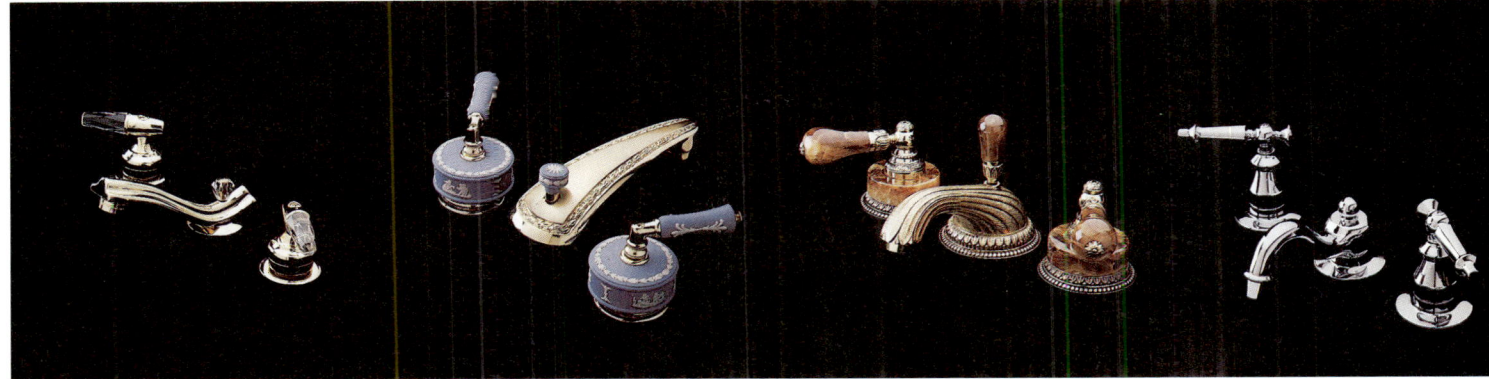

From left to right: Award Collection (model 3523BC) by Delta, simulated gold finish with crystal handles; Wedgwood from Artistic Brass, polished brass with Wedgwood; Onyx-460 series from Artistic Brass, polished brass with onyx; Antique Series from Kohler in polished chrome.

handles and an 8-inch-wide center set. The 8-inch-wide center set is easy to clean, attractive to look at, and simple to operate. Single-handle faucets are a popular convenience. A pop-up drain assembly should be part of any faucet set you choose.

The price of most faucets is determined by the quantity and quality of brass they're constructed with. Those constructed entirely of brass or finished with precious metals will obviously cost more. Ask your dealer for a written warranty for your new faucet; like other appliances and products, quality faucets have warranties to back them up.

If you are considering a foreign-made faucet, make sure you have access to a dealer in the United States who can supply you with replacement parts. You may have to use thread adapters to make the foreign-made faucet compatible with your plumbing system. Also check to see whether foreign-manufactured fittings meet plumbing standards for the United States.

### Tub and Shower Faucets

A tub faucet set includes a valve and fill spout; a shower faucet set features a shower head and valve. In combination fixtures, either the shower valve or the tub fill spout includes a diverter to route the water to the fill spout or to the shower head. Single-handle valves and separate hot and cold valve sets are available.

There is a great range of quality among shower heads. The best heads provide a wide water-spray pattern that is adjustable, pulsating, or both. Heads that restrict the flow of water but still provide a strong enough

### Do You Know ...

- that approximately 13,000 gallons of purified drinking water are flushed down the toilet of the average household each year? Installing a plastic dam around the flush valve will reduce the amount of water needed for each flush. (This inexpensive item can be found at a plumbing or building-supply store.)

- that putting bricks in your toilet tank can cause plumbing damage? They disintegrate, and particles get caught in the pipes.

- that up to 200 gallons of water can seep unnoticed into the toilet bowl through leaks in the tank? Identify leaks by putting food coloring into the tank. If after several hours the color has seeped into the bowl, you have a leak and need a new flushing device.

- that brushing teeth with the tap on uses 5 gallons of water, while turning it on just for a quick rinse uses just a quart?

- that insulating the hot water pipes and water heater tanks can save you up to $50 a year on your utility bill?

- that shower heads with push buttons that interrupt water flow while you soap up and restore it to the same temperature and pressure for rinsing save many gallons a year?

flow for a good shower are on the market and will help you save water.

The shower valve should do much more than simply mix the hot and cold water. Pressure-balanced valves monitor incoming hot and cold water volume and prevent surprise scaldings from pressure changes in the line. Newer, thermostatically controlled models have heat-sensing devices to maintain a preselected temperature of water.

For children's baths, you can get valves that will always turn on the cold water first; the handle moves through warm before reaching hot. For an extra safety measure, valves are available with high-temperature limits that let you preset the amount of hot water that flows through them.

Careful placement of the shower valve and head makes a big difference in the way the shower works. The ideal location for the shower valve is on the wall opposite the shower head, rather than directly underneath it. That way, you won't have to dodge the shower stream while trying to adjust it. You can even splurge on a "toe tester," a special minifaucet, located separately from the main shower head, that allows you to check the temperature of the water before you get doused.

The standard height for a shower head is 66 inches, but that may not be the best for you. If different-size people use the shower, consider mounting the head on a post so that the head can slide up and down.

If two people will need to get ready for work at the same time, consider putting in two shower heads, one on either side of the shower stall—each with separate controls. Hand-held shower heads can perform a variety of purposes—hair rinsing, cleaning of the shower stall—and consume less water than conventional wall-mounted models.

Consider a flow-restricting shower head. They are easy to install, relatively inexpensive, and come in many styles and finishes. A good one will reduce water consumption to between 2½ and 3 gallons per minute. That means a five-minute shower that previously sent 20 gallons of water down the drain will now use just 10 gallons. There are shower heads available with a spray of 1.6 gallons of water per minute, but the quality of the spray is questionable. Soft water means that it will take a *long* time to rinse shampoo out of the hair. And the expanded surface space of the water means reduced water temperature.

If you can't find a flow-restricting shower head that blends with your design, you can buy small flow-restricting devices that fit inside just about any fitting. Available at hardware stores, these devices are inexpensive and do an adequate job of reducing the flow. Remember, though, that it is better to install a shower head that has been designed for use with a flow restricter. The quality of the flow is more predictable.

## *The New Victorian Bath*

Antique fixtures and accessories can create—or re-create, as the case may be—a comfortable and romantic atmosphere in your bathroom. If you'd like to fill your bath with nostalgic charm, you'll be happy to know that you can bring back the past without sacrificing modern convenience.

Finding antique fixtures for an old-fashioned bath is a little like hunting for buried treasure—original pieces are hard to find. Garage sales are good places to look, as are salvage yards, antique shops, estate sales, and the classified sections of newspapers.

Vintage fixtures may have been beautiful in their day, but it often takes some elbow grease to make them sparkle again. Sometimes all they require is a good cleaning. But if the enamel is so badly worn that cast iron is showing through, you'll want to have the piece restored. Hairline cracks can add to a fixture's antique charm, but large cracks should be repaired.

Although it sounds easier, don't be tempted to spruce up a bathtub or sink surface with spray paint. Baked enamel, even in a state of disrepair, will be very moisture-resistant; not much will stick to it for long. If you truly cherish the item and wish to renovate it, take it to a professional.

There are a number of businesses that specialize in restoring antique bath fixtures. (See "Helpful Addresses.") Resurfacing a standard 5-foot tub will cost you anywhere from $350 to $500; a sink, about half that amount. It's always a good idea to inquire

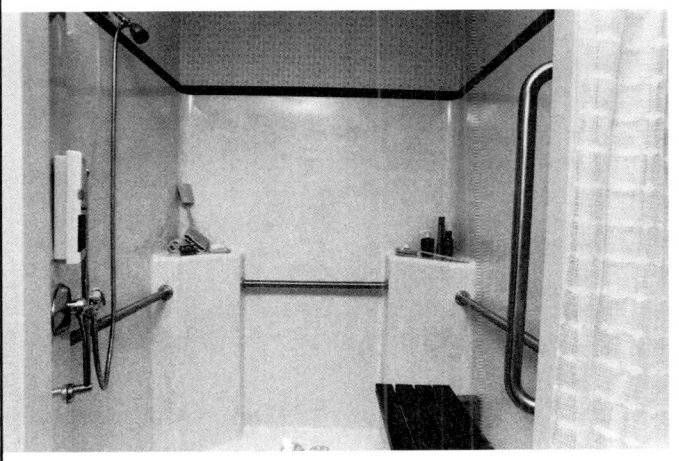
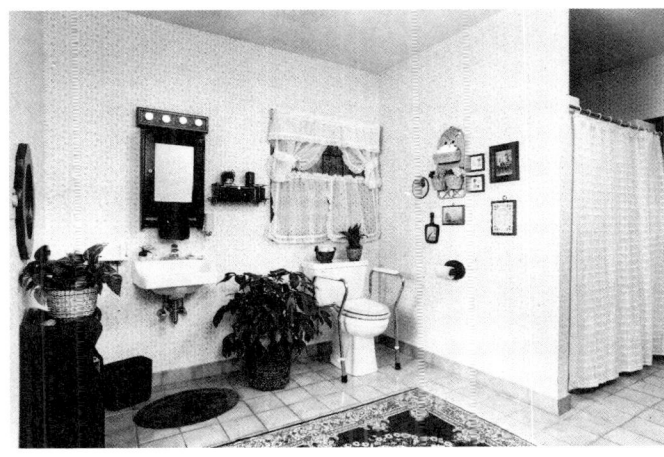
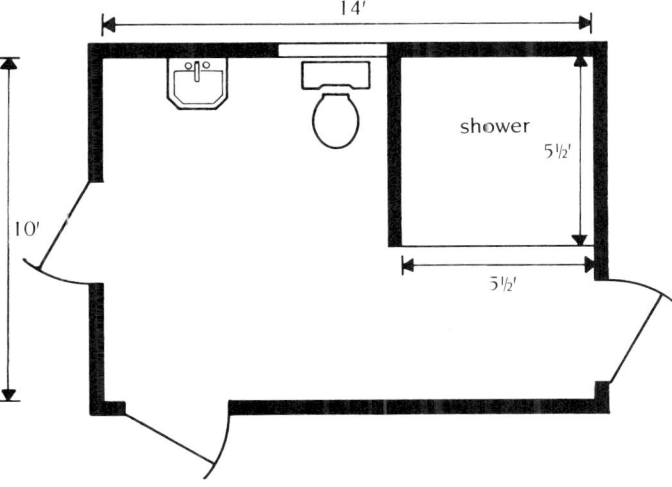

**David's Bath:** A bath designed for a person confined to a wheelchair should ideally be both accessible and comfortable. Such is the case with David Ziegenfuss's bath. The room is large, with extra-wide door frames that allow easy maneuvering of a wheelchair. The fixtures are all tailored to David's needs: The wall-hung sink allows plenty of knee space, and the toilet, which is about 4 inches higher than standard models, is equipped with safety bars. The shower is 5 feet square—big enough for a wheelchair—and has a hand-held spray attachment for more convenient use. But while it is functional, David's bath is certainly not institutional. The decorative touches added by his wife, Linda, make the room homey and comfortable.

about the reputation of the resurfacing company you choose; check with the Better Business Bureau about a company's reputation.

Make sure your genuine article will live up to present day wear and tear. Check drain assemblies and faucets to make sure internal parts are not too badly worn. Old-fashioned toilets can be equipped with modern flush mechanisms and oak water closets, but make sure the bowl is not of the outdated wash-down variety.

If you want the genuine look without the hassle of hunting down the genuine item, you can choose from the many "new Victorian" fixtures and accessories now available. These are well-designed reproductions made with modern, durable materials. Voluminous claw-foot tubs, pretty pedestal sinks, "antique" brass fittings, hand-painted porcelain accessories—even old-fashioned pull-chain water closets—are available from both specialty suppliers and conventional bathware manufacturers.

## Steam Adds Sizzle

A luxurious extra to consider for your new bathroom is steam. It can be gentle and relaxing and has long been known for its positive effects on the complex on of the skin—if used properly. For about $750 you can buy a steam generator small enough to be installed in a closet, basement, or attic. The cost for the total installation is about $1,500. Too pricey? For $50 or less, buy a shower head that creates a steamlike mist.

Before you invest in any kind of steam machine, examine your bathroom carefully to be sure that the tile grouting is in good repair. (It's a good idea to check your grout every year or so even if you don't install a steam bath.) Steam is pervasive. It can sneak through cracks that you can't see in the tile grout and can damage your walls. Also, be sure the shower is in good condition and that the shower door is sealed (but not airtight) to prevent steam leakage.

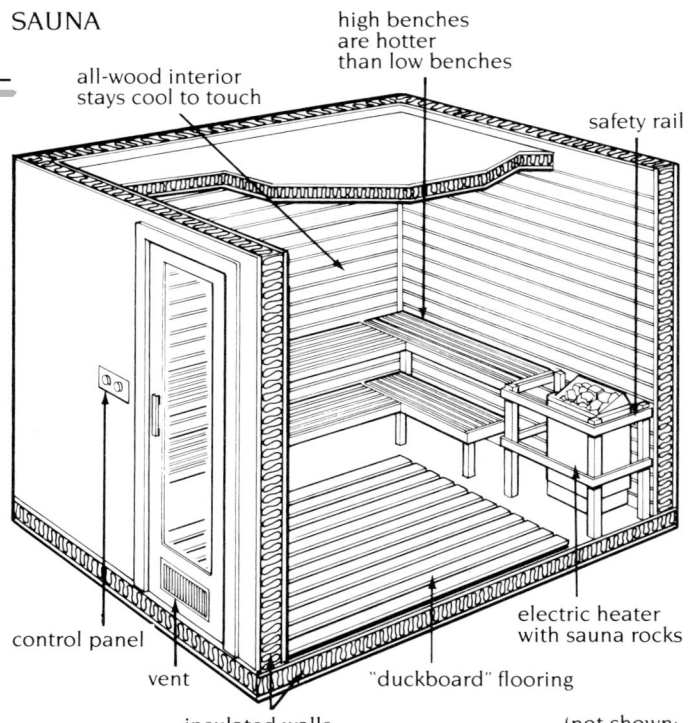

## Finish with a Sauna

For the total at-home spa experience, consider the sauna. The idea has been around for 2,000 years, and most aficionados agree that, as a source of mental and physical relaxation, it can't be beat.

A sauna is basically an insulated room, furnished with wooden benches and heated by means of a special stove to between 175 and 200 degrees Fahrenheit. A "sauna bath" consists of sitting in the dry heat for 10 to 30 minutes, taking a cold shower or bath, followed by another visit to the sauna. The second time around, a small amount of water may be ladled over hot coals to create a bit of steam. The second visit is again followed by a shower and cooling off period.

Though it sounds extravagant, a sauna really isn't. A one- or two-person sauna can cost under $3,000 installed—less than some of the new bathtubs. You may be able to further reduce the costs if you undertake some of the preparation work yourself; for example, you can get a spa heater for just under $1,000, then insulate and finish the room yourself. Your total outlay could be as little as $1,500.

A sauna doesn't have to take up much space, either. It can fit in a closet or be carved out of seldom-used space in an extra bedroom, basement, or even a piece of hallway.

## Making Hot Water

Adding or remodeling a bathroom is a time to evaluate your hot water needs and to be sure your existing system can carry the load. Particularly if you are installing high water consumers like whirlpools, look into improving your system's efficiency.

One simple way to get more mileage out of your existing water heater is to wrap the tank with fiberglass batts. Inexpensive insulating kits for tank and water pipes are available from utility companies and hardware stores.

If you have a gas heater, adjust the burner for proper combustion. If you have an old-fashioned pilot light, see if you can upgrade it to electric ignition. This not only saves fuel but is also safer—there's no open flame all the time. Also, if you are replacing a worn-out electric water heater, switching from electricity to gas is nearly always more economical.

In some cases, it might make more sense to heat water only when it's needed. (Use an automatic timer or a manual switch to turn on the system when you will need hot water.) This is particularly true for a large whirlpool tub that isn't used constantly.

Then there are tankless heaters, which don't heat a drop of water until a hot water faucet is turned on. They're available in numerous sizes from models meant to supply hot water to a single tap to whole-house water heaters.

The performance of tankless water heaters often is less than expected. They don't provide enough water for a shower unless a 1.7 gallons-per-minute shower head is used, and filling a tub can take longer than with a conventional water heater. A recent issue of *Consumer Reports* indicates that there is not much of a difference in operating costs between a gas tankless water heater and a conventional but highly efficient gas water heater.

## Your Heating Options

In their zeal to make their new bathrooms as pleasant as possible, many novice remodelers often forget about heat—the one factor that can turn a magnificently designed bath into the most undesirable spot in the house. Often bathroom renovation is done in the summer when heat is not required. But during the winter, a beautiful ceramic tile floor can get mighty cold unless you have an adequate source of heat.

If you are redecorating an existing bath, you may not need more heat than is already provided. Just make sure that new materials in your bath won't render your current heating system ineffective. Skylights, large windows, and extra doors to bathrooms often create drafts in cold weather.

If an addition will require that you extend heating, be certain that your present furnace can handle the extra load. You may need to consider supplemental heat sources.

Self-regulating wall heaters can be a nice alternative to rerouting central heating for a small bathroom; or they can work in conjunction with central heat in a large bath. Help the heater to work efficiently by installing it where it won't be blocked by doors or shelves. And don't locate it too near anything that may pose a fire hazard, such as linens or curtains. Electric heaters should be properly grounded to prevent electric shock, and gas models should have automatic pilot shutoffs.

Fan-assisted ceiling heaters are good for heating small areas of a large bathroom.

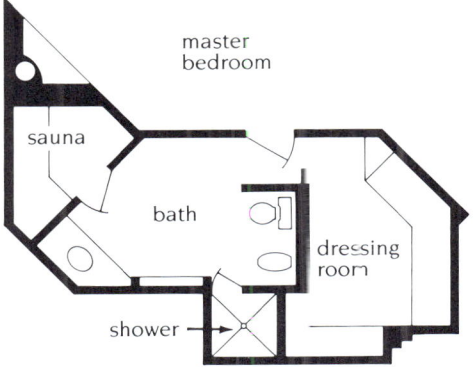

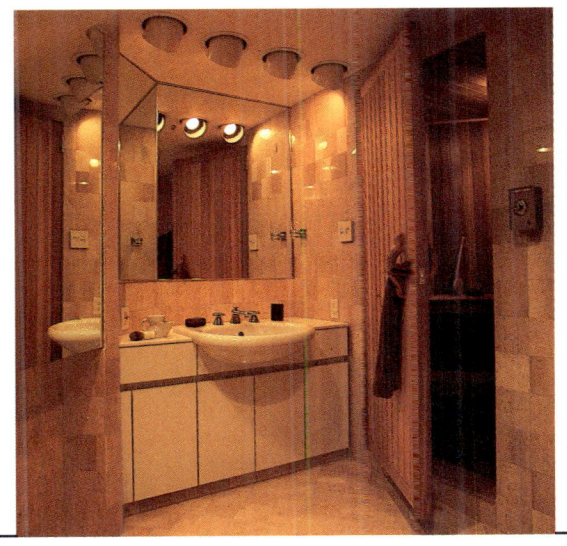

**A sauna bath:** With its new emphasis on relaxation and luxury, today's bath is a choice location for a sauna. With the right design and smart use of space, even a relatively small bath can easily house a comfortably sized sauna. And, as in this Toronto bath, a sauna can add an extra bit of flavor to the room. The bath design takes its lead from the warm, earthy wood of the sauna, which enhances the mellow tan, beige, and cream colors in the room and creates an inviting, soothing environment.

For safety reasons, never use portable heaters in the bathroom.

A unique way to heat your bathroom is with a radiant heating system (one example is Flexwatt, made by the Flexwatt Corporation, Canton, Massachusetts). This type of system heats people and furnishings directly; the air is heated incidentally, minimizing heat loss due to hot air rising to the ceiling. Electrically powered, the unit can be mounted on or in a wall, ceiling, or floor. Permanently mounted, quartz, infrared heaters are another option for bathroom heating.

## Heat Lamps

A heat lamp can re-create the sensation of basking in the tropical sun. The infrared bulb provides radiant heat—the kind that's given off by the sun. It warms you without overheating the room air.

The price of an infrared bulb is only about $10; it's the fixture that's costly. A practical way to incorporate a heat lamp into your bathroom is to buy a unit that combines a lamp fixture with an exhaust fan; the cost is about $120. A good place to install your heat lamp is right outside the shower. There, it will warm the toweling area and exhaust any steam that escapes from the shower.

For safety's sake, buy a heat lamp that comes equipped with a timer; you don't want to take chances with its overheating.

## What about Sunlamps?

If you're going all out with your new super bath, should you also consider installing a sunlamp? Certainly a sunlamp can help you to get a tan. And if you follow the manufacturer's instructions carefully and use common sense, you shouldn't get burned. Keep in mind that doctors aren't sure about the long-term effects of exposure to ultraviolet radiation (from the sun *or* a lamp). Tanning can lead to skin cancer, and the eyes are very vulnerable to ultraviolet light. Cut down on potential health risks by following these tips:

- Make sure your lamp comes with a timer that automatically shuts it off at a preset time, in case you fall asleep.

- Buy a lamp that's equipped with protective eye shields, or get goggles.

- Make sure the manufacturer provides clear and detailed instructions on the safe use of the lamp, especially about exposure times and how far from the bulb you should be.

- Avoid sunlamps that contain only a bare mercury tube in a metal reflector. Instead, get one with a filter that blocks most of the more hazardous short-wavelength radiation.

- Check with your doctor to find out if any drugs you're taking will increase your susceptibility to burning.

Finally, if you're a fair-skinned person, forget about using a sunlamp. The risks of sunlamps clearly outweigh any benefits.

For more information about the health risks of sunlamps, contact the Food and Drug Administration, Division of Consumer Affairs, HFZ-76, Center for Medical Devices and Radiological Health, 5600 Fishers Lane, Rockville, MD 20857.

## What about the Laundry?

In many houses, the laundry room is relegated to a cold, dark place far away from places where dirty laundry accumulates. In most households, dressing and undressing take place in or near the bathroom. So, today's homeowners are learning to lessen laundry inconveniences by locating their washers and dryers a little closer to the source of all those dirty clothes.

There are several ways to do this. One way is to put laundry appliances right in the bathroom. Standard-size washers and dryers, when placed next to each other, require a space that is 4½ to 5 feet wide and 3 feet deep. A large bathroom can easily accommodate standard-size appliances. They can be concealed behind bifold or accordion doors. If they are nice-looking and color-coordinated with the rest of the bath, they don't need to be concealed. If space is tight, one alternative is to invest in a set of stacked laundry appliances, which are now available in standard sizes. A closet can easily house stacked models. Another alternative is compact washers and dryers, which can be placed side by side or stacked. They are normally just 27 to 28 inches wide.

For a number of reasons, you may not want laundry appliances in your bathroom. If your laundry room and bath share a common wall, a two-way closet can be handy. One door opens into the bath, the other into the laundry room; a basket can be passed easily between the two rooms.

Often an existing floor plan makes it impossible to locate a washer and dryer next to the bathroom. A time-honored, effec-

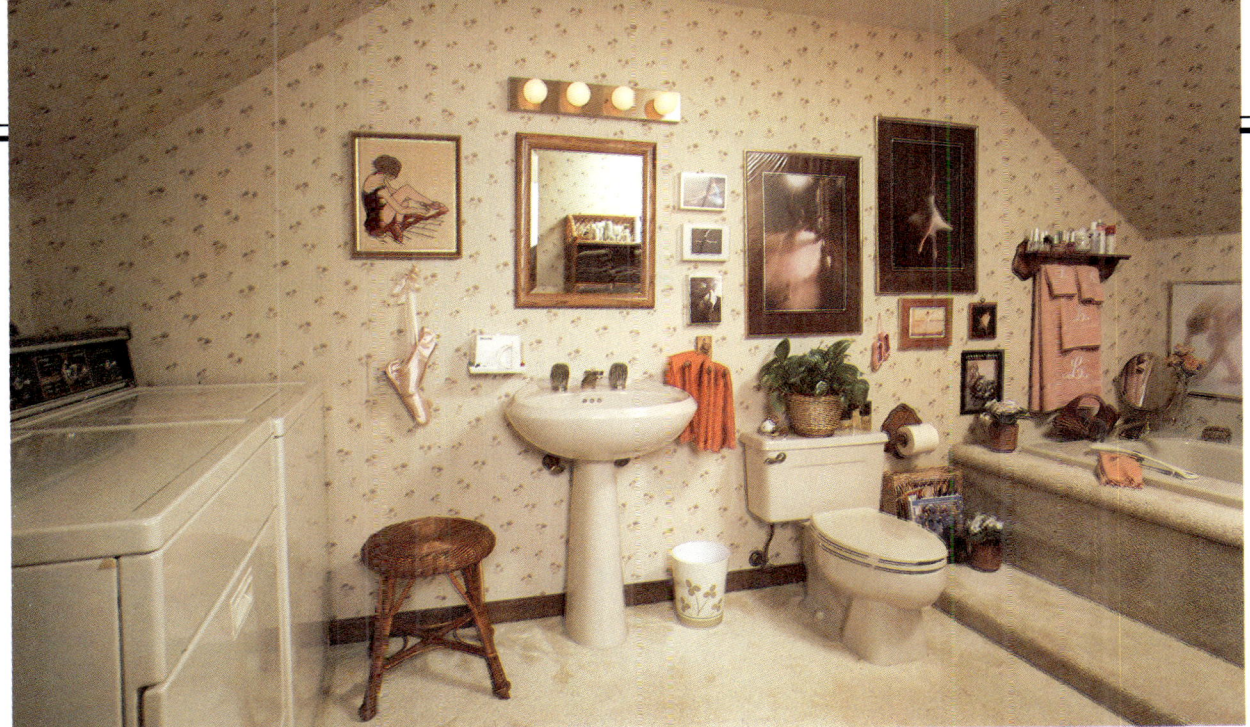

The off-white washer and dryer in this bath blend nicely with the room's decor.

tive way of linking bath and laundry room is with a laundry chute—often built right into bath cabinetry; clothes tossed into the chute end up downstairs in the laundry.

Sometimes it helps just to have a means to deal with dirty clothes and towels strewn around the bathroom. Many cabinet manufacturers now make laundry basket inserts that fit neatly into bath vanities. When ready to do laundry, you simply slip out the wire basket. It is important to provide for some sort of ventilation for the basket inserts, such as louvers at the top and bottom of the cabinet door. Otherwise, mildew will form.

It is often convenient to locate your laundry room close to the bathroom. In this design, the laundry and bathroom are connected by a two-way closet. Clothes to be washed easily find their way to the laundry room, and clean towels are always available to bathers.

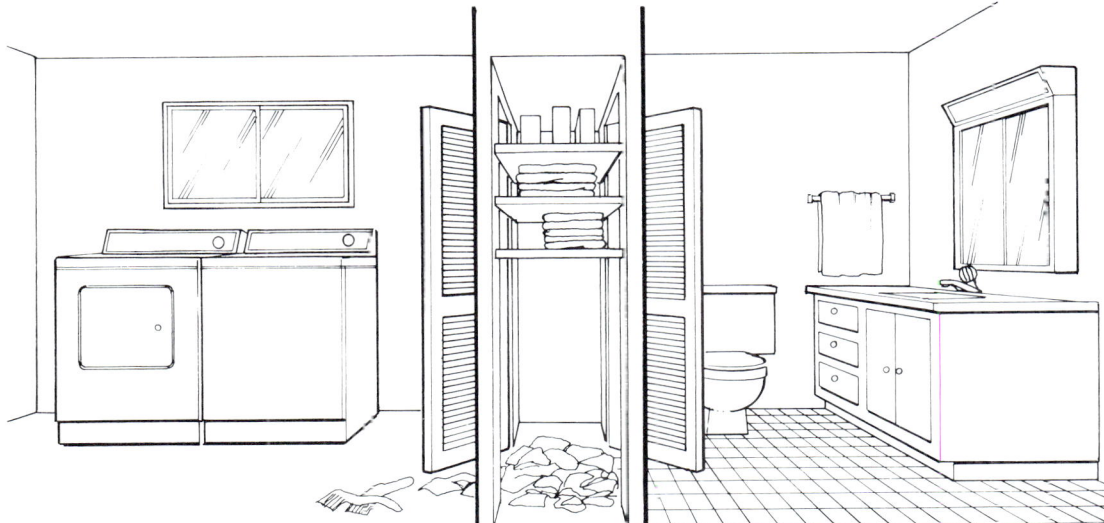

# Storage in the Bath

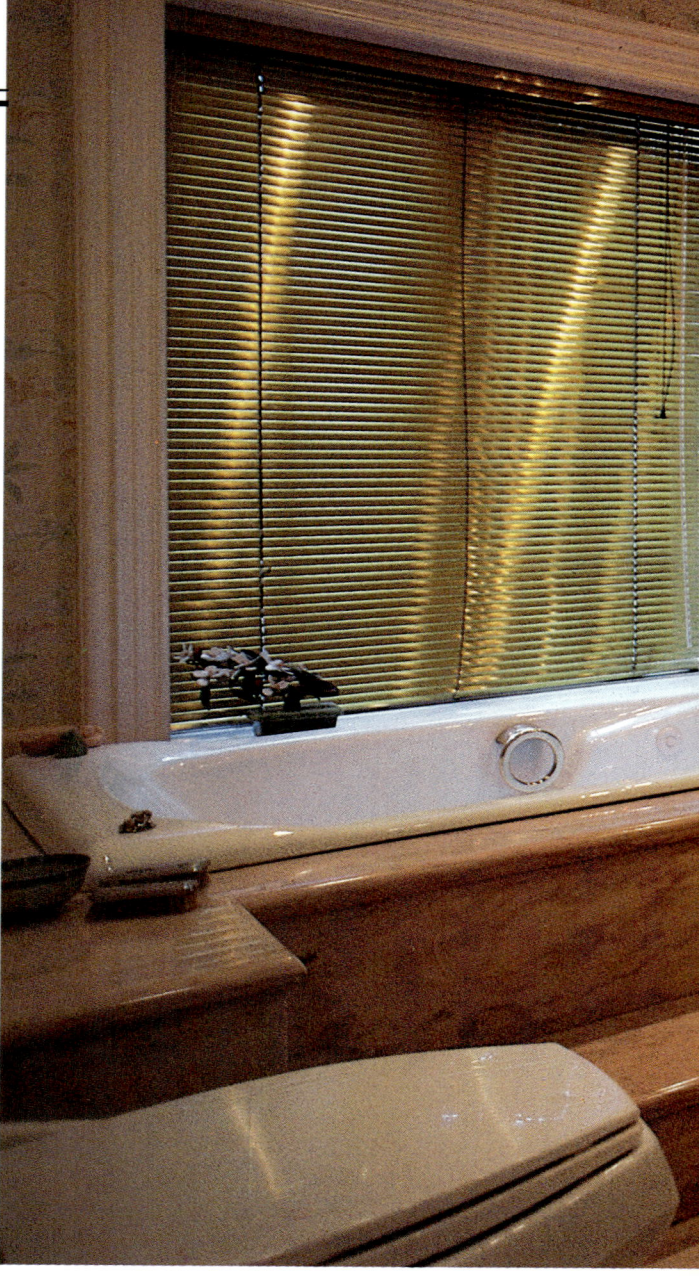

Imagine this scenario. Has it happened to you? You awaken from a restful sleep, jump out of bed, and head for the shower. Just as you are ready to step *out* of the shower and reach to grab a towel hanging nearby, you remember that the last clean towel was used up the night before. In the ensuing mad dash down the hall to the linen closet, you drip water on the hardwood floor.

Back in the bathroom, you riffle through a miscellaneous assortment of toiletries on the room's sole countertop in an effort to find a comb. The vanity drawer sticks when you try to open it to find some deodorant. Then you open the medicine cabinet, and a shower of small bottles, bars of soap, and dental aids falls out. By the time you leave the house for work—late, of course—you are exhausted. It's barely nine o'clock in the morning.

Well-planned bathroom storage can help your personal rush hours go much more smoothly. But because standard bathroom layouts generally allow for little flexibility, finding room for storage units in the bathroom is one of the designer's most challenging tasks.

You should begin thinking about the amount of storage you'll need in your bathroom right from the start of the design process, when you're still working out the layout. Simply having plenty of storage units will not guarantee that your bathroom will be an organized, efficient place. Making sure that all of your cabinets, drawers, and shelves are put where they're needed the most is equally important. Ideally, towel storage should be within reach of the bather the moment he or she steps from the tub. Grooming aids should be kept near a mirror and countertop. Extra rolls of toilet paper should be kept near the toilet, and so forth.

In "Workbook: The Basics of Bath Design," we emphasize the importance of drafting your bathroom floor plan on graph paper and studying it with an eye toward maximizing available space and allowing the proper clearances for fixtures. Once you've got a basic idea of the shape and size of the room and some possible locations for fixtures, take a second look at your prospective layout. The location of various fixtures will in part determine where you

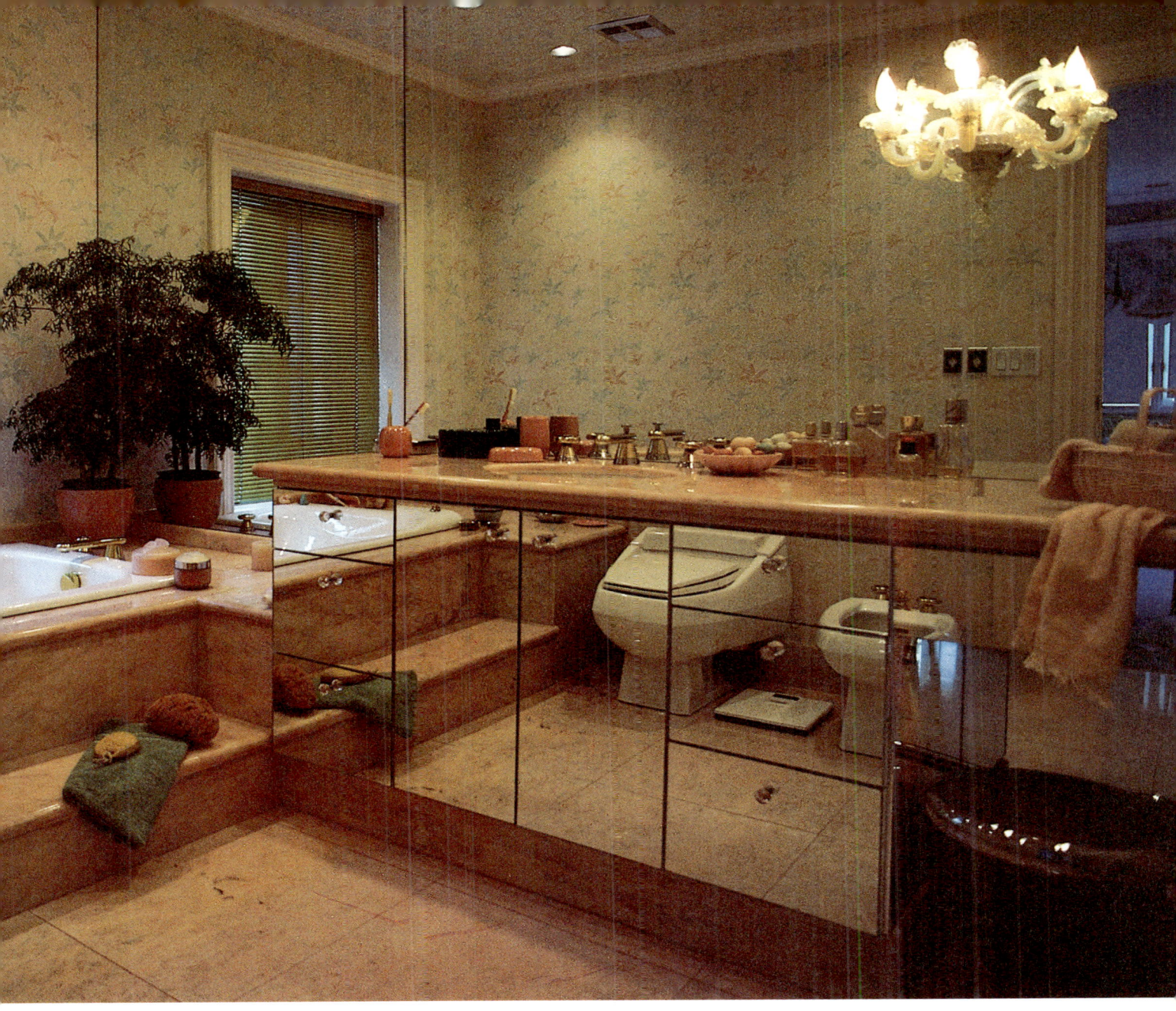

need to put some storage units. You need to find out whether your proposed layout will leave you adequate room for storage where you need it the most.

The easiest way to do this is to lay a piece of tissue paper over your floor plan and mark your probable activities with a pencil. For example, if you're likely to reach for a towel just as you step out of the tub, draw an arrow to the nearest possible location for a towel. If you're likely to reach for a hair dryer when you're standing in front of the mirror, draw an arrow from the place you're most likely to be standing to the spot that's the most convenient location for a hair dryer. This will give you a clear idea of where various items should be located. Once you know the most sensible place to put your storage units, you can make any necessary adjustments in your layout.

It's important to "walk through" a space like this, rather than just assuming that certain items will go best in particular locations. Many times design assumptions are based on what we, as people, have come to expect or been raised with, rather than what our activities dictate we really need. By feeling out what it's like to be in that space ahead of time, you might come up with some fresh ideas that really will help your new bathroom to operate at its functional best.

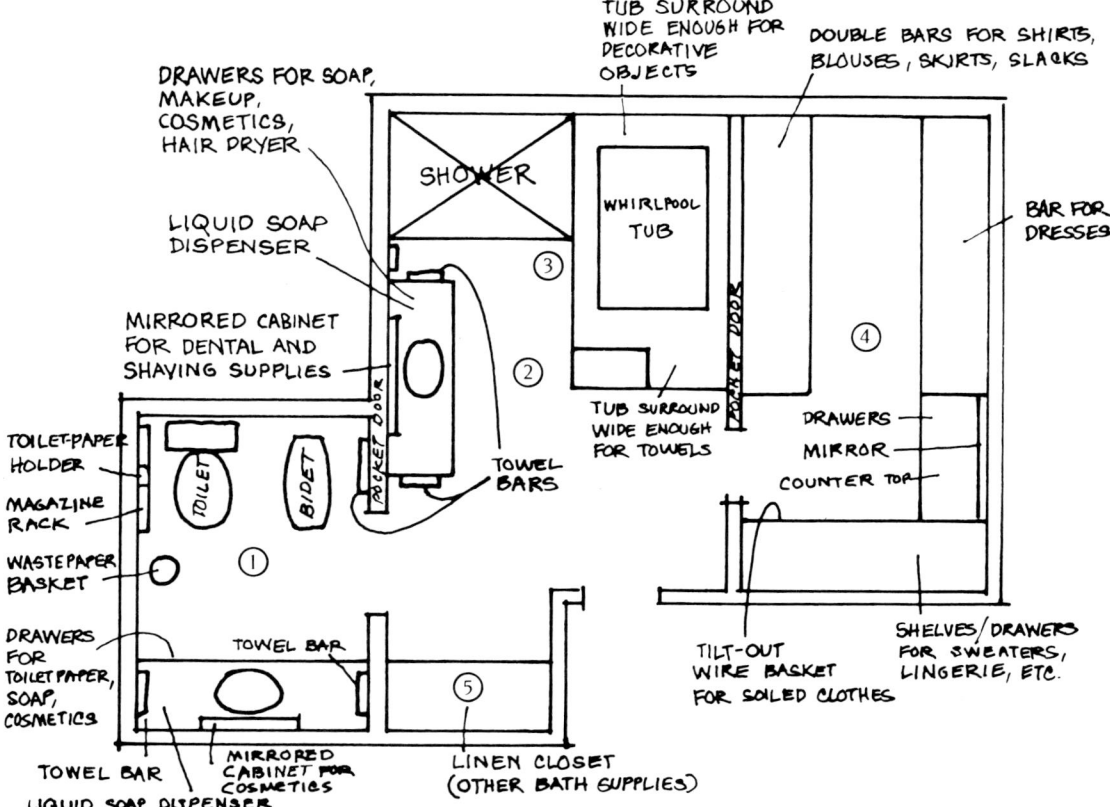

A good way to plan for storage in the bath is to indicate on the floor plan where certain activities will occur. In this bath there are areas for (1) personal hygiene, (2) grooming, (3) bathing, and (4) dressing, with additional space (5) for longer-term storage (extra towels, for example). The next step would be to add arrows to indicate specific activities. If you use a hair dryer as you stand before the mirror above the vanity, draw an arrow from the place you will stand to the place where you will store the hair dryer. If you do this for all of your activities, you can easily define your storage needs.

## Finding Storage Spaces

The size, shape, and kind of fixtures you choose will also affect the amount of space available for storage. Once you install bathroom fixtures, consider them permanent; they can only be moved at great expense. If you decide on a certain sink or tub without considering your need for cabinets or drawers, you will have already limited your options.

If storage is a priority in your new bathroom, look for fixtures that have storage units already incorporated into them. For example, look for bathtubs and shower stalls that have shelves, soap dishes, and the like molded into the plastic surround. Install a sink with a built-in vanity instead of a pedestal sink. Or consider a modern-day washstand: These European-style, all-in-one units come equipped with mirror, sink, towel racks, soap holder, and shelves.

Small-scaled fixtures are another option, because they free up space for built-in storage. Consider replacing that old clunker of a bathtub with a smaller shower or corner bath and use the space you gain for cabinetry.

Think carefully about where you plan to install your fixtures. Just shifting a sink a couple of feet can make a real difference in the way you end up using the space around it. For example, installing a sink off-center will free up counter space that can then be used as a dressing table or for clothes sorting. If your bathroom is going to feature an L-shaped counter, you might consider installing the sink in the corner of the "L." Cabinet corners are wasted space, unless you can somehow fit them with a lazy Susan. But, if you choose to install a sink there, the plumbing will take up most of the cabinet corner.

No matter what kind of fixtures you choose to use or where you plan to install them, there will probably be lots of areas in your bathroom that you can put to better use. Most items that need to be stored in the bathroom are small. Smaller dimensions mean that you can create storage places where you ordinarily wouldn't; for example, you can run a cabinet from floor-to-ceiling and practically across an entire wall, without bringing the wall in more than 4 to 6 inches. If you also tap space between the studs (roughly 4 inches deep), you'll lose even less space (or alternatively, increase the depth of the cabinet).

In many bathrooms, the ceiling above a tub is often much higher than it needs to be. Consider lowering the ceiling over the tub and incorporating shelves or a cabinet in that space.

If your plans call for retiling the tub surround, take the opportunity to include some narrow shelves and perhaps a towel bar at the far end. Extending the ledge around the bathtub itself is another option. Just three extra inches can make a shelf broad enough to put bath supplies at the bather's fingertips.

Are you planning to box in an old freestanding tub? Sliding doors can give you access to the space behind the tub apron.

Don't neglect the wall above a toilet seat. Extra towel bars, shelves, even a cabinet can fit in this space. (You can build your own storage units or purchase them readymade; cabinet manufacturers have started to make special cabinets just for this purpose.) As long as the plumber has access to the toilet bowl and tank, there's no reason why you can't build a storage unit around the toilet-bowl tank itself. Shelves should be at least 12 to 14 inches above the tank—high enough so you can see into the tank. Also, a shelf could be connected to the wall with hinges so it can be lifted up to allow access to the tank, or attach a shelf with shelf pins so that it lifts off.

In some houses, cabinet space is limited because of low windows. The height of most bathroom vanities is 36 inches; a window that has a bottom edge ending below the 36-inch mark effectively prevents the homeowner from utilizing that particular wall. By replacing the existing window with a shorter one, you'll keep a good amount of natural light and be able to install a roomy

---

### Finding Storage in Your Bath

Don't forget the "hidden" places in your bath when you plan for storage:

- Install tubs and showers with shelves molded into them.
- Select a vanity instead of a pedestal sink if you need extra storage space.
- Consider all-in-one-unit washstands because of their storage features.
- Install a sink off-center on a vanity top to allow more usable counter space.
- Install a sink in the corner of an L-shaped vanity.
- Install 6-inch-deep, ceiling-to-floor cabinetry.
- Utilize the space between studs for shelves or cabinets.
- Don't forget to use the space above the tub, sink, and toilet for cabinetry.
- Select window sizes that allow for storage units below windows.
- Use furniture with built-in storage compartments.

---

cabinet at the same time. Or, if your windowsill is deep enough, consider fitting the window with transparent shelves; they'll allow light to enter and can be just the place for pretty glass bottles of perfumes and bath oils, and so forth.

If you plan to borrow space from other rooms in the house, you'll probably end up building new partitions between the bathroom and at least one adjacent room. In designing the new partition, you have ample opportunity to incorporate some storage units into it. If you also plan to box in the toilet—install a partition between the toilet and the sink, for example—the partition should do double-duty as a storage unit as well.

Does your new bathroom plan call for a sitting area? Think in terms of a bench rather than a chair. The seat of the bench can flip up and you can use the space inside to store extra towels, hot water bottles, even the bathroom scale.

Use your imagination. A new interpretation of a conventional detail or a piece of trim—such as extending the wood edge molding on a countertop edge a few extra inches and outfitting it with a dowel so that you can hang towels on it—can make the difference between a bathroom that's well-equipped with storage and one that's not.

## Cabinetry for the Bath

Before you decide the exact number and kind of storage units to use in your new bathroom, you'll need to make a list of all of the things you want to store there. (See "Making Choices and a Budget" on page 139.) Include all the items that you'd like to store, given the chance, even if you've never previously stored them there before.

Keep in mind that special activities have special storage requirements. If, for example, you plan to incorporate a spa in your new bathroom, you may need a place to store specialized cleaning equipment. If you're designing a bodyroom, you'll need a convenient space to stash free weights and a scale. Do you want to equip your bathroom with a washer and dryer? Then it also makes sense to include a cabinet that can house laundry soaps, an ironing board (maybe a pull-down, wall model), and a counter for sorting clothes.

Next to each item on your list, describe the kind, amount and size of the space you need to store that item. It's a good idea to be as specific as possible here: Most shelves, cabinets, and other factory-made storage units come in standard dimensions that might not suit your real needs, in which case you'll have to either modify a store-bought unit or improvise on your own a storage system that's altogether different.

Cabinets are made from a number of different materials and are available in a wide variety of finishes. For the bathroom look for cabinetry made from materials that resist moisture, fingerprints, staining, and general wear and tear.

### Vanities

Once you have your master list, you can start thinking about actual storage units.

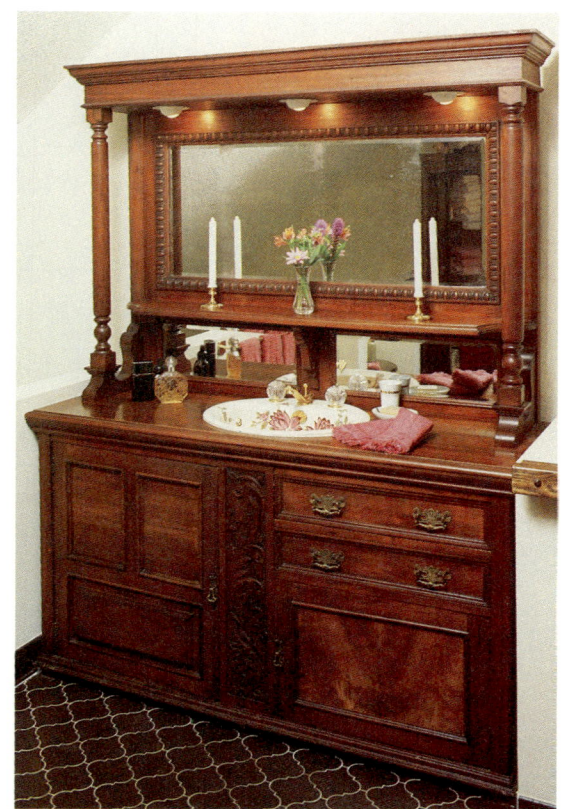

The vanity is the most common type of storage unit in the bath. This one-of-a-kind vanity has a sink (with a floral pattern) set into an antique dresser.

The most common bathroom storage unit in America is probably the vanity, a cabinet or cabinets typically located under the bathroom sink.

If you have a vanity cabinet (or any other cabinet) in your bathroom, now is the time to reassess it. Are you satisfied with it? If not, why? Does it lack storage space? Take a look behind the doors. Bathroom cabinets are often little more than four walls with a counter above and a floor below—in other words, an empty box. By adding shelves or drawers, you could more than triple the available storage space.

Some vanities are well-equipped with shelves, but the shelves are too deep or too wide to be useful. Storing bathroom necessities in baskets or deep-sided trays before you put them on the shelf will give you immediate access to the full depth of a single shelf; instead of rummaging blindly in the back, all you'll have to do when you're looking for something special is pull out the needed tray and rest it on the counter. All of the contents will be visible.

If your cabinet just needs a face-lift, consider refinishing it. In most cases, giving a cabinet a cosmetic make-over is a lot cheaper than replacing it with a brand-new one. Or, if you're pleased with the cabinet, but you're unhappy about its location, consider moving it.

### American-style Cabinetry

If you prefer to (or, in the case of new construction, must) purchase new cabinets, the first question to ask yourself is whether you want to purchase a traditional American-style cabinet or a more modern European-style cabinet.

The classic American-style cabinet has a wood face frame on the cabinet front onto which the drawers and cabinets are fastened. The drawers and doors are rarely flush with the face frame; in fact, they generally close against the frame.

**Stock, Factory, or Custom.** The cheapest cabinets are "stock" cabinets. Stock cabinets offer the least number of options to the homeowner. They come in a limited number of styles and colors and are manufactured in standard widths and heights only. Stock cabinets may be purchased separately and pieced together to create more of a custom look.

*Factory-built* cabinets are the next step up. They are made to order for your particular needs. Most manufacturers offer you a range of cabinet styles and finish materials from which to choose.

The cream of the crop, of course, is the *custom-built* cabinet. Custom-built cabinets offer an endless range of options. They are the best choice—and sometimes the only one—for awkward or unusually shaped spaces.

### European-style Cabinetry

"European-style" refers to how a cabinet is made and not where. European-style cabinetry can be made anywhere—Pennsylvania or Germany. A typical European-style cabinet, in contrast to an American-style cabinet, has no face frame. The doors and drawers cover the entire front of the cabinet opening, creating a smooth, clean look. The good thing about European-style cabinets is that all of the storage components—baskets, drawers, cabinets, and so forth—are designed to be modular. This means that if you get tired of the color of a cabinet door, you can easily replace it with the same model in another color; you don't have to replace the whole cabinet. If your storage requirements change, you can replace a cabinet door with drawer units just as easily. Such flexibility saves the consumer time and money.

European-style cabinets are ordered and specified in metrics, as opposed to feet and inches. This is a fact you'll need to keep in mind when the time comes to order.

### Wood Cabinets

Many people prefer the warm look of natural wood cabinets. However, solid-wood cabinets do have a few disadvantages. First, they tend to be expensive, costing a third or more than their laminate-finished counterparts. Cost needn't be a deterrent if you plan to do much of the work yourself. If you don't have the time to build your own cabinets and you like the look of wood cabinets, there are some options. You can get cabinets imported from Europe that are made of particle board, finished with a wood veneer. These cabinets are a fraction of the cost of solid-wood cabinets and can be bought and installed yourself, thus holding down expenses even more. Or, you can take the path of colonial poor folk, who could rarely afford quality wood furniture, and use paint to create a *faux finish* in the form of an imitation wood grain.

If you do opt for natural wood you will have to apply a sealer to the surface of the cabinet to protect the wood from moisture. Polyurethane, spar varnish, or bar sealer have all been used successfully to waterproof wood furniture. Liquid polyester, which gives the cabinet a glossy surface akin to lacquer, is another moisture-resistant finish that is being used more and more on wood cabinets, but it is more expensive than the other sealers.

Many cabinets are made of particle board coated with some type of surface, usually a laminate. In general, particle-board cabinets are quite sturdy. But because particle board itself is much heavier than solid wood of the same dimension, it can be difficult to handle. The particle-board edges can also be smashed, crushed, or broken off if they are handled carelessly during shipping or transporting, so it behooves the consumer to check out all parts before purchasing.

Generally speaking, particle-board cabinets covered with melamine are the least expensive of any cabinets, and many of the inexpensive cabinets from Europe (commonly called *knock-down cabinets*, because they come ready to assemble in a box) are made of this combination of materials.

The melamine finish is durable and easy to clean. However, it can be scratched with a sharp instrument. Also, melamine-finished cabinets come in only a few colors, and many are available only in white.

### Laminate Cabinets

Another option is cabinets finished with a decorative laminate. Decorative laminates are made from layers of paper impregnated with a plastic resin and treated with pressure and heat until the separate layers chemically bond into a single sheet. Laminate itself is a nonstructural material. A laminate cabinet is really a plywood cabinet that has been covered in laminate for a decorative effect.

Although laminate cabinets are generally more moisture-resistant than untreated wood cabinets, you still must be careful not to subject laminate cabinets to excess water. Because the laminate is glued to the wood, it can loosen and raise up with repeated soakings.

### Mixing Materials

The trendiest of today's cabinets are made from a combination of materials. You can find wood cabinets with glass fronts (usually reinforced with a wire grid); wood or laminate cabinets with cloth or rattan inserts in the doors; laminate cabinets edged with wood; and much more. If you choose to design or build your own custom cabinets, a look at these designer combinations will serve to inspire and delight.

## Cabinets as Design Elements

In most bathrooms, the cabinets are second only to the fixtures in influencing the atmosphere of the room and suggesting a decorating theme. Elegant wood cabinets will inspire a colonial or Victorian theme, while sleek, streamlined metallic laminates tend to suggest a more modern approach. But you needn't be hostage to the material you choose, either; laminates, for example, can be routed to create a lacy, Victorian

Dark chocolate penny tile covers the countertop and forms the sink of this vanity, handcrafted of redwood.

effect. Textured laminates can give a room a back-to-basics, "natural" flavor. The rule: Be creative; experiment.

### Color

Color is another important design element to consider when choosing cabinets. In the old days, most bathroom cabinets were available only in natural wood tones, white, or beige. All of that's changed today, however, as designer colors have invaded the marketplace.

New wood stains tint ordinary wood gray, yellow, cranberry-red, and more, while allowing the grain to show through. You can find laminates in any color from deep jewel tones to metallics, to primaries, to bright pastels. Even neutrals have become more exciting. In the new neutrals' palette, you'll find grayed roses, orchids, greens and blues, pinky beiges and peachy tans. You'll also find neutral-colored laminates decorated with subtle patterns, like grids and stripes. Textured laminates also give the neutrals and pastel palettes a boost.

The style and color of storage you elect to install in your bathroom can affect how small or large your bathroom appears. In small bathrooms, streamlined cabinetry in the same color as the walls and/or the floor makes a small bathroom seem larger. Cabinets with space-saving sliding or bifold doors and flush hardware (instead of raised handles) also help make the most of a small space. Coordinating the bathroom color scheme with an adjacent bedroom or dressing area is a good idea if you want to give your interior spaces a sense of continuity.

No matter what style, color, or shape of cabinet you choose, inspect the cabinet hardware carefully. On any cabinet, smoothly operating hardware is a must; bathrooms see a lot of rush-hour traffic, and it can be irritating when drawers don't slide smoothly or cabinets don't open easily.

### Countertops

Many people assume that cabinets automatically come with counters. Actually, counters are usually sold separately, although most cabinet manufacturers do offer some

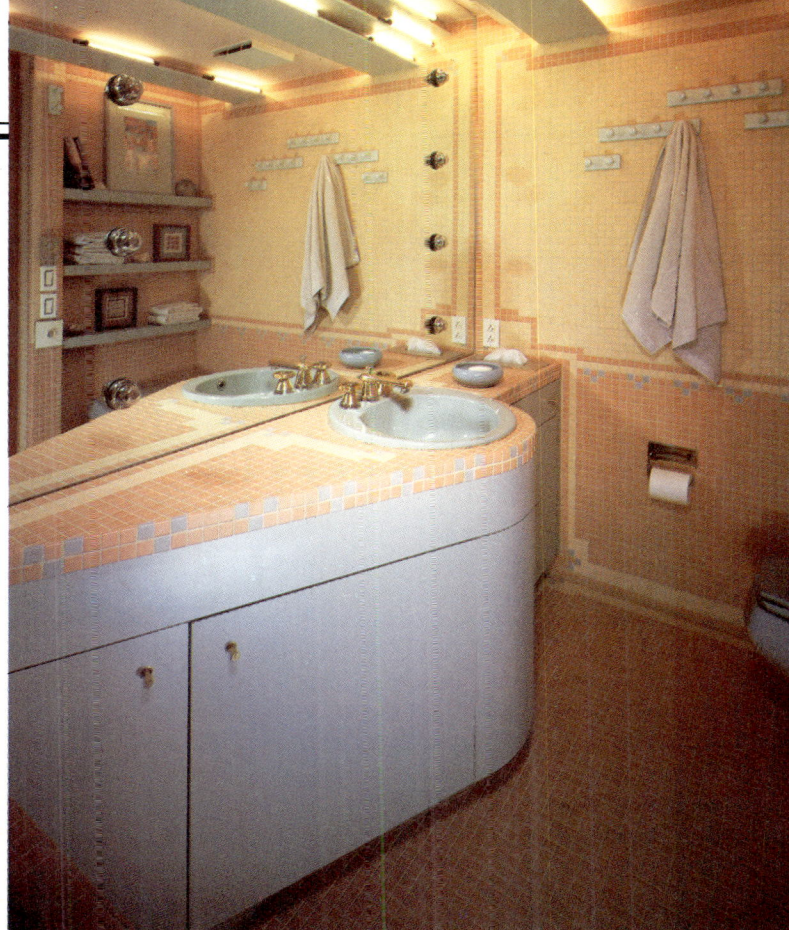

Color is an important consideration when selecting bathroom cabinetry. Laminate cabinets, such as this one, are available in just about any color you can imagine. Give your creativity full rein in selecting fixtures and tile to complement the color of cabinetry.

sort of package deal for those homeowners who want to buy their cabinets and counters together.

If you're happy with your cabinets, but you want to replace your counters, you can get countertops custom-made to your specifications from a local cabinet shop. Just be prepared to give the overall dimensions of the counter you need and the type of edge and backsplash you want.

You can also make your own countertops. Building a countertop is a relatively simple project; the only type of counter that is out of the do-it-yourselfer's league is a curved laminate countertop with a radius over 6 inches. Although laminate is fairly easy to cut with a router or handsaw, curving or bending laminate requires special tools, since the laminate must be heat-formed. The only exception to this rule is tamboured laminate, which is grooved and

## DESIGN TIP

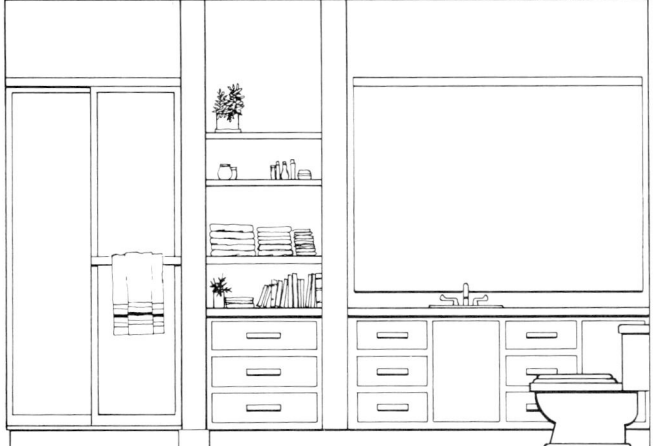

Lining up various elements in a bathroom will help pull together the overall design. Look at the countertop or shower door when choosing the height for a shelf or towel bar, for example, or at the top of a window when hanging a mirror.

highly flexible. However, because it's grooved, it's probably not a good idea to use it on a counter where it's likely to receive a lot of wear and collect dirt.

If you intend to build your own countertops, plan carefully. Most materials come in standard widths, and you'll want to make the most of your purchase. Before you cut that sheet of laminate or lay that tile, plan your use of the material on paper.

A well-designed bathroom countertop will have a minimum of seams. (They tend to collect dirt and standing water.) The edge of a counter will often overhang a base cabinet by a few inches, to protect the cabinet face from accidental spills. On some tile countertops, the edges are raised slightly, to prevent water from spilling onto the floor.

The most common countertop materials are laminate-surfaced plywood or particle board; ceramic tile; Corian and 2000X, both synthetic materials; and cultured marble. If you're creatively inclined, you can make counters out of a host of other materials as well—wood, natural marble, stone, slate, and ABS (acrylonitrile-butadiene-styrene) plastic, to name a few. Copper, brass, stainless steel, and aluminum can be used for small areas. As long as the material you choose can be effectively protected from water and can withstand wear and tear, it can be used on a bathroom counter.

### Laminate Countertops

Conventional laminate is made from a decorative sheet of paper backed with layers of kraft paper impregnated with resin and fused together under heat and pressure. When a piece of laminate is installed on a countertop, the kraft paper is visible, creating a dark line along the countertop edge. The new solid-core laminates—made of multiple layers of colored paper—have the same color throughout, so there are no dark edges.

When you choose laminate for your bathroom countertops, look for one that is slightly thicker than the laminate used on walls. A laminate that has a matte finish is also a better choice for countertops than one with a glossy finish, because a glossy finish will wear sooner.

The least expensive edging for a standard laminate countertop is a metal molding. You can also finish laminate countertops with a plastic "T" that you insert into a groove in the countertop edge. Covering the countertop edge with a strip of laminate (a process often referred to as a "self-edge") is an inexpensive and attractive possibility.

A solid-core laminate can do even more to create interesting effects. Layer several different-colored laminates to create striped edges; route or bevel layers of the same laminate to create a finished edge that's a single color; or edge the countertop with wood.

### Ceramic Tile Countertops

Ceramic tile is another popular bathroom countertop material. Ceramic tile is known for its durability, and it is water- and fire-resistant. You can get tiles in just about any color, pattern, or style you want. There are tiles that are patterned after antique quilts; tiles embossed to look like lizard and snakeskin; tiles imprinted with leaves; tiles with raised triangles, squares, dots, and half moons applied to the surface; tiles with softened surfaces that imitate suede; checkerboard tiles; striped tiles; hand-painted floral tiles—the choices are endless.

If you choose to cover your counters

with ceramic tile, size is an important consideration. You'll have to choose between tiny, delicate mosaic tiles; standard 4-by-4-inch tiles; large 8-by-8-inch tiles; even larger 12-by-12-inch tiles; as well as oblong, hexagonal, and other odd-shaped tiles.

In the past, most people preferred the standard 4-by-4-inch tiles; nowadays, consumers are showing a preference for larger tiles, which tend to give bathrooms a cleaner, more streamlined look. But the size of your bathroom will have a lot to do with the size of tile you choose to purchase. Generally speaking, though, tiles slightly larger than standard 4-by-4-inch tiles help to expand small spaces. A 12-by-12-inch tile is best-suited to a large bathroom.

*Installing Tile.* Installing a tile countertop involves applying a chemical adhesive (often called mastic) to a clean, level surface, placing the tiles on the mortar base, tamping them down, and grouting them. In the past, white grout was the norm, but today, grout has become a design element. It comes in a rainbow of colors—anything from turquoise blue to dusty rose. The variety of colors enables the homeowner or designer to have more control over the way a countertop looks. For example, a dark grout can help camouflage dirt; a grout that matches the tile will give the countertop a smooth, unified appearance; a grout that contrasts with the tile will emphasize the grid as a design element.

How you set and grout the tile will also affect the countertop design. You can install some tiles edge to edge, with hardly any grout showing at all; or you can set them far apart and use up to ¼ inch of grout between them for an entirely different look. You can even use strips of wood around tiles, in lieu of thick grout, if you want a wider separation between the tiles. But whether you choose grout or wood strips, make sure to seal the material between the tiles. Grout, like wood, can discolor and mildew from excess moisture.

For a finished look, you can fit the corners of your countertop with mitered tiles (tiles with one edge cut at a 45-degree angle) and fit the edge that meets the wall surface with tile that curves into a backsplash.

*Corian Countertops*

Another countertop option is a type of synthetic marble, such as Corian by Du Pont or 2000X by Formica. Unlike laminate and tile, Corian and 2000X are not "finish" materials; they are solid. It's safe to scrub them with household cleansers, and, because the color goes all the way through, most surface nicks and scratches can be sanded out. Corian is available in four colors, with others forthcoming; 2000X is available in six colors.

*Cultured Marble Countertops*

Cultured marble is a popular countertop material because it's inexpensive and easy to clean. You're somewhat limited when you opt for cultured marble, however, since most countertops made from this material are preformed and include a molded-in sink.

This cultured marble vanity top in a rich brown is a natural match for the laminate cabinets in cream. Cabinets over the sink provide extra storage.

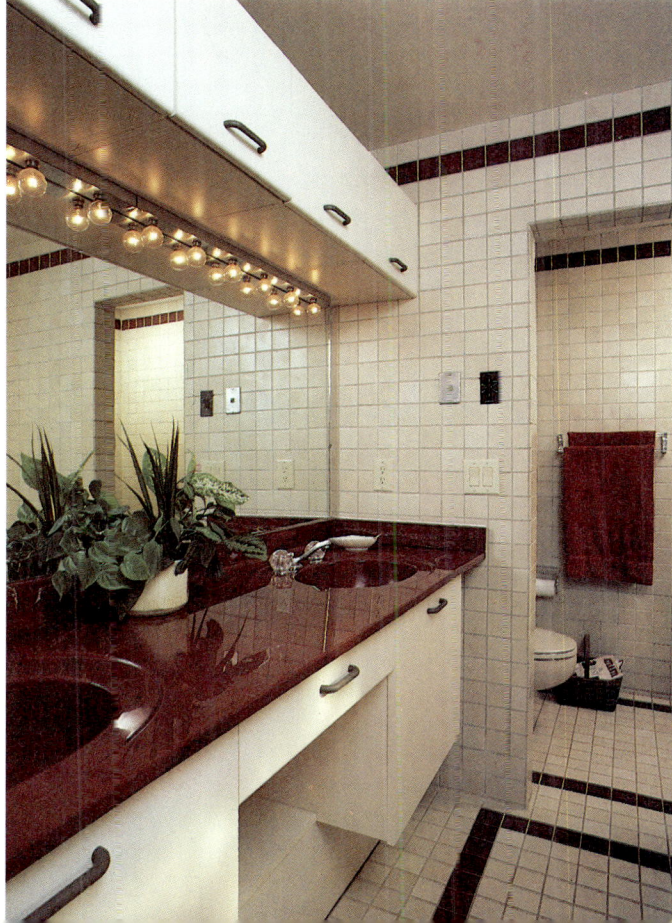

## Backsplashes

Backsplashes are a useful addition to bathroom countertops and cabinets. Their purpose is to keep water from splashing the wall behind the cabinet, ruining the wallpaper, or causing other moisture damage to the wall.

A countertop that's designed with an integral backsplash has a smooth, seamless look, but is more difficult to build than a countertop with a separate backsplash. It's also more difficult to install because the wall that the counter is going up against must be fairly straight and even.

A separate backsplash can compensate for small irregularities in cabinets and walls. Also, a separate backsplash offers many more design possibilities, since it can be made from a different material or in a different color from the countertop itself.

In general, backsplashes run 4 to 5½ inches above the countertop surface. Of course, there's no reason why you can't extend the backsplash if you prefer to use a larger tile or if you're designing a bathroom to be used by children. (After all, kid-size splashes tend to be larger than adult-size splashes.)

## Other Storage Options

For inspiration, study the displays in your favorite home center or department store or your nearest bath-fixture showroom. Most commercial space is extremely expensive to rent and to operate. Display people are constantly coming up with new ways to store goods attractively without taking up a lot of space.

One trick you can learn from department store displays is that the most mundane objects can be kept accessible at all times and still not detract from the attractiveness of a "room" if the storage unit itself has character. So don't be afraid to experiment.

For example: If you live in a big, old house and you're fortunate enough to have a roomy bathroom, consider foregoing conventional bathroom cabinetry altogether and use an antique sideboard or hutch to store your beauty supplies and linens. Instead of using a countertop as a vanity, convert a writing desk into a dressing table. For a country look, collect unusual handmade baskets and fill them with brightly colored towels. An old-fashioned quilt rack also makes an attractive towel holder.

If your bathroom is small, you won't have quite as many options, but even a lack of space is no excuse for not trying something different. Many sink manufacturers today are showing delicate, bowl-shaped sinks recessed into tables and desks that formerly were to be found only in the living or dining room. A smaller, recycled bureau, writing or end table, or antique washstand give a tiny bathroom the same old-time elegance.

And don't be afraid to "steal" ideas from other rooms in the house: Stainless-steel grids—the ones that many industrial kitchens use to hold pots and pans—can be put to use in the bathroom holding mirrors, hairbrushes, anything that hangs. Ordinary pegs are another option. (They take up less space than conventional towel racks but hold more towels.)

## Accessories

Storage accessories designed especially for the bathroom include towel bars and rings, toothbrush and tumbler holders, soap dishes, and toilet-paper holders. These accessories are available in either surface-mounted or recessed versions. Surface-mounted models are made from a variety of materials, including plastic, iron, brass, and wood, and typically attach to the wall with screws. Recessed models are anchored to the structural parts of a wall with adhesives or with screw mounts.

You can buy these accessories either together in sets, or individually. Buying them in sets will help to give your bathroom a finished look. In a small space, especially, a set of matching accessories prevents a sense of clutter.

It's been said that style is defined by an attention to detail. That's certainly true in the bathroom, where small items like toothbrush holders and towel racks are the center of attention for most activities. By replacing these bathroom accessories, you can almost change the entire atmosphere of your bathroom, and at very little cost.

If you are designing a bathroom from scratch, you'll want to make sure that your accessories reinforce the style of cabinets you choose. Fortunately, towel bars and the like are available in a variety of styles, from elegant brass designs to more rustic-looking wood designs. You should have no trouble finding storage accessories that will work with your decorating theme.

When you install any of the above accessories, keep in mind that toilet-paper holders, soap dishes, towel racks, and so on, are designed to hold paper, soap, and towels—not people. Try to avoid installing these items in areas where people will be tempted to use them as grab bars; or install a grab bar that will safely support the weight of a person in a convenient, nearby location.

### Mirrored Cabinets

Another accessory found in most bathrooms is the mirrored cabinet. Mirrored cabinets are also available in either surface-mounted or recessed models. Recessed models contribute to the streamlined look of a bathroom by helping to retain a smooth, uninterrupted wall surface.

Mirrored cabinets are fitted with shallow shelves (usually 4 to 6 inches deep). They come with sliding and swinging doors. Some are equipped with an additional vanity shelf or cabinet below the mirrored surface, outlets for hair dryers and shavers, and lights. On some cabinets, the mirrors are slanted, enabling you to see yourself, even though the cabinet itself is mounted above eye level. Others have three-way mirrors that enable you to see yourself from a number of different angles.

While the most common mirrored cabinet is trimmed in aluminum, manufacturers are increasingly producing bathroom cabinets that are as stylish and decorative as they are practical. You'll find mirrored cabinets with carved oak frames, beveled-glass edges, and trim in bright colors.

These decorative cabinets tend to cost a bit more. They are worth it, however, if they look good and are well made. To make sure you're getting your money's worth, examine the cabinet carefully. Door hinges or rollers should operate smoothly, so that the door swings or slides open at the touch of a finger. Finishes should be moisture-resistant. (An anodized aluminum finish is usually the most durable.) And, ideally, these more expensive bathroom cabinets should come equipped with a swing-out tray or other, similar container on the inside that's designed to hold small items, like razor blades, safely and conveniently.

In addition to the accessories listed above, you might want to consider equipping your bathroom with some less common, but equally useful items. Towel warmers that hold towels and keep them at a cozy temperature are one option. (If you can't afford a towel warmer—they tend to cost a couple of hundred dollars or more—you can achieve almost the same results by positioning an ordinary towel rack so that the towels hang over a hot-air vent or a radiator. Also, you can make a towel warmer by running the hot water pipe through an exposed loop on the way to the shower. Hang a towel over the loop to get warm while you shower.) A retractable clothesline allows you to hang wet bathing suits and freshly washed clothes directly over the tub, where they can drip-dry without creating a puddle of water on the floor.

### Dressing Room Inserts

If you plan to locate your new or renovated bathroom near a dressing area, or to use the bathroom as a dressing room, it makes sense to design some clothing storage units into these spaces. Before you incorporate a closet or wall storage system into your bathroom, take an inventory of your wardrobe so that the new closet space reflects your needs.

Dividing part of your closet space in half and installing a hanging bar at the top and another midway down will help you to use that space to its fullest by allowing you to hang shirts or blouses in the top half of the closet and skirts or pants below. Drawers and shelves are your best bet for storing sweaters, shorts, underwear, and lingerie. A shallow tray keeps socks neat and imme-

*continued on page 58*

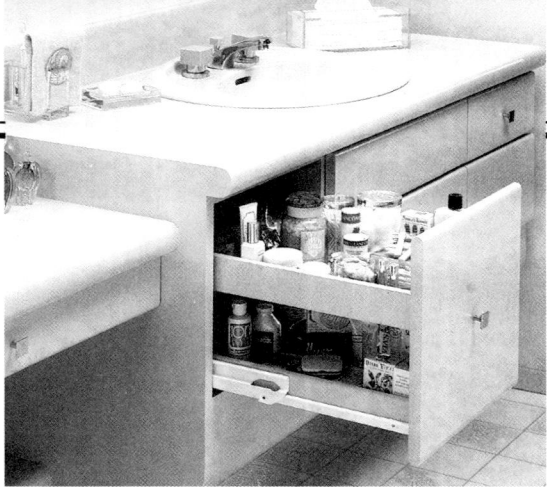

This drawer does double duty by keeping lots of supplies organized. More frequently used items are stored on the top shelf, and items used occasionally are on the bottom.

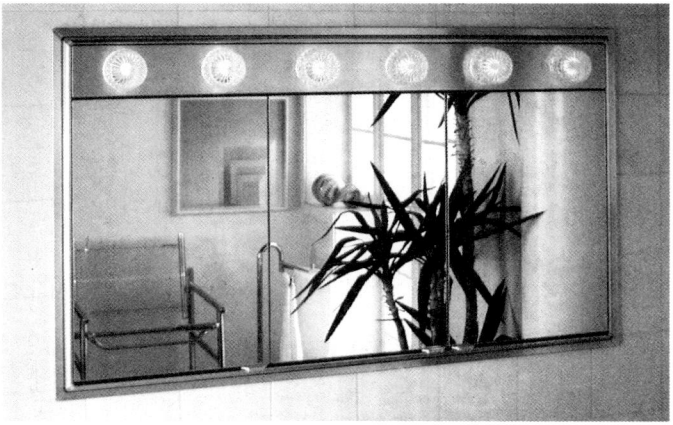

The mirrored doors on this recessed cabinet easily glide open with the touch of a finger. Swing-out storage trays inside keep small objects such as razors handy.

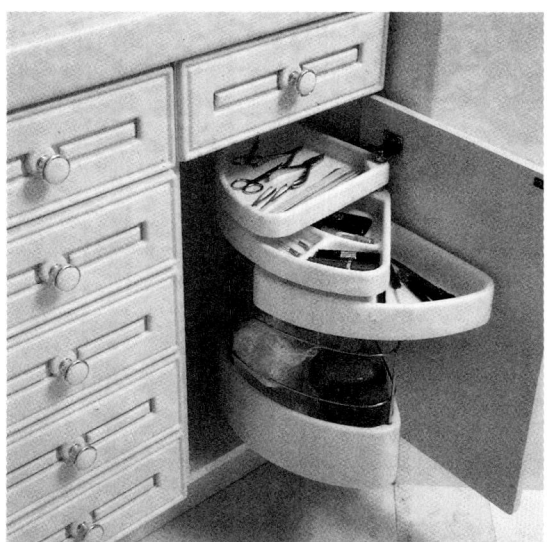

Swing-out shelves keep your health and beauty aids easily accessible.

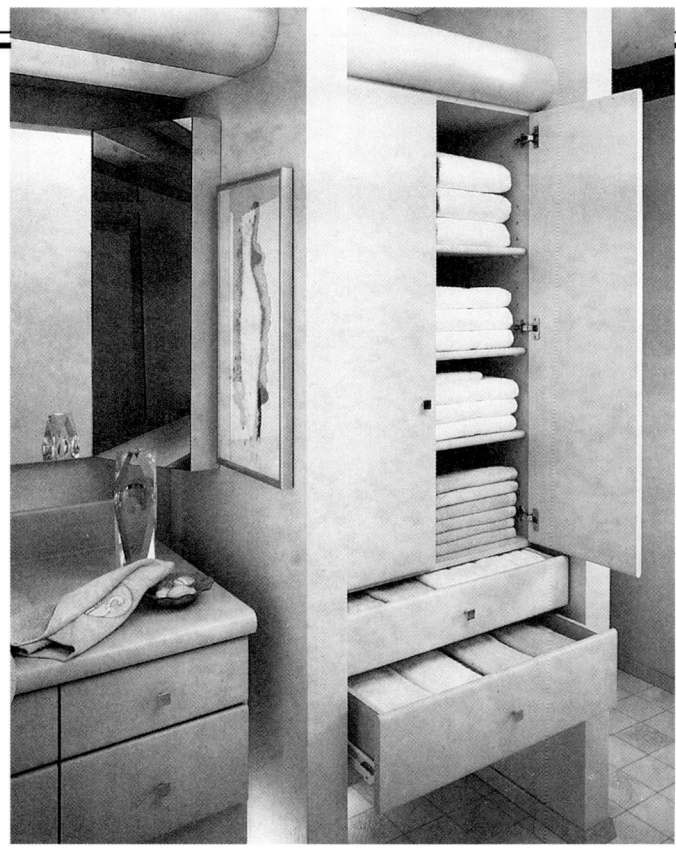

If you need to store lots of towels and linens in the bath, install a storage unit that can do this. With European-style cabinetry, drawers can be replaced with cabinet doors (and conversely) if your storage requirements change.

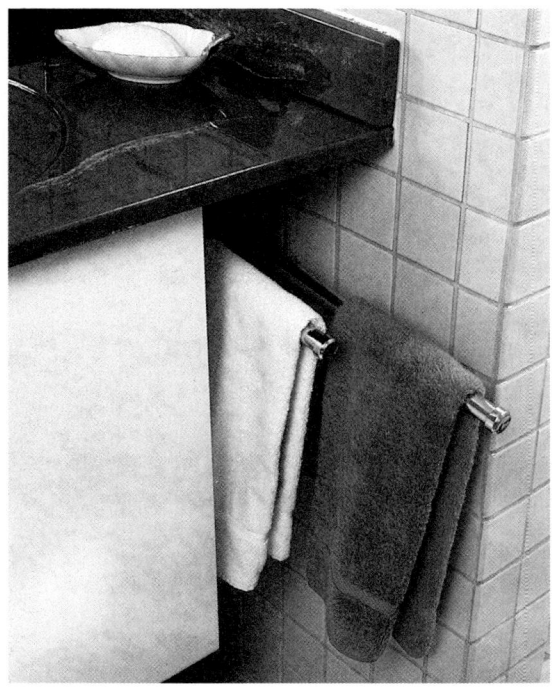

This towel bar slides out when needed and out of sight when not in use.

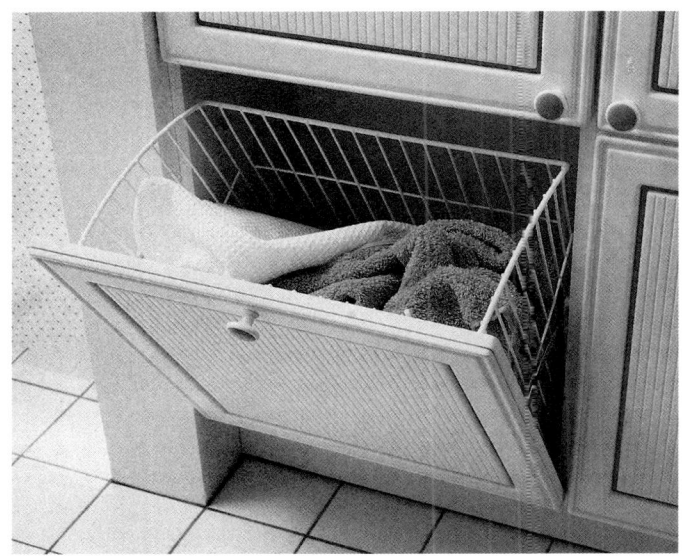

This wire basket hidden behind the cabinet door is a great place to collect clothes to be washed. Don't store *wet* towels here unless you make allowances for ventilation.

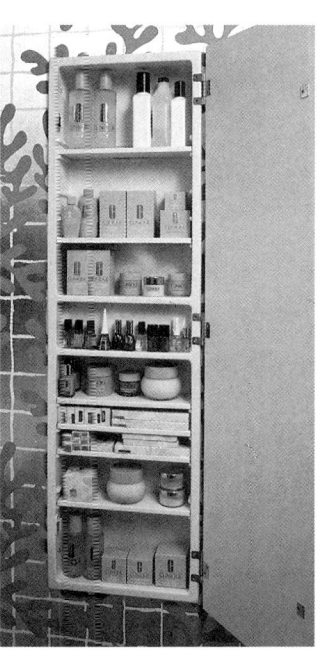
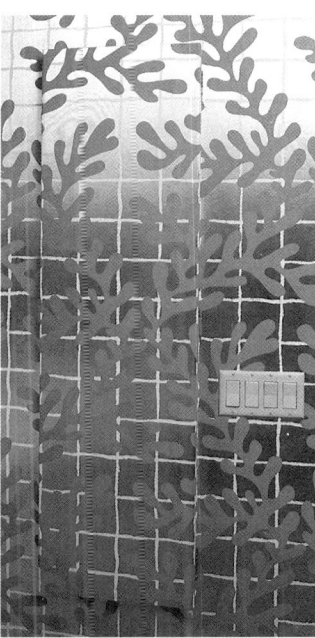

This cabinet for cosmetics is installed between the studs. It is out of view when the door is closed.

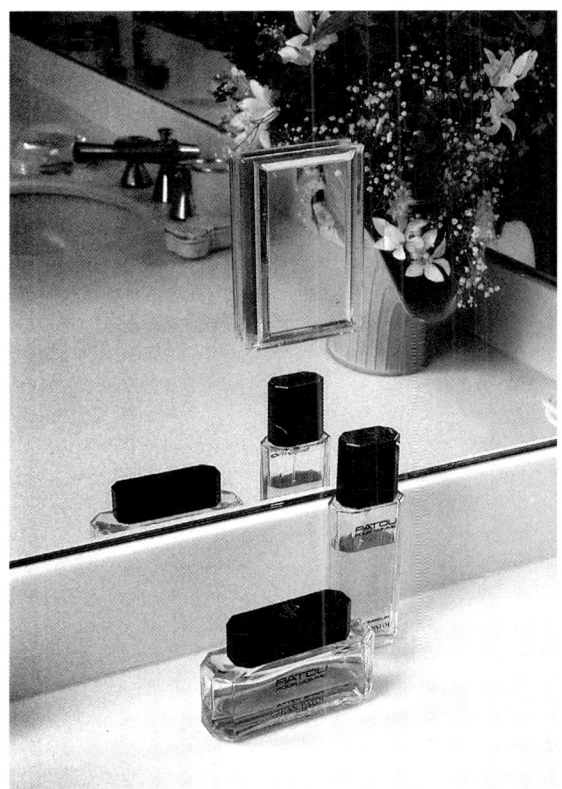
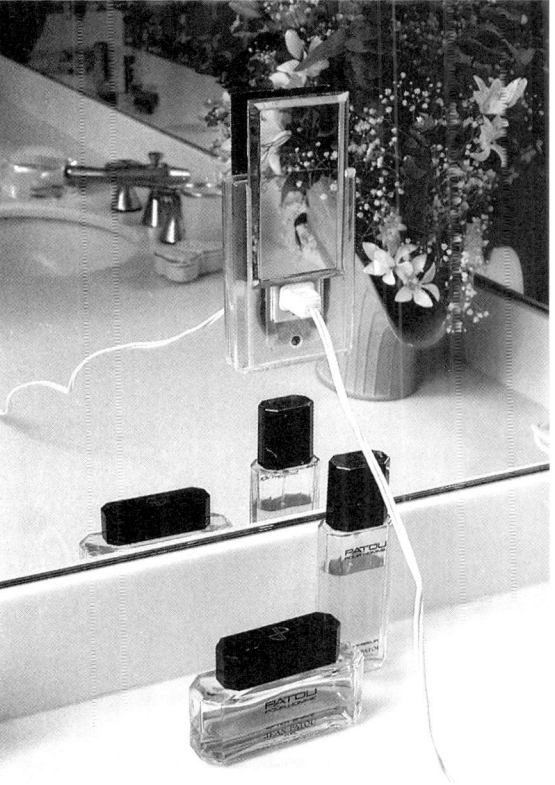

Disguise electrical outlets in a vanity mirror with mirror-clad plastic when they are not in use.

diately visible; a slanted board or rack made from dowels keeps shoes organized.

You can build such a storage unit out of plywood; or you can purchase a prefab storage system. The cheapest, and least permanent, prefab system is made from cardboard. More expensive units are made from vinyl- or melamine-coated particle board.

Many people prefer closet inserts made from vinyl-coated or enameled steel wire. Such systems offer a number of advantages over other closet storage systems. The vinyl-coated steel is strong, but lightweight. It's also durable and rust-resistant. Because it isn't solid, air can circulate freely through the clothing, discouraging mildew and odors from accumulating. Best of all, it's easy to install and to add or subtract units as your clothing storage needs change.

In addition to designing a space to store clothing that's ready to wear, you might also consider including a hamper for clothes to be washed. You can get a wire-basket hamper that attaches to a pull-down door front; a conventional freestanding hamper; or—perhaps the best solution—a wooden bin on wheels that you can easily roll to your laundry room.

## Store It Safely

Nearly every homeowner has a mirrored cabinet hanging on the bathroom wall, a cabinet commonly referred to as

## Cabinets and Countertops

| Material | Installation | Design Trends | Special Considerations |
|---|---|---|---|
| Ceramic tile | Used on countertops and backsplashes; must be installed on a supporting structure (usually plywood); level of difficulty depends on tile selected: new pregrouted and self-stick tiles cater to the novice; can be laid in wet concrete | Larger 6-by-6-inch and 8-by-8-inch tiles are increasing in popularity over the traditional 4-by-4-inch tiles; new manufacturing processes give factory-made tiles a handcrafted look; recent innovations include three-dimensional tiles, tile "chair rails," and mosaic tapestries | For the most part, a highly durable material; cold on the feet; does not absorb sound; tiles not rated Class II or better for durability can scratch easily; grout can mildew—must be sealed |
| Corian (Du Pont) 2000X (Formica) | Used mostly for countertops and countertops with integral sinks but can be used for trim and tub surrounds; can be cut with a table saw and router; difficulty of installation varies with complexity of project | Corian available in white, almond, beige, gray (others forthcoming); 2000X available in blue, pink, yellow, white, almond, beige; can be routed for special effects | Solid throughout; scratches can be sanded away; resists stains, chipping, cracking; expensive |
| Cultured marble | Polyester material cast in a mold to form sink and countertop; although cultured marble is a heavy material, it is easy to install (since the washbasin is already molded into the counter, no cutting or routing is necessary) | Trend toward gray, platinum, black and white "marble look"; away from pastels, beige, and tan | An off-the-shelf item, available in limited designs; inexpensive |
| Laminate | Used on countertops, backsplashes, and cabinets; easy to | More colors and styles to choose from than before; | Solid-core laminates show fewer nicks and |

"the medicine cabinet." This label is actually a misnomer. In fact, most professionals don't recommend storing medicines in the bathroom. The moist, warm, humid environment can affect the stability of many drugs.

Furthermore, the typical medicine cabinet, with its hinged front, is a safety hazard: It has no lock, so children have easy access to potentially deadly contents. Prescription drugs aside, ordinary over-the-counter medications (aspirins, for example) can cause convulsions, even death, if swallowed by a child.

If you insist on storing drugs in the bathroom, even temporarily, *don't* store them in the "medicine" cabinet. Keep them in a separate cabinet or drawer that is equipped with a childproof latch or a lock. (You can also get plastic cabinet inserts that are lockable with a key.) Make sure the name of the medicine and the patient and the expiration date are typed clearly on the label. *Never* mix different pills together in the same bottle. And once the illness has disappeared, throw out any leftover medicine.

Household cleaners are another potential hazard. (Drain cleaners, for example, can cause burns.) However convenient it may be to have a washer and dryer in the bathroom, keep in mind that bathroom cleaners and laundry aids don't mix. (When mixed together, chlorine bleach and ammonia, for example, can create a noxious chlorine gas.) To avoid danger, store these items separately.

| Material | Installation | Design Trends | Special Considerations |
|---|---|---|---|
| Laminate *(continued)* | install; must be glued to a supporting structure of plywood or particle board; can be worked with conventional woodworking or metalworking tools | bright primaries; sherbet pastels; grayed colors; subtle patterns; grooved, scored, and textured surfaces; special designer edge treatments; solid-core laminates | scratches than traditional laminates; use a thicker laminate on a horizontal surface than on a vertical surface; also look for coatings that resist scuff marks; hair dyes, laundry bleaches, and toilet bowl cleaners can stain |
| Natural marble | Available in tiles or slabs, natural marble is mostly used on countertops and backsplashes, although a washbasin could possibly be made out of marble; difficult to work with; can chip easily | Marble is becoming more popular as manufacturers find new ways to make it accessible to the public; new thin marble tiles are easier to install; new pastel colors; inlaid, patterned floors | Cold material; does not absorb sound; can chip, stain, and discolor; expensive, quality look; waterproof; can last for years; classic material; never goes out of style |
| Wood | Used to build countertops and cabinets; easy to work with; homeowners with workshop experience will find it easy to customize; prefab kit cabinets (made of a combination of solid wood and plywood) are easily assembled by the novice | Trend toward light wood tones—like ash and light oak—and away from dark tones; also, more wood is being stained with colored stains (mauve, cranberry, or yellow); very glossy, polyester-lacquered wood cabinets with curved corners and cabinets give bathrooms a designer look | Must be treated with waterproof finish (polyurethane, bar varnish) or will rot; feels warm on the feet; helps absorb noise; cedar gives off natural fragrance |

# The Finishing Touches

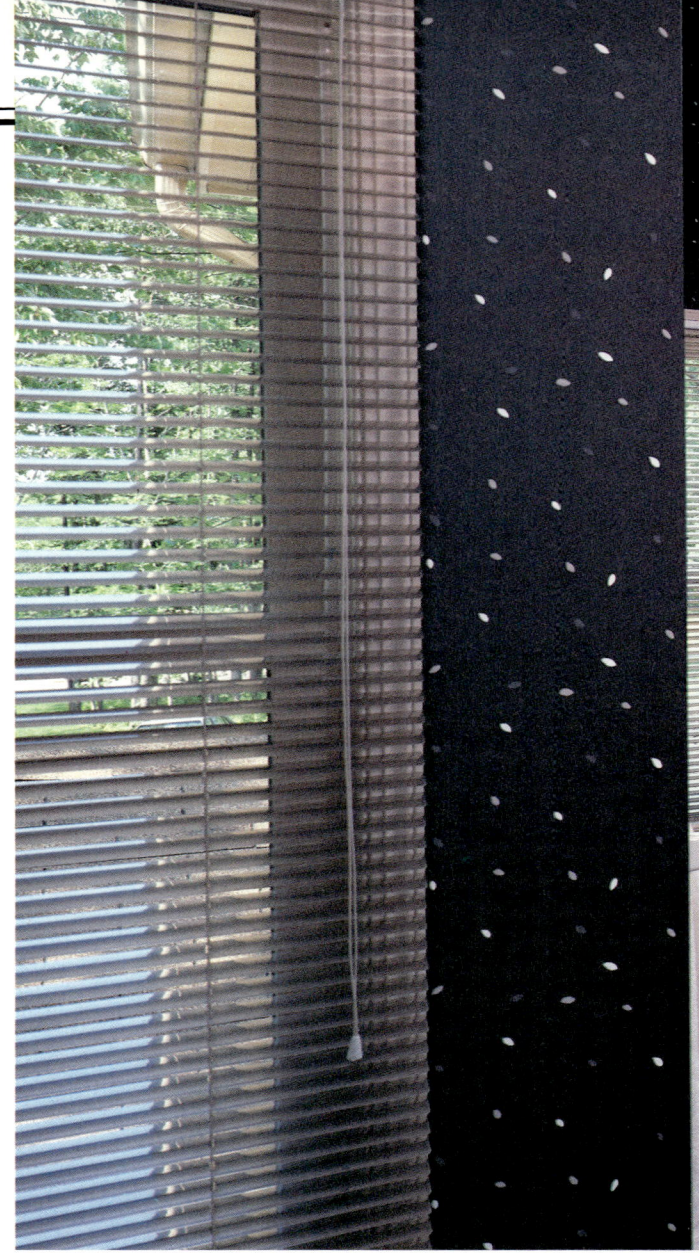

Walls, floors, lighting, and decorative accents might very well be the last step in your bathroom renovation. But think about your options, and your head will soon start spinning. Will it be marble for the tub surround, or ceramic tile? Pretty wood to warm your walls, or a high-gloss enamel? Durable vinyl for the bathroom floor, or the soft texture of carpeting? Skylights or sconces? What about plants and furniture for your new bath?

You'll quickly realize that you've got a myriad of choices to make in this department. And your selections will have a profound effect on the look of your bathroom. It's probably safe to say that these so-called "finishing touches" are the most important elements in solidifying your bathroom design. They pull the room together visually and conceptually.

Look to the walls to add color and texture to your bath. Let the materials you choose for them offset the cold, clean lines of your fixtures. By picking the right shades, patterns, and textures for your walls, you can transform your bath into anything you want it to be—rugged and rough around the edges, sleek and sophisticated, country cottagelike and romantic.

Don't feel trapped into working with just one material for walls. Using a blend of materials is one of the best ways to add dimension and character to your bath. You can start with redwood paneling at the floor and take it halfway up the walls, and then finish the rest with an interesting wallpaper. Or combine ceramic tile with paint or laminate. Teaming up different surfaces broadens your design horizons tremendously—and it can cut costs, too.

Bathroom floors take a tremendous beating and so need to be durable. But that doesn't preclude them from being attractive. Again, consider using different kinds of flooring. A central island of carpeting paired with tile or vinyl around fixtures and tub/shower area offers comfort as well as utility.

When selecting wall or flooring materials, keep in mind the primary users of the bathroom. The floor of a heavily trafficked children's bath needs a tough, kidproof surface. But you might want to splurge on something more elegant for a master-bath retreat.

Don't forget the ceiling when planning a bath renovation. It's as important as the

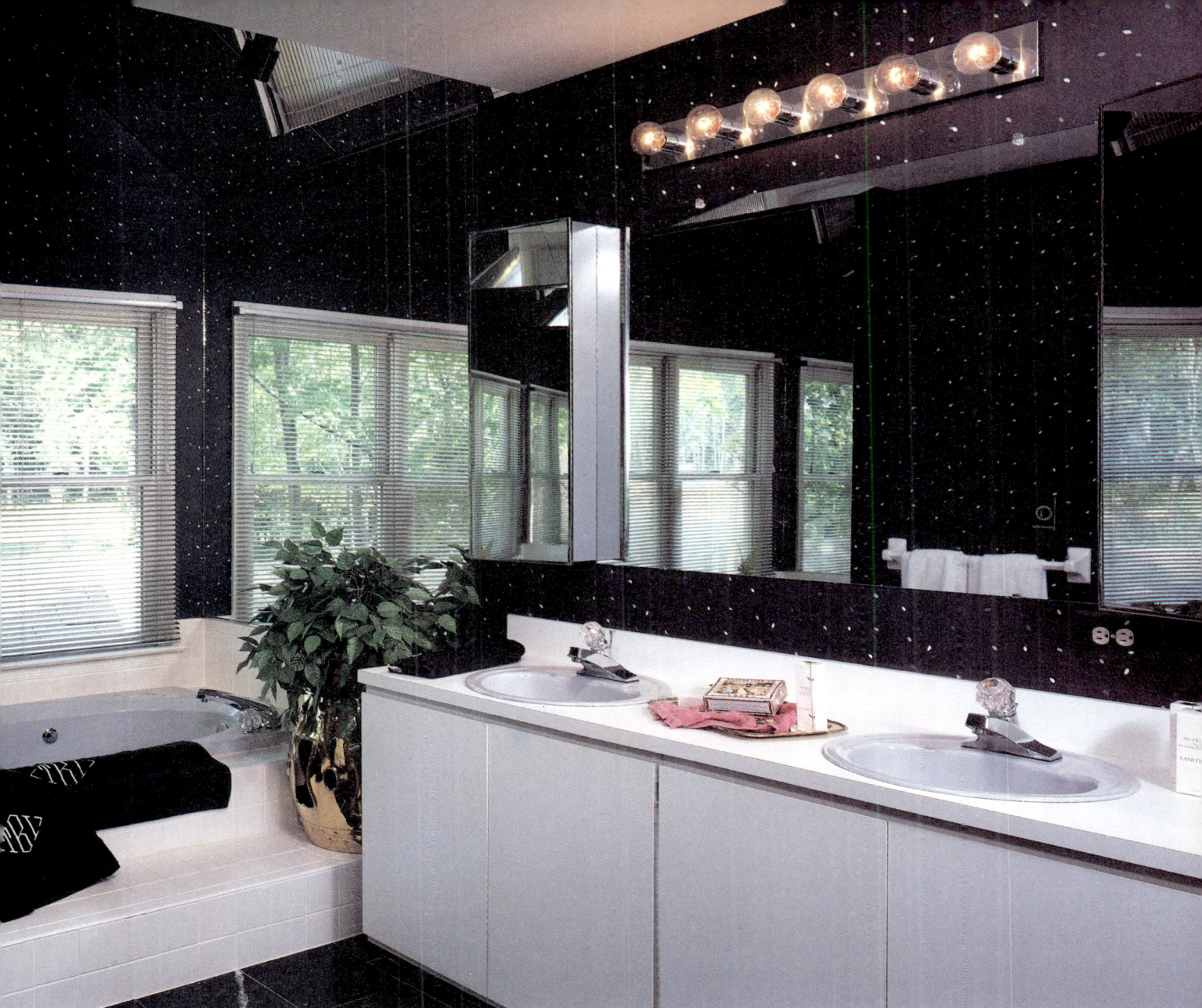

walls or floor in defining your bath space and should receive as much attention. You can choose to paint it, panel it, paper it, or perk it up with a number of exciting lighting options.

Remember when choosing materials for floors, walls, or ceilings that darker colors will absorb light and diminish space. If you plan to use dark colors in your bath, you may need additional lighting sources.

Prices for various wall, flooring, and lighting options and other final touches vary greatly—some are very expensive. But remember that you can pare down the damage to your pocketbook if you're willing to supply your own labor. Most building-supply stores that sell these materials offer guidelines for easier do-it-yourself installation.

Gone are the days of bathrooms with pasty-looking walls and nondescript floors, strewn with a few ragged mats. No longer is it necessary to groom by the unfriendly glare of a cold, fluorescent bulb. Plants and furniture are now as much a part of a bath's decor as fixtures. The finishing touches you put on your new bath are important steps toward making it a more inviting room. And the following information will help you to execute those final touches with polish.

## On the Walls

Any material you use to cover the walls in your new bath should be water-resistant

61

(waterproof in the shower stall) and washable, since moist bathroom environments often promote mildew growth.

In "The Working Parts" we told you about sinks formed from Corian, 2000X cultured marble, and cultured onyx, four elegant synthetic options. You can use those materials to cover bathroom walls or choose from a number of other surface alternatives.

## Marble

Besides offering a look of total luxury, real marble is durable and waterproof. It's available in a wide range of colors and naturally occurring patterns to use on your floors, walls, or countertops. It's one of the most expensive surface treatments you can buy and, because of its considerable weight, can be tricky to install.

Real marble is very slippery when wet. And while it lasts for years—even decades—marble scratches and stains. White marble, softer than colored versions, absorbs stains more readily. But scratches are more noticeable on the darker surfaces of colored marble. Once cracked or chipped, marble is difficult to repair.

To enjoy the luxury of real marble without all the headaches, consider using it only in light-use bathrooms where a visual statement is your top priority. To keep costs and installation problems down, choose marble tiles rather than marble slabs.

Marble is a very porous material, which makes it somewhat difficult to clean. Don't use abrasive cleaners or soap on marble—they'll make marble surfaces appear dull and lifeless.

## Ceramic Tile

Ceramic tile is another material that suggests long-lasting quality in a bathroom. It's durable and easy to maintain, and beautiful as well.

Ceramic tile comes in a stunning selection of shapes, sizes, colors, and finishes and is available with slip-resistant surfaces for floors. Individual tiles that get scratched or broken can be replaced.

Since it is completely waterproof, ceramic tile is wonderful for a tub or shower surround. Many homeowners surface sunken tubs with tile, or create "doorless" showering rooms out of tile. Tile also works well as a backsplash on the wall behind the sink area.

Although ceramic tile is expensive, you can save money by installing it yourself. Tile is now available on a flexible backing so you don't have to set individual tiles by hand; tiles even come pregrouted on boards. Another time- and effort-saving product is Wonderboard, a prefabricated sheet of mortar sandwiched between fiberglass. It supports the tile, provides a good bond for the

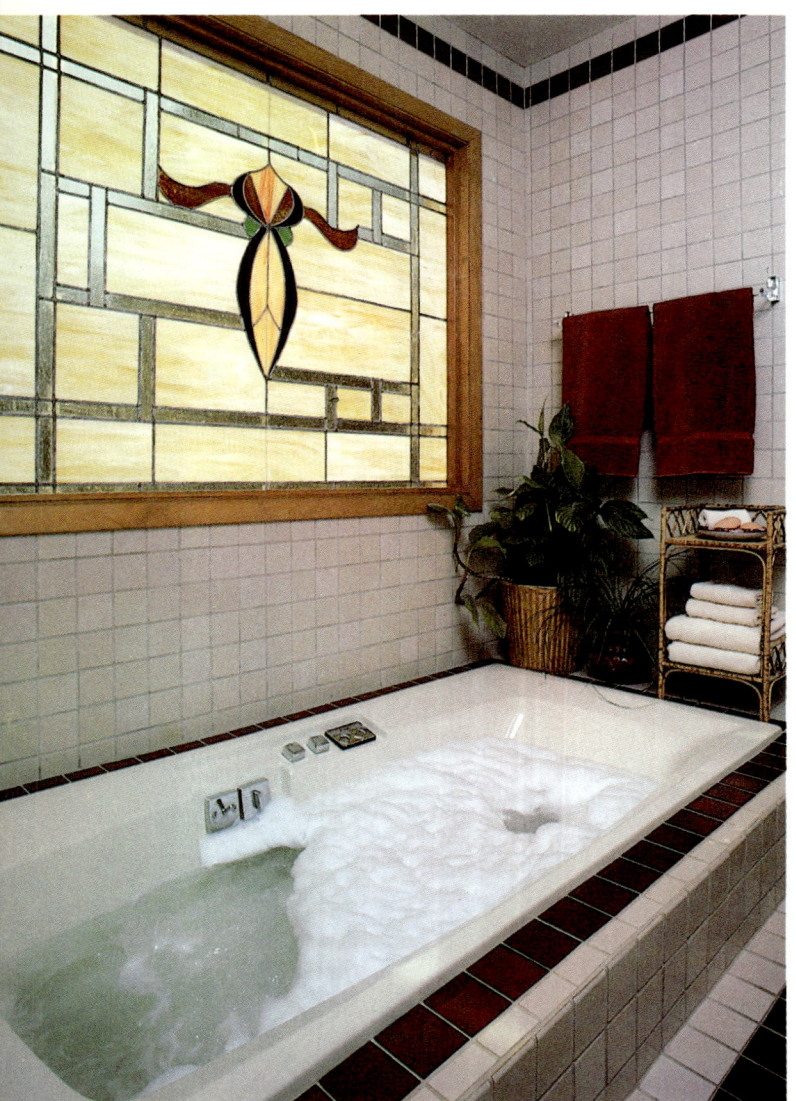

The use of unique and unexpected treatments—like the large stained-glass window and deep red ceramic tile in this bath—gives the room an added dimension.

mortar, and resists moisture decay that can loosen ceramic tiles.

One problem with ceramic tile is the grout. Mildew grows easily in grout and discolors it. Discoloration is less of a problem with medium-color grout than with light or dark shades. Regular maintenance will also help to minimize grime buildup.

## Paint

In contrast to marble and tile, paint is one of the least expensive ways to cover the walls in your new bath. Paint is easy to apply and maintain and is available in any color that suits your fancy. The solid, patternless appearance painted walls create is a good way to stretch the visual space in a room.

Paint is ideal for family and children's bathrooms in which maintenance should be minimal and wall surfaces durable. One advantage of painting is that if you aren't completely satisfied with the results, you can simply repaint without a huge expense.

In bathrooms, it's best to use a high-gloss, oil- or alkyd-based enamel for a durable, washable finish. If you've had a mildew problem in the bathroom, mix a mildewcide in the paint before you brush it on. Alkyd-based paint will adhere well to latex paint, provided the latex isn't glossy—you might have to sand it a bit first. But you can't paint over alkyd with latex paint. You'll have to sand and prime the alkyd layer before applying the latex.

## Wallpaper

Wallpaper can also be an inexpensive treatment for bathroom walls, although fancy designer patterns and colors can cost twice as much as generic versions. Wallpaper is easy to install and comes in almost unlimited colors and patterns.

Because of the moisture in most bathrooms, wallpaper will almost always come loose a bit at the seams—plan on periodically repasting them. For the same reason, wallpaper is not as durable as other wall coverings and will probably need to be replaced sooner than other types would have to be. Vinyl-backed wallpapers last longer than paper-backed types. Avoid foil wallpapers; the foil often develops rust spots because of moisture.

## Mirrors

Because bathrooms are often small rooms, they need visual expansion. Mirrors do the job beautifully. They stretch space and let you see yourself from many angles for grooming. Mirroring the ceiling not only heightens the room but helps to brighten it as well.

For safety, you should use tempered glass or mirrorlike sheet plastics rather than a regular window-glass mirror. The standard mirror thickness is ¼ inch, but you can save money by choosing a 3/16-inch thickness; just be sure the thinner mirror is flat and doesn't reflect a distorted image. You don't want to feel like you're in a fun house every time you enter the bathroom.

## Decorative Laminates

Although generally considered a counter and cabinet surface, versatile decorative laminates can double as a wall covering. Laminates—color surfaces bonded to base materials, usually plywood or particle board—are durable, inexpensive, and easy to install. They resist stain and abrasion and come in a wide variety of colors and finishes—from bright jewel tones to textured pastels to wood grains, and other subtle patterns.

Laminates work well in a European-style bath. Their smooth surfaces and clean colors complement the simple, elegant accessories and curvilinear shapes that are typical of the continental bath design. Because they're waterproof, laminates also make good shower and tub surrounds.

Until recently, laminates always had dark lines along the edges where plastic met plastic. Several companies, however, have introduced solid-color surface materials (Solicor and ColorCore) that show no dark line.

## Wood

For a bathroom wall covering that is naturally warm and beautiful, moderately priced, and easy to install, try wood. It provides some soundproofing and can help insulate your bath space. Remember, though, that unless wood is painted or treated to resist moisture, it may rot in your bathroom's steamy environment. An excess of wood in the bathroom can also darken the space, making it seem smaller.

Two good wood choices are redwood and cedar. Both are naturally water-resistant and can be left untreated. Periodic sanding freshens the surfaces. If you choose another kind of wood, be sure to treat all of its surfaces with a waterproofing agent to prevent warping and water damage.

## The Ceiling

Many of the same treatments used for walls will work nicely on the bathroom ceiling. Laminate or ceramic tile, of course, are not practical choices, but a number of others produce good results. Whatever you use, though, it should help to define your bath space without attracting too much undeserved attention.

Paint is the least expensive and most popular option. It can either be the same color as the walls, or a different shade to blend with the walls or create a new look. As with the walls, you will need to use a high-gloss enamel that will resist moisture and prevent rotting.

Wallpaper is another common choice. Like paint, it is not too expensive for the most part. And since many bathrooms now have skylights and irregular angles on the ceiling, a ceiling treatment needs to be versatile. Like paint, wallpaper easily accommodates a unique design.

Wood is very pretty on a bathroom ceiling, as long as the bath space is not too small and the wood is not too dark. Mirrors work as well up top as they do on the walls; mirroring a couple of walls and the ceiling produces startling, space-stretching results.

## The Floor

The material you choose for the floor of your new bath needs to be a waterproof, nonslip surface that's easy to clean. If you have a large bathroom, you can mix flooring materials, putting nonslip or waterproof material near the shower or tub and water-resistant materials in other areas.

Ceramic tile works as well on floors as it does on walls. If you do choose this material, save the highly glazed, slippery tiles for the walls, and opt for a textured surface for the floors, especially for the tub and shower area.

Marble and other stone surfaces can also be used, but they are quite expensive and difficult to care for—they're best left on walls and countertops unless you have time for fastidious care. For the look of marble without the tricky maintenance, try using ceramic or vinyl tiles in a "marbleized" pattern. In fact, it is also possible to create a "marbleized" effect with paint.

Vinyl tiles and sheets are also good floor coverings. Vinyl is cheaper than tile

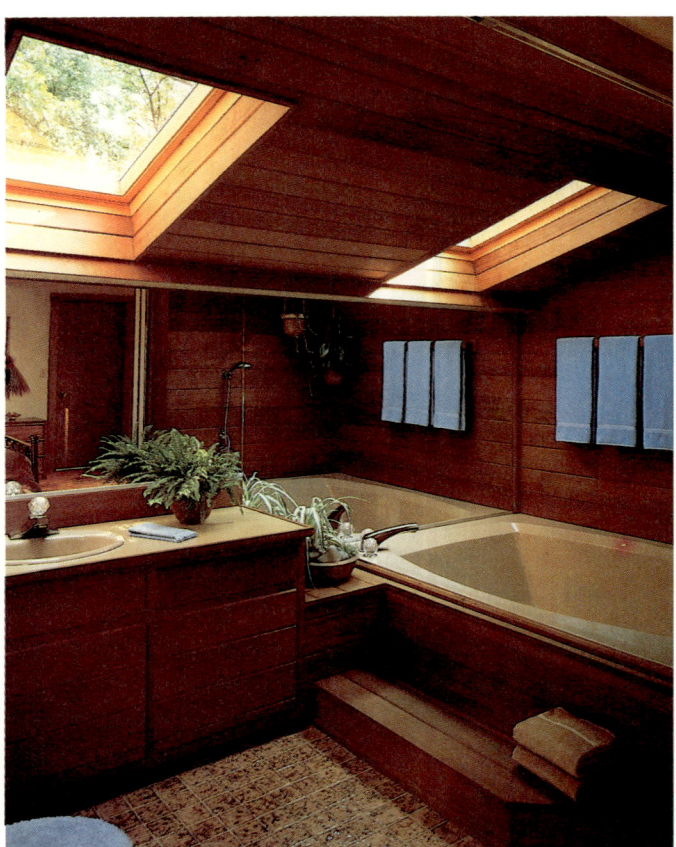

The durable beauty of redwood sets a warm tone in this bath. Redwood is one of several woods that work well in a humid bathroom atmosphere.

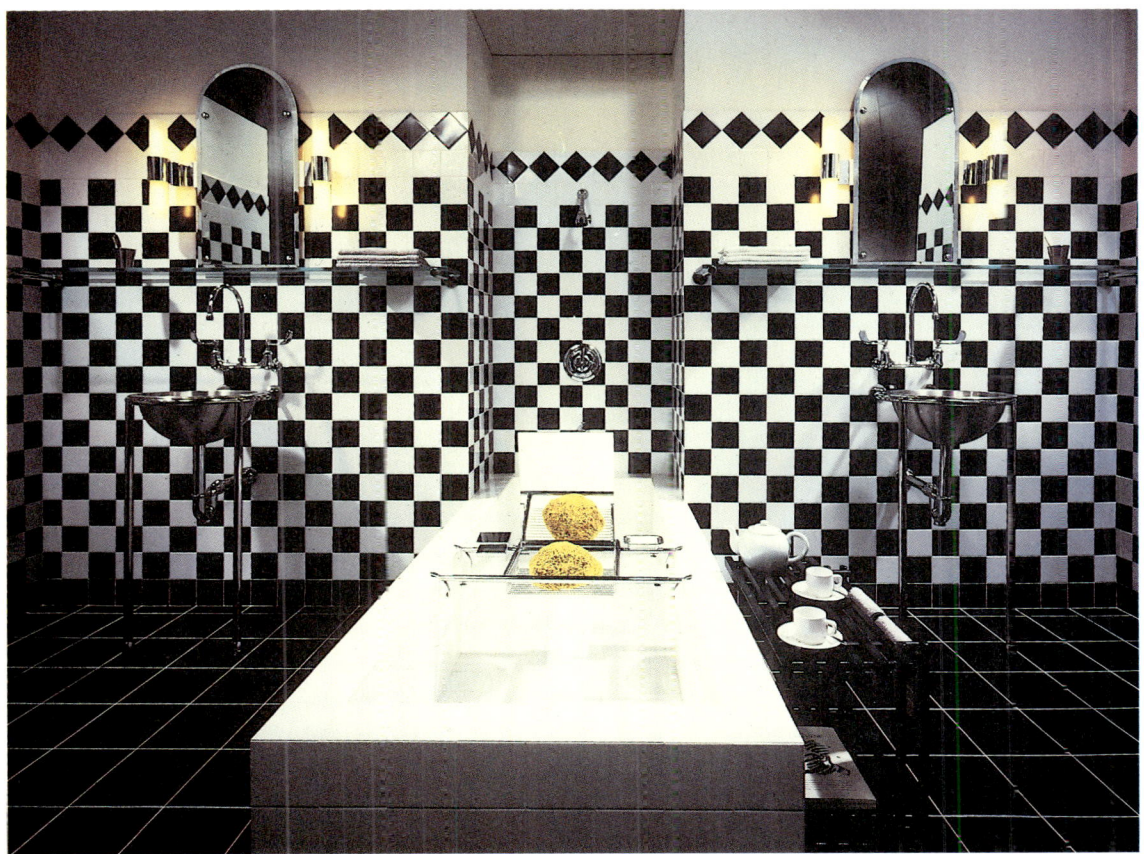

The classic combination of black and white provides an arresting backdrop for this European-style bath. While neutrals are popular, bright bold colors can also complement a bath design.

and marble; it's relatively easy to install. You can buy vinyl tiles and sheets in kits intended for the do-it-yourselfer. Vinyl isn't as durable as ceramic tiles, but it is easy to maintain and comes in a wide range of beautiful colors and patterns.

Wood also works as well for bathroom floors as it does for walls. Proper sealing and finishing is necessary to prevent water damage, but once sealed, wood is fairly easy to maintain. Several companies now offer a wood flooring bonded with a thin top layer of clear vinyl for longer wear and lasting beauty.

For an extra touch of comfort, consider a resilient or cushioned sheet vinyl. These surfaces give slightly when you walk on them and feel much warmer underfoot than tile, marble, or regular vinyl. They're easy to care for, and the inner material helps to absorb sound.

More and more people are using carpet in the bathroom; it provides a warm, comfortable, nonskid surface for bare feet and adds a feeling of luxury to this personal room. Carpeting offers you an incredible palette of colors to choose from: brights, pastels, and blends in as many patterns and textures.

Bathroom carpet does require extra care, though. It's not easy to clean, and, if it gets wet, it can remain soggy for days. To prolong the life of bathroom carpet, lay it loose—don't nail it down—so you can remove it for cleaning. You may want to cut a separate section to fit around the toilet bowl so you can clean that section more often. Stitching or chemical sealing around the edges of these carpet sections will prevent unraveling. Rugs of synthetic fibers will resist rot and other kinds of water damage.

## Lighting

Proper lighting isn't always easy to achieve in today's modern bathrooms. The white sinks, tubs, and toilets always found in bathrooms years ago actually helped to light the room, although that was not their primary purpose. Today's bathrooms are much more aesthetically pleasing, but those elegant dark woods, tiles, and colored fixtures absorb incredible amounts of light.

This makes the job of designing your bath's lighting tough, because lighting is more important in the bathroom than in almost any other room in your house. Your choice of lighting systems must provide good grooming light, accentuate your bathroom design, and achieve that delicate balance between too dark and too light. It's a tall order, but it can be done.

The darker the colors in your bathroom and the more contrast you introduce, the more lighting you will need. Instead of attempting this with brighter bulbs, use more light fixtures. Also, take advantage of "bounce light," the bonus light reflected from light surfaces in a room. If you're planning a dark color scheme for your bathroom, consider adding a light-colored sink, vanity, or ceiling.

Light-colored walls, tubs, sinks, and toilets—like those old-fashioned white tubs and toilets—don't necessarily increase the amount of light that enters a room, but they make the best of the light that is available. If you are making use of a number of shiny, reflective surfaces, be careful that the wattage of the lights you use is not too powerful.

### Electric Lighting

If your primary source of illumination in the bath will be electric lighting, you have a number of choices. In most bathroom situations, however, good overhead lighting, combined with localized lighting of

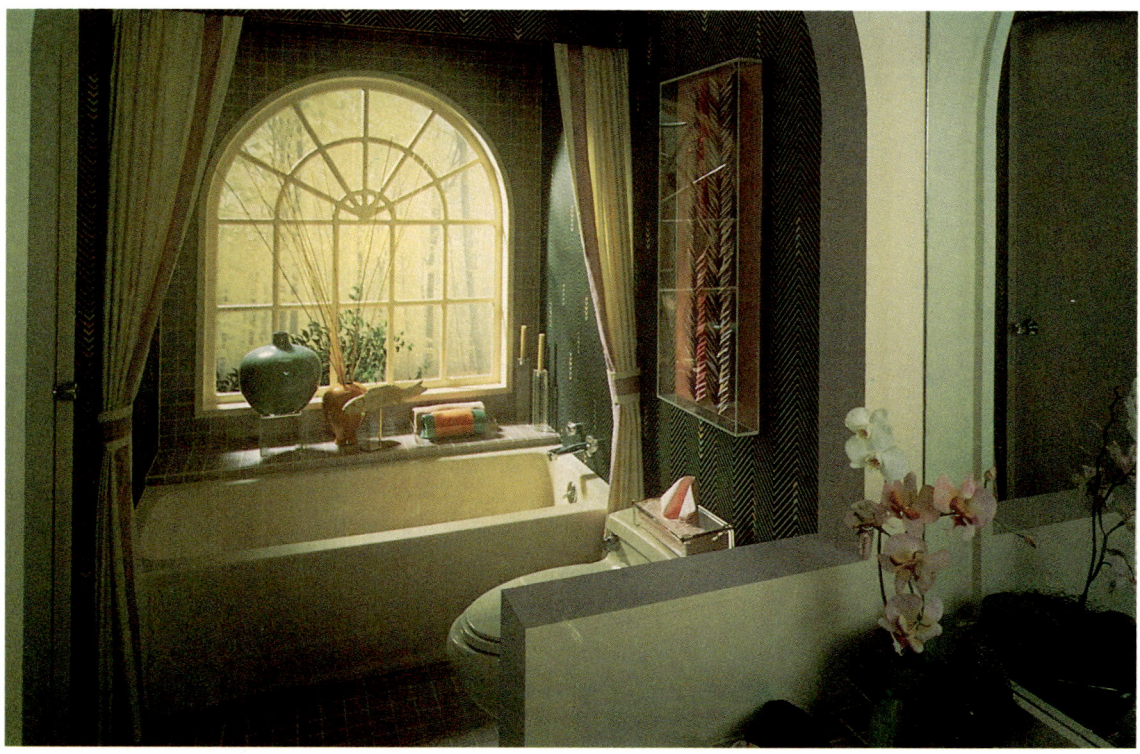

Your finishing touches will be the key to setting the mood in your bath, whether it's bold and bright, quiet and pretty, or somewhere in between.

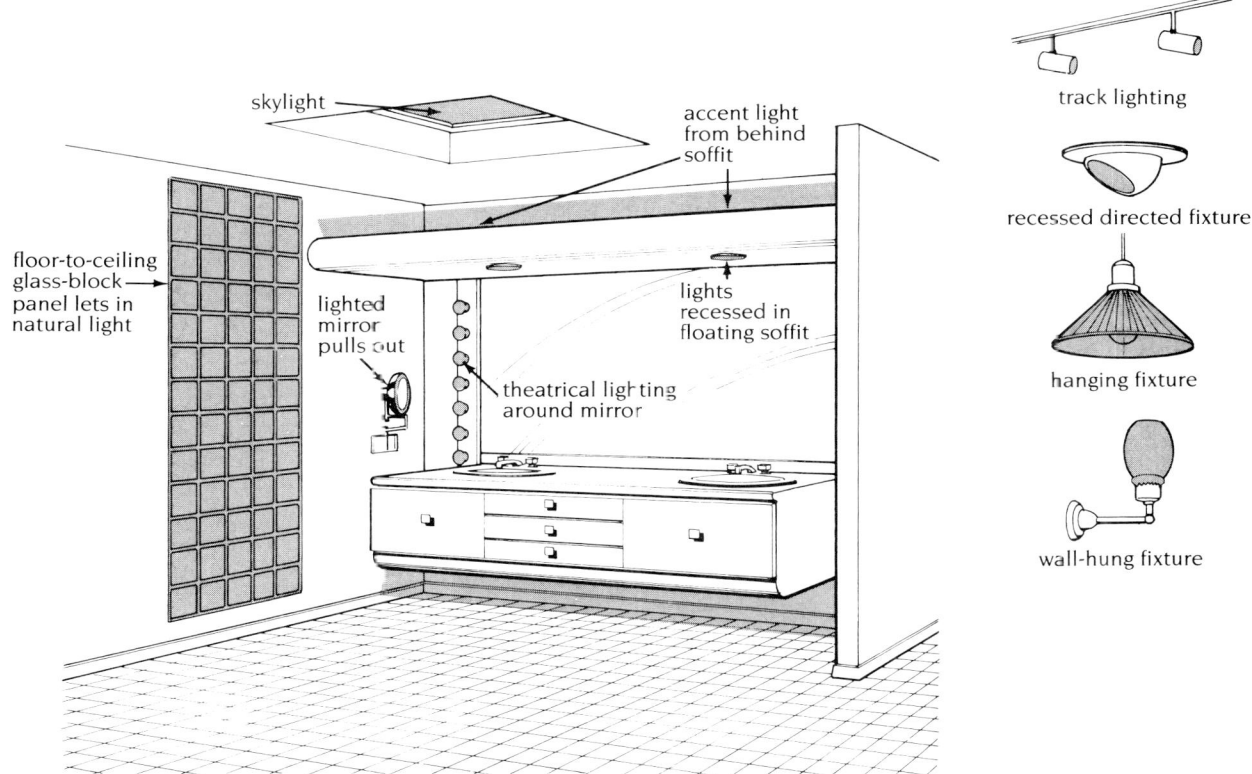

Windows, skylights, and glass-block walls allow natural lighting in the bath. Electric lighting provides good overhead illumination while other fixtures provide task lighting for grooming and toilet areas and storage spaces. Dimmer switches help to create mood lighting.

grooming stations, toilet areas, and storage spaces, works very effectively.

Using diffused overhead light is an excellent way to strike a balance between too much and too little light. It softens the harshness that is often the result of overcompensating to brighten a dark room. To provide diffused light, simply cover light fixtures with highly translucent (milky white) plastic or glass.

Another good way to effectively light the entire bathroom area without creating shadows is with a luminescent ceiling. This can be achieved by covering ceiling fixtures with a piece of translucent plastic or glass paneling. A luminescent ceiling creates a "skylight" effect, and, since light is dispersed evenly, it allows you to utilize much less wattage.

When planning task lighting, make sure to provide adequate light for the grooming area. To eliminate shadows on your face, light should come from both sides of the mirror as well as from overhead. Sidelights can be close to the mirror, but don't position them so that they shine directly on the mirror itself, since this will produce a harsh glare. Use your height as a guide when positioning the sidelights. Also, make sure that swinging cabinet doors clear all your light fixtures.

Theatrical lighting supplies a true, shadowless reflection and is therefore a good choice for grooming light. You might also consider several fluorescent tubes, track lights, or other decorative fixtures. For a very large vanity area, you may want to install your light fixtures on a soffit above the mirror; recessed lights work very nicely in this case. Recessed fixtures can be placed so that their light shines straight down or pinpoints certain spots in the room.

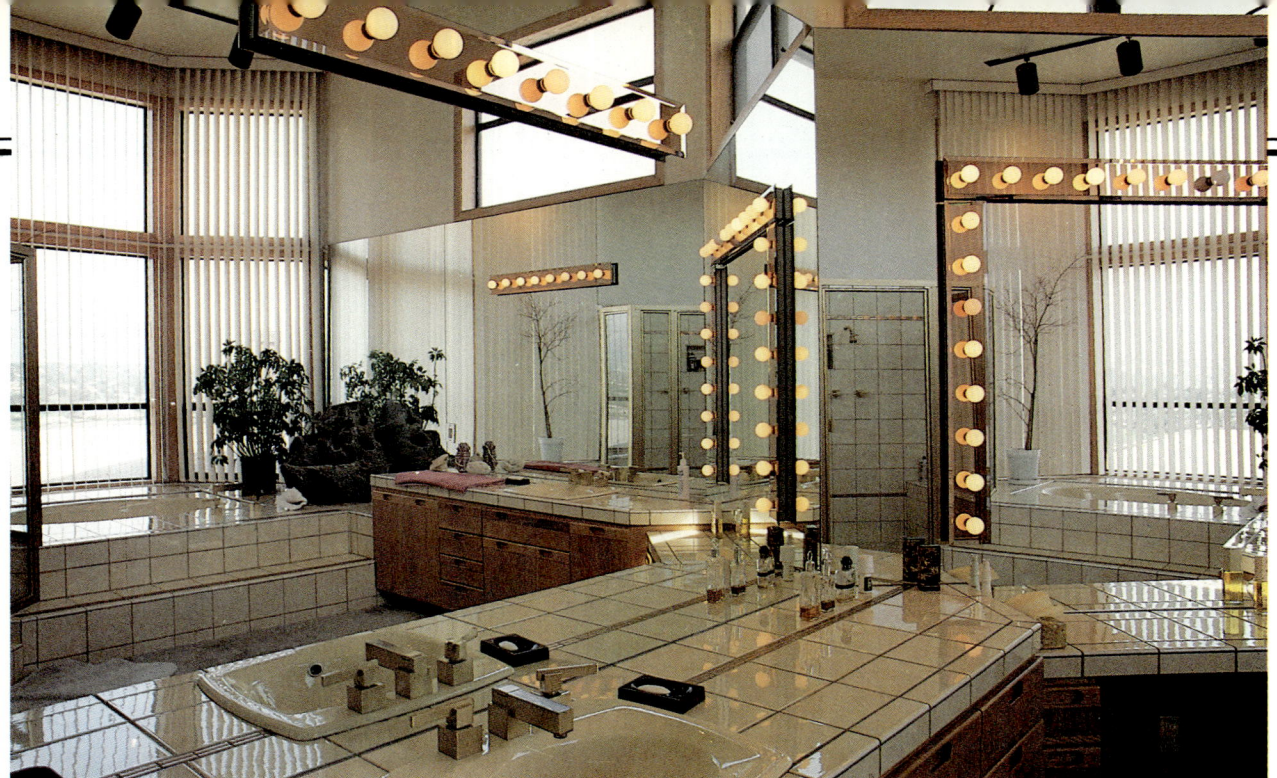

Filling your bath with natural light will make it appear larger as well as more pleasant. With its many skylights and windows, this bath lets the sun shine in.

Incandescent bulbs produce a light that is similar to sunlight. It's much more flattering than conventional fluorescent light and is usually the best choice for the vanity area. However, fluorescent light uses much less wattage than incandescent light.

If you are considering fluorescent light fixtures, or if your bathroom is already equipped with them, investigate the new color-corrected or full-spectrum fluorescents. The light they produce is much truer and warmer than what conventional cool-white fluorescent tubes emit. Both incandescent and fluorescent bulbs can be used—and work well—in recessed light fixtures.

If the toilet is contained separately from the rest of the bath, you will need an additional light for that area. A separate light over the shower/tub area is a good idea if a heavy curtain is keeping the space darkened; the light fixture should be approved by Underwriters Laboratories for use specifically in a highly moist area. Make sure the light switch is at a safe distance—out of reach of wet hands.

To create mood lighting for luxurious soaks in the tub, put some of your lights on dimmer switches. Dimmers control the amount of heat as well as the amount of light lamps emit—an important consideration in a hot climate.

Night-lights are very practical for any bathroom, but especially for children's bathrooms. They use very little wattage and can be equipped with dimmer switches that adjust the level of light emitted.

If you are remodeling your bath, try not to change the position of existing light fixtures unless they are completely unacceptable—rewiring can get costly. Make provisions for lighting in a new bath in the early planning stages, because it will become more difficult and expensive to add light fixtures later on.

A word about electrical outlets: Just make sure you have enough of them. Most codes usually require a minimum of one outlet near the basin for each bathroom, but, depending on your family's bath habits, you may need more. Consider all of the electrical appliances you will be using in the bathroom—electric razors, lighted makeup mirrors, curling irons, hair dryers, electric toothbrushes, contact-lens boiling units, and so forth—and plan outlets for them. Codes also require ground-fault circuit interrupters (GFCI) on all bathroom receptacles. (See "Codes" on page 128.)

### Natural Lighting

One easy way to take your bathroom beyond the ordinary is to provide some indoor sunshine. Natural light is the most pleasing kind of light; it's flattering and makes us feel good, and it brings out the best in almost any design or decor. You can bring in the sunshine several different ways.

The most obvious is with windows. Windows bring the outdoors inside. They let in cool, fresh air; they afford pleasing views of gardens, skies, and surrounding landscapes; and they bring in natural sunlight that warms the room as well as illuminates it. Windows can be important design elements in the bath and, when positioned properly, can also help expand space.

If you are constructing a new bath or thinking of repositioning the windows of an existing bath, make sure you place them properly. Don't position a window so that bright sunlight hits the grooming mirror. And if you locate one in the tub/shower area, make sure all family members will be able to bathe in privacy.

It's always nice to have a bathroom window that opens to allow fresh air in. But if your design calls for a permanently closed one, make sure the room is equipped for it. You may, for instance, need extra ventilation and cooling for hot summer days.

**Decorating Your Windows.** Plan to decorate your windows as specially as you would the rest of your bath. Use your imagination. There's no rule in home design that requires windows to be square or rectangular; you can make them any size and shape you wish—round, oval, triangular, hexagonal, or octagonal.

Give them a luxury treatment—a Japanese shoji screen perhaps, or stained glass, frosted glass, patterned glass or beveled glass for windows. These treatments are a bit more expensive, but may be the ticket to round out your bathroom design.

Unless your bathroom window opens onto a private yard or garden, you'll need some way of shutting out the world when you need a little privacy. Curtains work nicely when they are made of durable, washable fabric; because of moisture buildup in the bathroom, you'll want to launder them occasionally. Laces, sheers, and other delicate fabrics are much harder to care for.

Colorful pull shades or shutters can provide pleasing design accents in your bath, as can blinds. Blinds are no longer the ugly, rusting white blades you remember from schoolrooms and old public buildings. Today's blinds come in an attractive array of sizes and colors, open horizontally or vertically, and can lend a decidedly European touch to your bath. Shades and shutters (especially ones with insulating or reflective qualities) also help to keep your bath warm in winter and cool in summer.

### Insulating and Reflective Windows

Clear glass is the least expensive and the most common type of windowpane. It admits up to 90 percent of available light into the room, and it has essentially *no* insulating or reflective properties. If you live in a warm climate, you may want to consider installing reflective glass that can provide some relief from intense heat and brightness. Conversely, if you live in a cold climate, you will want to consider insulating windows.

Reflective glass is regular glass, coated on the outside with a substance that decreases the amount of heat transmission by as much as 70 percent. It also reduces glare and ultraviolet transmission. Coating existing windows with a special polyester film provides the same result without your having to replace the windows altogether.

A double-pane window consists of two panes of glass between which a dry gas or airspace is sealed. This setup reduces heat loss on cold days and keeps the bathroom cooler on hot days. It also prevents the buildup of condensation, a common problem in bathrooms during cold winter weather. There are even triple-pane windows, but keep in mind that each layer decreases any benefit you might get from the warming rays of the sun. A solution to this problem is to use low-iron glass, which transmits more sunlight than regular glass. Other types of windows with good insulating qualities have layers of high-transparency plastic film between the panes.

### Skylights

Another way to flood your bath with sunshine is to install a skylight, or a roof window. Skylights are one of the most popular lighting treatments used in new baths today, and they are often the highlight of a room. A skylight brings in daylight when a conventional window might not be practical. It can make your space feel bigger and look brighter.

Skylights are excellent sources of overhead light. In a small bath, a skylight often provides all the light you need during the day—a nice savings on your utility bill, since you'll only be flicking the switch at night. Skylights over the shower/tub area can eliminate the need for extra lighting there.

There are several different types of skylights. They can be big or small, dome-shaped or flat, clear, translucent, or colored. Some can be opened during good weather to allow fresh air in; others remain sealed. You will need to check the building codes in your area to determine the types of materials approved for use, how much space the skylight can cover, and any other requirements or restrictions.

Plastic domes are the most popular choices for residential skylights. The domed shape is desirable because rainfall helps to keep it clean, and the shape inhibits "ponding," the buildup of water on a skylight that can cause leaks.

You may have read or heard about homeowners' complaints of leaking skylights, but most manufacturers and contractors will tell you that if you follow the installation instructions to the letter, you will not have a problem. Most leaks, they assert, occur when corners have been cut during installation. It might save you time and money in the long run to have your skylight professionally installed.

### Glass Block and Sunspaces

There are other ways to let the sun shine in. Opening up part of an exterior wall and installing glass block is an expensive but fantastic one. Glass block allows light to enter but maintains privacy. Glass block comes in a variety of sizes, patterns, and even colors. For the more adventurous, a sunspace bumpout can make an elegant enclosure for an oversize tub or spa. Keep in mind, though, that a sunspace will generate a fair amount of heat.

## Ventilation

Excessive moisture is a potential problem that energy-efficient housing experts are recognizing more and more. As houses are tightened up, indoor humidity levels can climb. (A typical family of three can produce 20 pounds of water vapor a day.) Problems range from mildew, rust on fixtures, and condensation on windows to more serious structural damage as moisture condenses in wall cavities and attics. Here moisture can cause extensive wood decay, degradation of insulation materials, and peeling of paint on exterior surfaces.

Bathrooms in particular are prime areas for the generation of moisture, odors, and even air pollution from spray cans and cleaning chemicals. Because the bathroom represents a concentrated source of moisture vapor, it's important to plan for adequate spot ventilation during new construction or remodeling. Hot tubs and spas call for even greater consideration.

Natural ventilation is one way to deal with moisture buildup—just open a window, ensure good cross flow through the bathroom, and let the breeze flush out the humidity. The trouble is, this method is so dependent on variable factors like the weather that it's obviously unpredictable and inconvenient in most cases, and it wastes valuable heat energy in winter.

### Ventilating Fans

The best solution is to install a ventilating fan in your bathroom and duct it to carry the moisture outside of the house. Properly sized and installed, a fan can very effectively handle the temporary humidity load from showers and other bathroom activities.

The difference a ventilating fan can make in a bathroom is shown in the graph on the opposite page, which presents the results of research done at the Texas Engineering

Experiment Station, Texas A & M University, as reported by the Home Ventilating Institute Division of the Air Movement and Control Association. Note how a shower caused the relative humidity to rise almost immediately to near 100 percent, when the air was saturated with moisture. In an unventilated bathroom the humidity stayed very high, decreasing only a few percent in over a half hour. In contrast in a bathroom with a ventilating fan of recommended capacity, relative humidity peaked during the shower but began to fall quickly and reached a level near the starting point 25 minutes after the shower stopped. The researchers found that even 2 minutes after the shower ceased, the moisture content in the ventilated bathroom was lower than that of the unventilated bathroom 20 minutes later.

*Selecting a Fan*

How do you select a fan of the right capacity for your particular situation? The American Society of Heating, Refrigerating and Air-Conditioning Engineers (ASHRAE) has recommended minimum ventilation levels specified as a certain continuous amount of air entering each room in a house. The rate for bathrooms is given as 50 cubic feet per minute (CFM). This recommendation, put forth in ASHRAE Standard #62, adopted in 1981, doesn't account for different *sizes* of bathrooms, however.

A second standard is put forth in the United States Department of Housing and Urban Development (HUD) minimum property standard. The 1979 version of this standard describes the ventilation capacity in terms of complete exchanges of *all* the air in each room (independent of room size). Eight air changes per hour is the ventilation rate recommended for bathrooms. This standard originates with the Home Ventilating Institute (HVI), a consumer communication group of the ventilating industry.

To determine the correct capacity for a ventilating fan (rated in CFM) the HVI recommends this simple calculation: multiply the area of your bathroom floor by 1.1 (assuming an 8-foot ceiling height). That is: length × width × 1.1 = fan capacity in CFM.

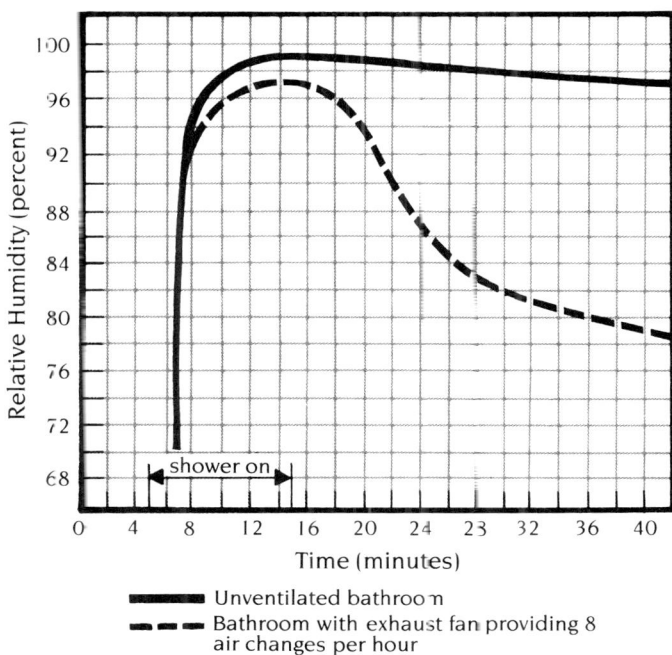

Redrawn with the permission of Home Ventilating Institute, Division of AMCA.

An exhaust fan keeps moisture in the air lower during a shower and rapidly reduces it after a shower.

For example, a 6-foot-by-9-foot bathroom would require an exhaust fan with a rating of 6 × 9 × 1.1 = 59.4 or about 60 CFM.

All fan motors make noise, so it's important to select a unit that is as quiet as possible. The sound level of fans is rated in *sones*. Quality ventilating fans of typical bathroom capacity usually have a rating of about 2 to 4 sones. Once you've narrowed your selection to the correct air flow, choose a fan labeled with the lowest sone rating.

There is a wide variety of ventilating fans, and they are readily available from local heating contractors, electrical-equipment suppliers, or some hardware and home centers. It's wise to plan and purchase an entire ventilation system—fan and ceiling grille, ductwork, controls, and exhaust vent with backdraft damper. A good damper is important to ensure that the duct is closed off to the outside when the fan is not operating, which prevents undesirable drafts. For hints on problems to avoid during installation see "Installing Ventilating Fans" on page 134.

Expand your options by using ventilating fans with lights and heaters in a ceiling-mounted unit. Also, choose a simple on-off manual switch, a timer switch, or a humidistat that senses moisture buildup and switches the fan on or off automatically.

### Air-to-Air Heat Exchangers

Operating a ventilating fan unfortunately exhausts precious warm air in winter. Just how much is lost in terms of dollars is highly variable, depending on the frequency of fan use and local fuel costs. In situations where a large fan is operated often—for example, in a spa room—it might pay to design a ventilation system using an *air-to-air heat exchanger*. This device transfers most of the heat that would be lost in the exhaust air stream to a fresh air intake. An air-to-air heat exchanger costs much more to purchase and operate than a ventilating fan.

Most air-to-air heat exchangers are designed to be part of a whole-house ventilation system. Sizing such a system is a job for an architect or heating engineer. But remember that, although the unit might produce a ventilation rate of only about 0.5 air changes per hour for the rest of the house, the bathroom still requires 8 air changes per hour. Thus the machine must have the additional capacity to handle this intermittent extra ventilation. Using booster fans in the bathroom ductwork of a whole-house ventilation system is one way to gain the extra capacity.

Recently two companies, Des Champs Laboratories and NuTone, have developed small, wall-mounted air-to-air heat exchangers suitable for use in bathrooms or spa rooms alone. They have a maximum fresh airflow of around 75 CFM and cost roughly the same—about $330. An air-to-air heat exchanger will produce condensation from exhaust air, so be sure that any model you select has drain capability. Also, keeping the cover on a spa when it's not in use will help to control moisture in the room.

## Furniture in Your Bath

Furniture in the bathroom? "But there's not enough room!" you say. And that might be the case. But if you can be imaginative and create room, there is no better way to make your bath look more comfortable than to include a few special pieces of furniture.

An old but treasured desk or chest can make a wonderful vanity, adding a special, intimate touch to your bathroom that no laminate could. Remember that plumbing requires a considerable amount of space inside a vanity; so a piece of furniture might not yield as much storage space once it is converted. A cabinetmaker can probably retrofit new shelves inside if you will need them.

Because there are so many different kinds, chairs, too, can help to round out your bath design and give it the look and feel of a special room. If you'll be lowering a portion of your countertop to serve as a makeup table, you'll want a small chair to make grooming more comfortable.

A little creativity goes a long way. A brass coatrack makes a stylish towel holder for a Victorian-style bath. A small, glass coffee table near the tub provides a place to put bath oils, sponges, and small decorative items. Or instead of the usual bath hardware, try using a nice wood shelving unit for towels and other bath linens.

If you do decide to include furniture in your bath, make sure that it can withstand high levels of humidity. Woods should be treated with a waterproofing sealer, and fabrics on chair seat covers or divans should be sprayed with Scotch-Gard or some other kind of waterproofing agent.

## Personal Touches

You will want to add special items to the bath to make it your own room: a collection of seashells, sculptures or paintings, special soaps and towels, decorative perfume bottles, towel rings and bars, and so forth. The key is to keep the look simple, though. Don't fill up all the available spaces with objects.

Also, you will want to consider items that make life in the bath easier *and* fun: bathtub vanity trays, foam headrests for relaxing in the tub, water-resistant clocks, floating telephones, precision scales, towel warmers, and extension mirrors. Such items are available in specialty bath shops and through mail-order houses.

### Keep Your Bath Bright

Installing beautiful materials in your bath is really just the beginning, though. The loveliest tile and the most modern of fixtures will quickly lose their luster if they're not maintained properly.

To keep your bath looking its best, you'll need to take care of it. (See "Keep Your Bath Bright" on pages 142-43.) Bathroom cleanup does not have to be dreaded. Rather, think of it as a way to protect your investment. If done regularly, it's fairly painless; only when the job is neglected for a long time does bathroom cleaning necessarily become a loathsome chore.

Make routine cleanup a group effort. Every family member can get into the habit of doing a little something each time he or she uses the bathroom—whether it's toweling down the shower curtain or door, mopping up spills on the countertop, or wiping splashes off the mirror. This will reduce the amount of major heavy-duty cleaning you'll need to do.

You will, of course, have to do some scrubbing and polishing from time to time. Most manufacturers of bathroom surface materials and fixtures supply cleaning instructions with their products, so it's wise to read up on them. A commercial cleaner that works well on vitreous china and ceramic tile might damage fiberglass.

Maintenance, too, is important in the bathroom. Keep an eye on drippy faucets, gurgling toilets, noisy fans, and other quirks in the plumbing and electrical accessories. Anything with moving parts is prone to giving out every once in a while, but careful attention to and correction of minor problems will spare you the inconvenience of a major, expensive repair job.

Before you run out and start replacing washers, ball cocks, switches, or other parts, however, make sure you check the warranty on the fixture or appliance. Small problems are often caused by normal wear and tear, but some are the result of improper assembly and faulty parts. These repairs may be the responsibility of the manufacturer.

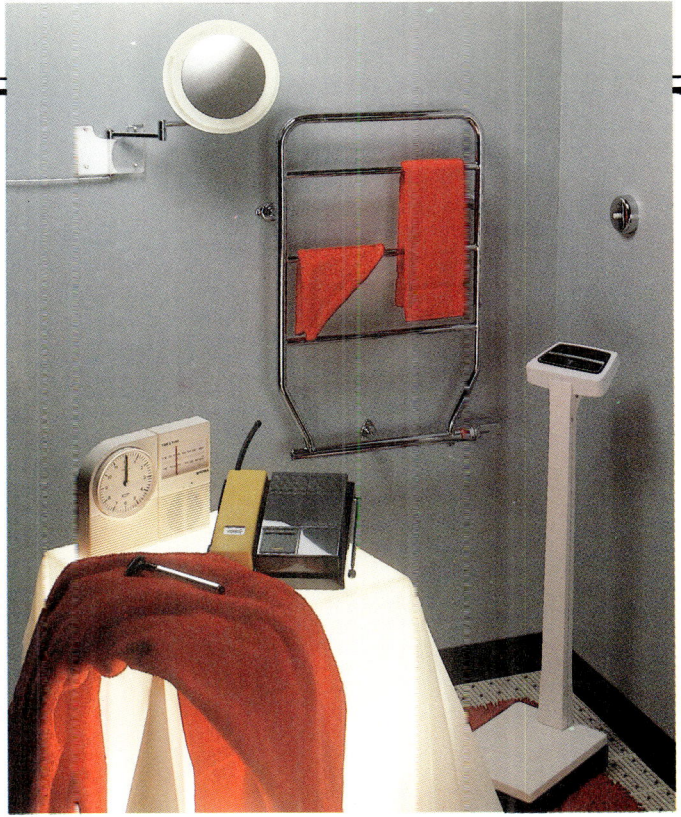

Accessories add to a bath's decor and can be a fun part of the room. Some neat items to consider for your bath include (clockwise from the top left): an extension wall mirror; an electric, wall-mounted towel warmer; a retractable clothesline; an electronic scale with digital display; a cordless, floating phone for your bathtub or spa; and a water-resistant shower clock radio.

### Plants in Your Bath

Plants and baths belong together. Of all the rooms in a house, the bath is where plants feel most at home. The warmth and humidity levels are perfect for healthy, luxuriant growth. As the plants thrive in this ideal environment, you'll find that having them there is good for you as well. Surrounding yourself with an arrangement of lush greens heightens the feeling of being in an oasis or a luxurious retreat. Plants are living accessories that soften expanses of tile, laminate, and marble and beautify the bath setting in a natural way. A well-chosen pot of greenery can add just the right finishing touch to a bath's decor.

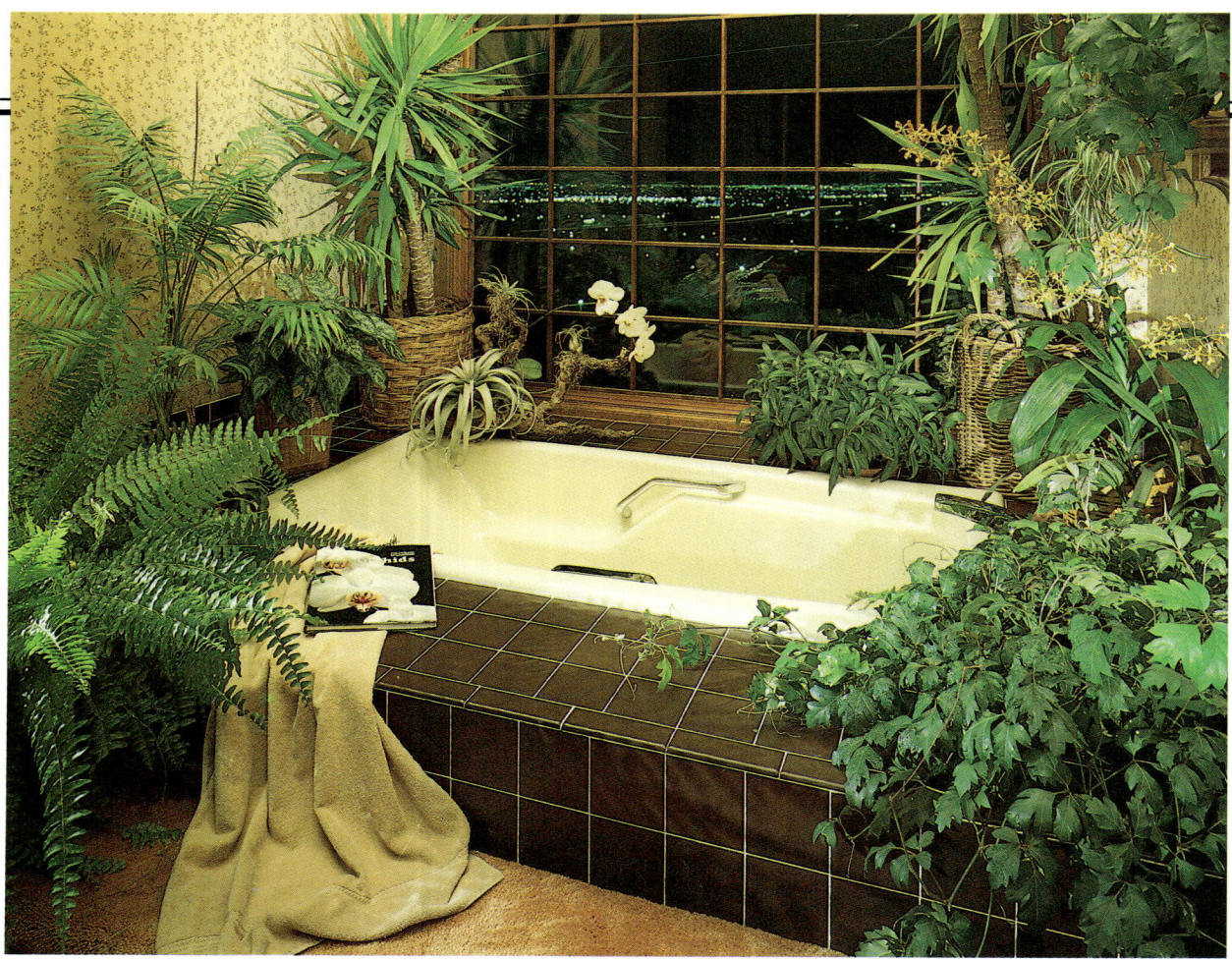

Plants love the moist air in the bath; even people without green thumbs can turn their bath into a paradise of greenery. Great plants for the bath include (clockwise from the left bottom corner): Boston fern, palm, Chinese evergreen dragon tree, bromeliad, orchid (with white flowers), wandering Jew, dragon tree, orchid (with yellow flowers), spider plant, grape ivy, corn plant, and grape ivy.

There's a wide array of foliage and flowering plants from which to select. See "Great Plants for the Bath" on pages 76-77. In general, ferns, palms, bromeliads (such as earth-star, living-vase plant, and queen's tears), and certain orchids flourish in the bath. Keep cacti and succulents in other parts of the house, since the bath environment will be too moist for them to do well.

Choose plants to complement your decor as carefully as you select the wall treatment, floor covering, and shower curtain. Take advantage of their rich variety of textures, colors, and patterns to heighten the drama of the decor, add accents, or carry through a color scheme. Foliage textures range from frilly, feathery, and lacy, to bold, sleek, and smooth. Leaves come in every shade of green imaginable, sometimes with highlights of white, cream, silver, burgundy, rose, or yellow. Flowers bloom in every color of the rainbow. Leaf patterns include marbling, geometric bands, irregular stripes, and networks of contrasting veining. This means that there is a plant for *every* decor.

### Special Effects with Plants

The effects you can create with plants are limitless. A graceful, fluffy Boston fern in a wicker stand helps evoke the right mood in a Victorian or country-style bath. A living-vase plant with the silvery sheen of its broad, sleek leaves and the dramatic slash of its fiery red flower stalk is an eye-catching accent in a modern European-style bath with stainless steel sinks. The cool elegance of a pastel orchid is an appropriate touch in a bath with marble or one with white or pastel laminate. Add the deep green of a lush palm or a stately Norfolk Island pine to a bath with lots of wood and brick and you enhance the earth-tone color scheme. The rich coloring of a caladium, its emerald leaves punctuated with ruby red veins, is striking against a backdrop of dark green, red, or black tile. You can even find wallpapers and floor coverings with plant motifs; include real plants in the setting to carry out the theme.

Keep a sense of scale in mind as you select your plants. A large area, a master suite, spa, or bodyroom for example, can support large specimens. In a spacious bath a 5-foot-tall dragon tree would command attention and become a focal point, creating far more impact than a 6-inch, potted prayer plant. But the same dragon tree would be overpowering and ridiculously out of place in a small powder room. In large spaces it can be more effective to let a large specimen stand alone. In small areas, mass small- to medium-size plants for more drama, but don't go overboard so they create the undesirable effect of clutter.

Tuck small plants on shelves, windowsills, or countertops. Strategically place them in front of a mirror to double their impact. Medium-size plants can fit on a countertop or shelves or sit on the floor. Mass them on a tub surround, assembling a group of plants with a pleasing contrast of heights, leaf shapes, textures, and colors.

Small- and medium-size plants are suitable for hanging, a good solution to the problem of cramped floor space. Suspend them from around a skylight, hanging at different levels for a more interesting look. Install a track with movable hooks in the ceiling in front of a window. Hang pots of viny plants or bottles filled with water and plant cuttings to form a leafy curtain. Certain ferns and bromeliads can be mounted on pieces of cork or driftwood and hung on the wall. Fill a window with glass shelves, and line the shelves with potfuls of fluffy ferns. These tiers of cascading greenery can take the place of blinds or curtains. Consider bumping out a conventional window to create a greenhouse window. These are available as kits or can be custom-built.

Large plants demand floor space. Master-suite baths, spas in sunspaces, and outdoor baths offer plenty of room. Consider building waterproof planters either sunken, floor level, or raised. These can hold an array of tall plants that act as a functional but fun room divider or screen. For instance, surround a bath in a sunspace with a border of potted palms and you've instantly created your own oasis of privacy.

A bath that opens onto a private courtyard gives you an opportunity to create an inviting plantscape to view through a door or window. If this area is exposed to the outdoors, choose plants that are suited to your climate. (In all but the warmest, year-round growing areas, these will need to be different from the plants you grow in your house.) Create a scene that makes you feel like you're bathing in a mountain stream in your own secret hideaway.

---

## *Tips on Growing Plants in the Bath*

- Keep a plant's light requirements in mind and match the plant to the available light. For low- or no-light areas, use an "itty bitty" GroLite (see "Helpful Addresses") that attaches directly to a plant's pot and provides the essential 12 to 16 hours of light.

- Feed, water, groom, and check plants for pests and diseases on a regular schedule.

- Never spray plants for pests and diseases while they're in the bath. Remove and treat; return them to the bath when they've recovered.

- Place plants, in particular hanging ones, where they won't interfere with daily use of the bath.

- Anchor hanging plants securely. Screw hooks into a stud or joist, or install with an appropriate-size molly bolt.

- Don't let a declining plant mar the looks of your bath; replace it with a vigorous, fresh specimen.

- For complete growing information and color photographs of the plants discussed here, see *Rodale's Encyclopedia of Indoor Gardening* (Emmaus, Pa.: Rodale Press, 1980) or *The Good Housekeeping Encyclopedia of House Plants* (New York: Hearst Books, 1985).

## Great Plants for the Bath

| Plant | Light Preference | Comments |
|---|---|---|
| African violet (*Saintpaulia* spp. and cultivars) | Filtered moderate to bright | Delicate flowers in lovely pastel shades; mass these small plants for more color impact |
| Aluminum plant (*Pilea cadierei*) | Bright | Small plant with puckery foliage with silver and deep green pattern |
| Anthurium (*Anthurium* spp.) | Bright to moderate | Small- to medium-size plant with exotic red, pink, or white heart-shaped flowers with prominent spike rising from the center |
| Areca or butterfly palm (*Chrysalidocarpus lutescens*) | Bright | Elegant palm with arching fronds; grows to 5 ft tall |
| Arrowhead vine (*Syngonium podophyllum*) | Bright | Trailing vines can be grown in water; green leaves may have yellow or white markings |
| Bird's-nest Fern (*Asplenium nidus*) | Filtered moderate | Medium- to large-size plant with bold, glossy fronds; makes nice contrast to lacy, more delicate ferns |
| Boston fern (*Nephrolepis exaltata* 'Bostoniensis') | Filtered bright | Frilly, arching fronds perfect for country or Victorian decors; medium-size plant suitable for hanging |
| Brake or table fern (*Pteris* spp.) | Filtered bright | Small- to medium-size fern with erect, feathery fronds |
| Caladium (*Caladium* spp.) | Bright to moderate | Medium-size plant with eye-catching foliage coloring; leaves feature combinations of white, silver, pink, red, and green |
| Chinese evergreen (*Aglaonema* spp.) | Moderate to low | Small- to medium-size plant for low-light situations; can be grown in water |
| Corn plant (*Dracaena fragrans* 'Massangeana') | Bright to moderate | Statuesque plant with bold leaves, sometimes striped with gold; tall specimens make dramatic accent plants |
| Dragon tree (*Dracaena marginata*) | Bright to moderate | Treelike form with narrow, spiky leaves edged in red; can grow to 5 ft tall; makes bold accent plant |
| Dumbcane (*Dieffenbachia* spp.) | Bright to low | Interesting leaf patterns, white or yellow on green; specimens up to 6 ft tall make striking floor plants |
| Earthstar (*Cryptanthus* spp.) | Bright | Petite plant with distinctive rippled leaves in rosette form; comes in shades of green, pink, copper, and bronze; can be mounted to hang on wall |
| Fishtail palm (*Caryota urens*) | Bright | Distinctive-looking palm with broad leaves that resemble fish tails |
| Flaming sword (*Vriesea splendens* 'Major') | Moderate to low | Medium-size plant with sword-shaped leaves with striped bands; dramatic 2-ft red flower spike looks like a torch |
| Grape ivy (*Cissus rhombifolia*) | Bright | Cascading branches of bright green leaves perfectly suited to hanging containers |
| Hare's-foot fern (*Polypodium aureum*) | Bright to moderate | Arching, broad, ruffled fronds appear on small- to medium-size plant |

| Plant | Light Preference | Comments |
|---|---|---|
| Lady's-slipper orchid (*Paphiopedilum* ×*maudiae*) | Filtered bright | Leaves are marbled in yellow-green and blue-gray; single flower is white with green stripes and has yellow-green pouch; easy to nurture |
| Living-vase plant (*Aechmea fasciata*) | Bright | Medium-size, sleek plant with broad, gray leaves; torchlike flower comes in shades of rose and blue |
| Maidenhair fern (*Adiantum* spp.) | Filtered moderate | Lush, small- to medium-size plant with masses of delicate, arching fronds; perfect for hanging containers |
| Mosaic or nerve plant (*Fittonia verschaffeltii*) | Low | Small plant that adds interest with dark green leaves, punctuated with network of pink veins |
| Moth orchid (*Phalaenopsis* spp. and hybrids) | Bright | Graceful, arching stalk carries series of elegant flowers in shades of white, pink, or yellow; easy for home grower |
| Norfolk Island pine (*Araucaria heterophylla*) | Moderate to low | Tiers of branches with soft needles give delicate, lacy effect; can grow up to 6 ft tall |
| Parlor palm (*Chamaedorea elegans*) | Low | Medium- to large-size, upright palm with lacy fronds; tall specimens make pleasing focal points |
| Philodendron (*Philodendron* spp.) | Filtered bright to moderate | Leaves may have shadings of green and bronze; mass of vines perfect for filling empty corners; excellent for hanging |
| Prayer plant (*Maranta leuconeura*) | Moderate | Petite plant with satiny leaves, veined with red or gray |
| Queen's tears (*Billbergia* spp.) | Filtered bright | Exceptionally striking flower stalk is lined with small, tubular blooms in shades of green, red, lilac, or blue |
| Rabbit's-foot fern (*Davallia mariesii*, *D. fejeensis*) | Filtered moderate | Light, airy mass of delicate, lacy fronds makes nice appearance in hanging basket; small- to medium-size plant |
| Rex begonia (*Begonia* ×*rex-cultorum*) | Filtered bright | Medium-size plant with striking foliage patterns in rich shades of green, red, purple, silver, or white |
| Rubber tree (*Ficus elastica*) | Bright to moderate | Bold, sculptural plant with large, glossy leaves; tall specimen makes a striking focal point |
| Sentry or paradise palm (*Howea belmoreana*, *H. forsterana*) | Bright to low | Deep, spiky fronds appear on plants that can grow to a dramatic 8 ft tall |
| Staghorn fern (*Platycerium bifurcatum*) | Filtered bright | Gray-green fronds that look like antlers fall attractively when plant is mounted and hung on wall |
| Wax plant (*Hoya bella*, *H. carnosa*) | Bright to moderate | Viny plant with delightful waxy, star-shaped flowers that give off a sweet fragrance to delicately scent the bath |
| Wandering Jew (*Tradescantia* spp.) | Bright | Viny plant with showy leaves striped in green, white, purple, or pink; meant to be displayed in hanging containers; can also be grown in water |

# GALLERY
## A Tour of Fine Baths

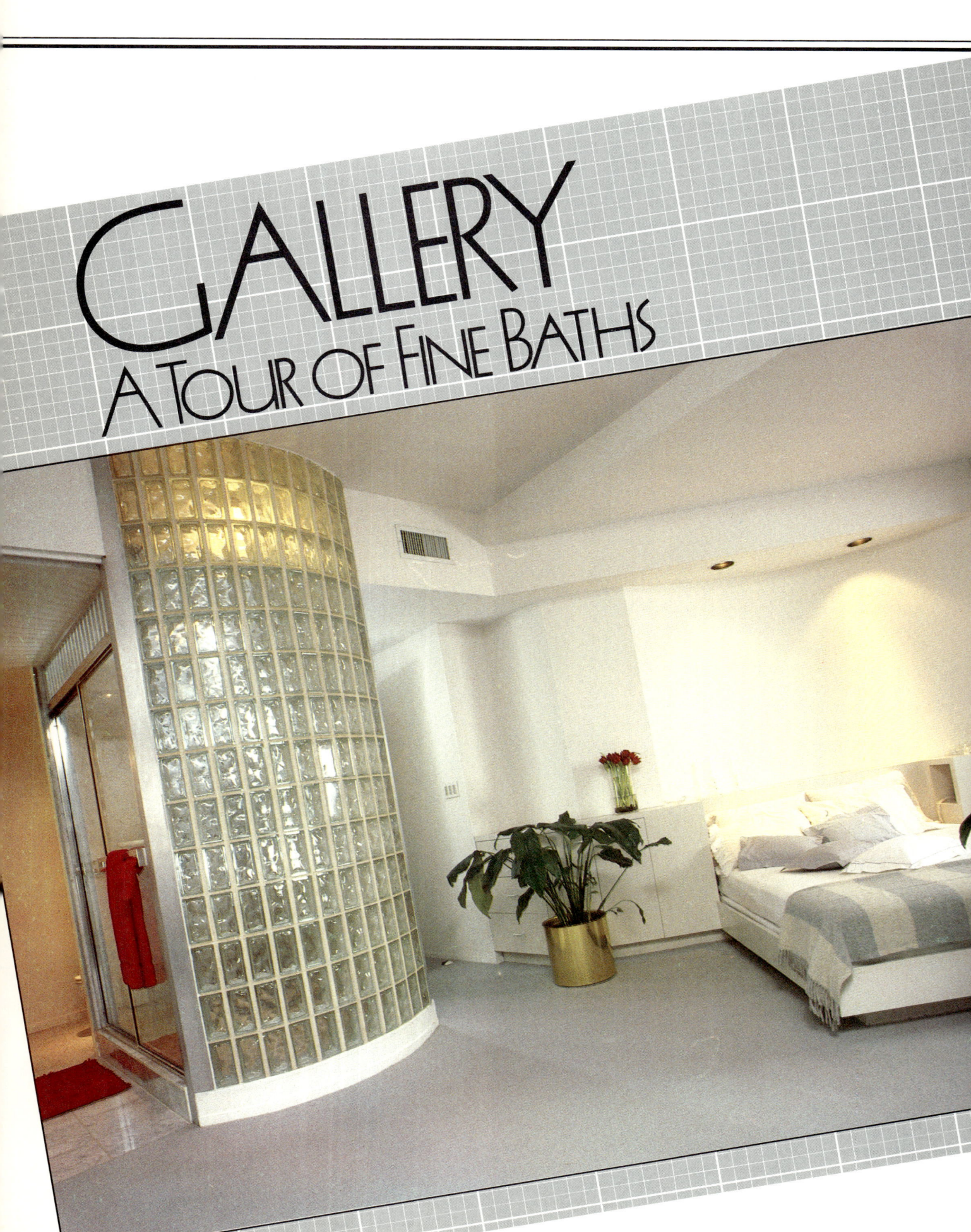

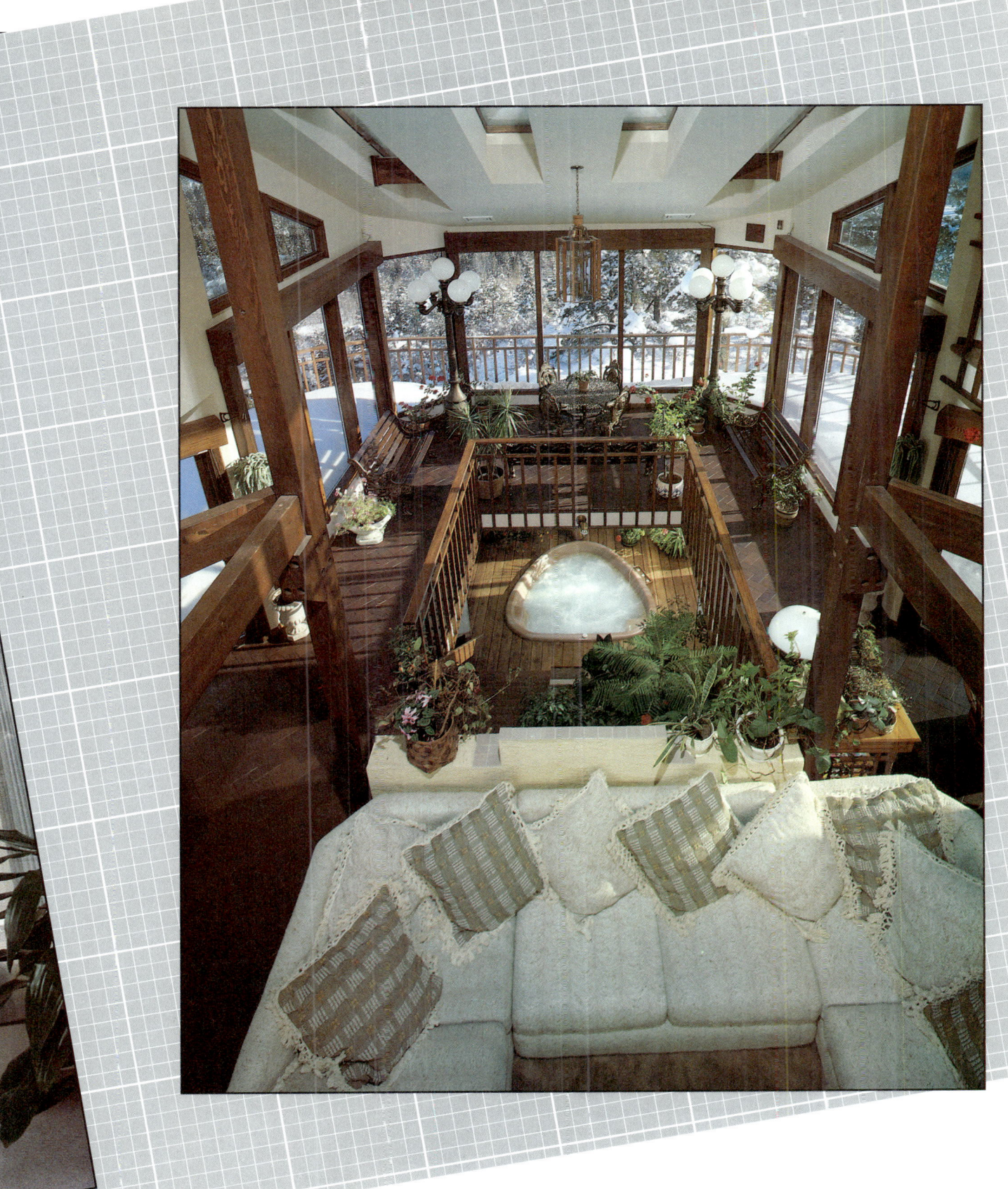

# Windows on Their World

The new home of Anna and Art Fisher sits in the middle of a spacious meadow in the mountains of Colorado. The master-bedroom suite in their house reflects the beauty and simplicity of those natural surroundings.

In keeping with the clean, contemporary look of the rest of their two-story solar home, the Fishers wanted a master-bedroom suite of understated elegance in a space that was open and functional. To accomplish this, architect Sears Barrett, of Equinox Design Group, employed clean, simple curves and lines and lots of natural light.

The result was a spacious set of uncluttered rooms (bedroom, bath, sunspace spa, and walk-in closet) that the whole family feels comfortable in. The abundance of windows and skylights makes the area open and fresh and affords breathtaking views of the Colorado landscape. There are no window coverings in the master-bedroom suite. "The area we live in makes it possible to do without," says Anna, "even when you're taking a shower."

The windows as well as the doors of the sunspace spa area are trimmed in an earthy, light oak. The wood paneling in the

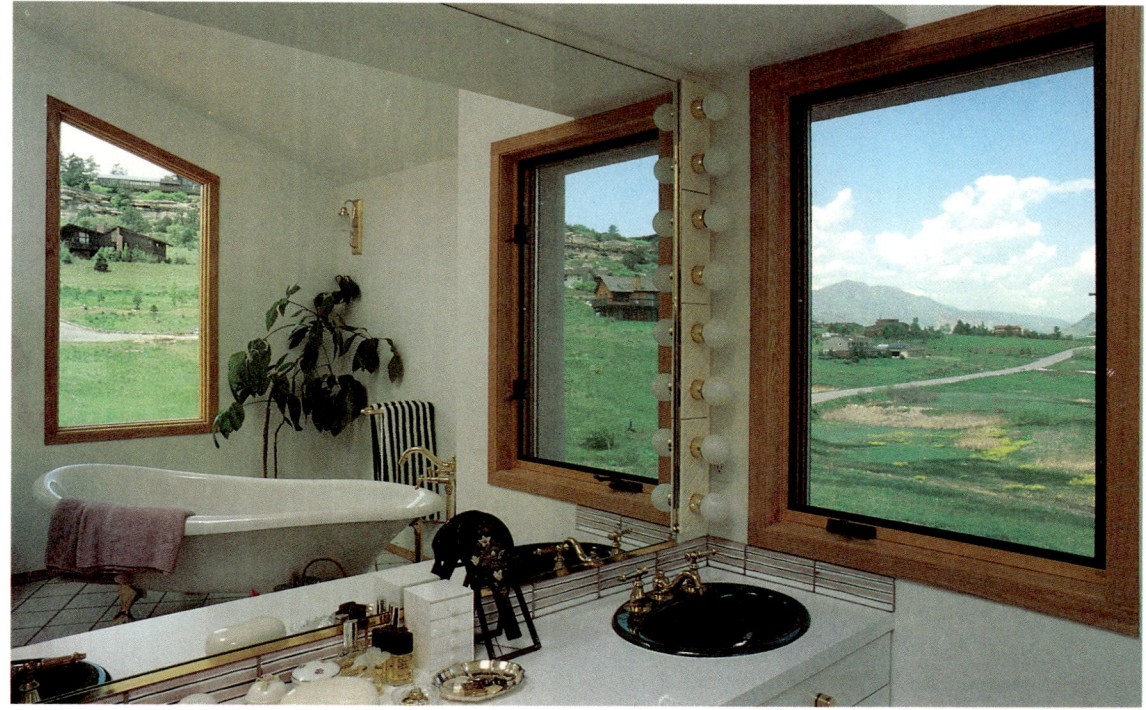
Windows in the bath let in lots of fresh air and sunshine and provide an unobstructed view of the lovely countryside.

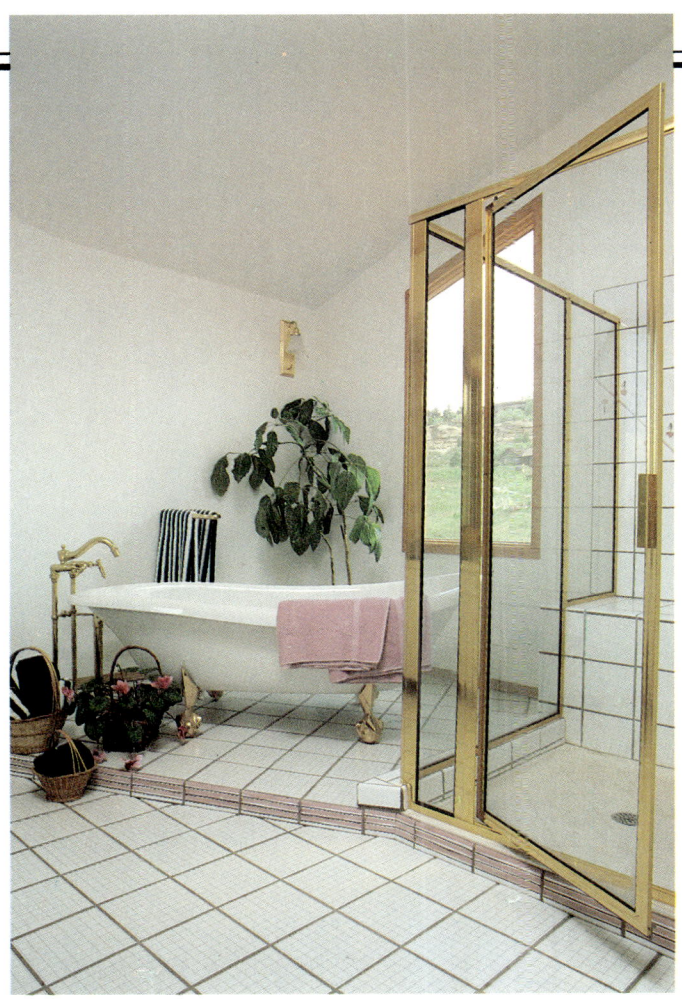

Anna Fisher's claw-foot tub (the Birthday Bath by Kohler) lends a touch of old-fashioned charm to this modern bath.

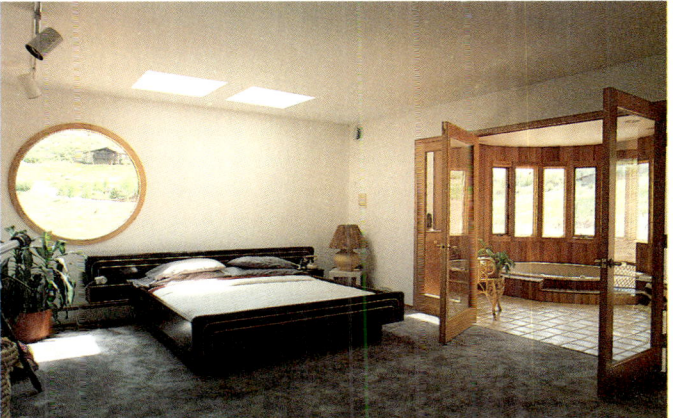

The Fishers' master suite is elemental in design; neutral colors, earthy wood, and natural light from the spa room set the tone in this suite

spa area and the trim around the spa are also oak, treated with an oil sealer to prevent moisture damage. The sunspace is a Fisher family favorite, says Anna; the whole family is active in sports, and the whirlpool provides soothing hydrotherapy as well as relaxation after a hard day's work or play. The long, rectangular windows of the room's rounded enclosure take full advantage of the sun's warming power.

Walls, tile, cabinets, and vanity top in the bathroom are white, expanding the space and increasing the amount of light in the room. An ebony black sink and toilet serve as bold accents; brass, wicker baskets, and flowering plants soften the effect. Very few objects adorn the walls, which exaggerates the bath's linear look—it's a no-fuss, no-frills room.

Anna really enjoys her bathtub—it's a sparkling white, old-fashioned, claw-foot tub with brass fittings. It adds a wonderfully romantic touch to this otherwise contemporary setting. The original bath floor plan had called for an oversize sunken whirlpool tub, but when Anna found this one, she quickly had the plans changed. "It's so pretty and comfortable," she says.

Anna reports that there really isn't anything about her master-bedroom suite that she'd change. With its many windows on their world, it's the perfect place to retreat any time of day.

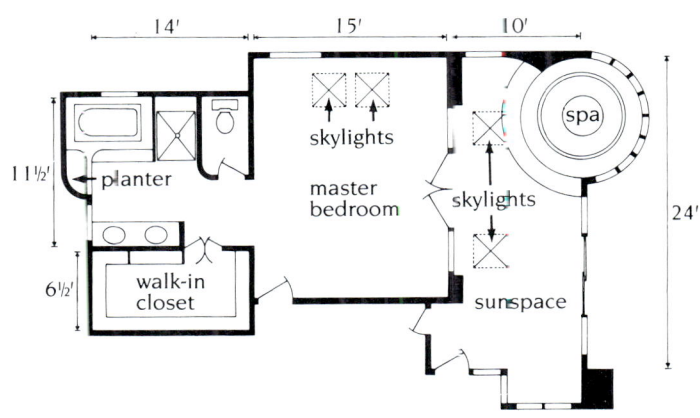

# An Unplanned Oriental Bath

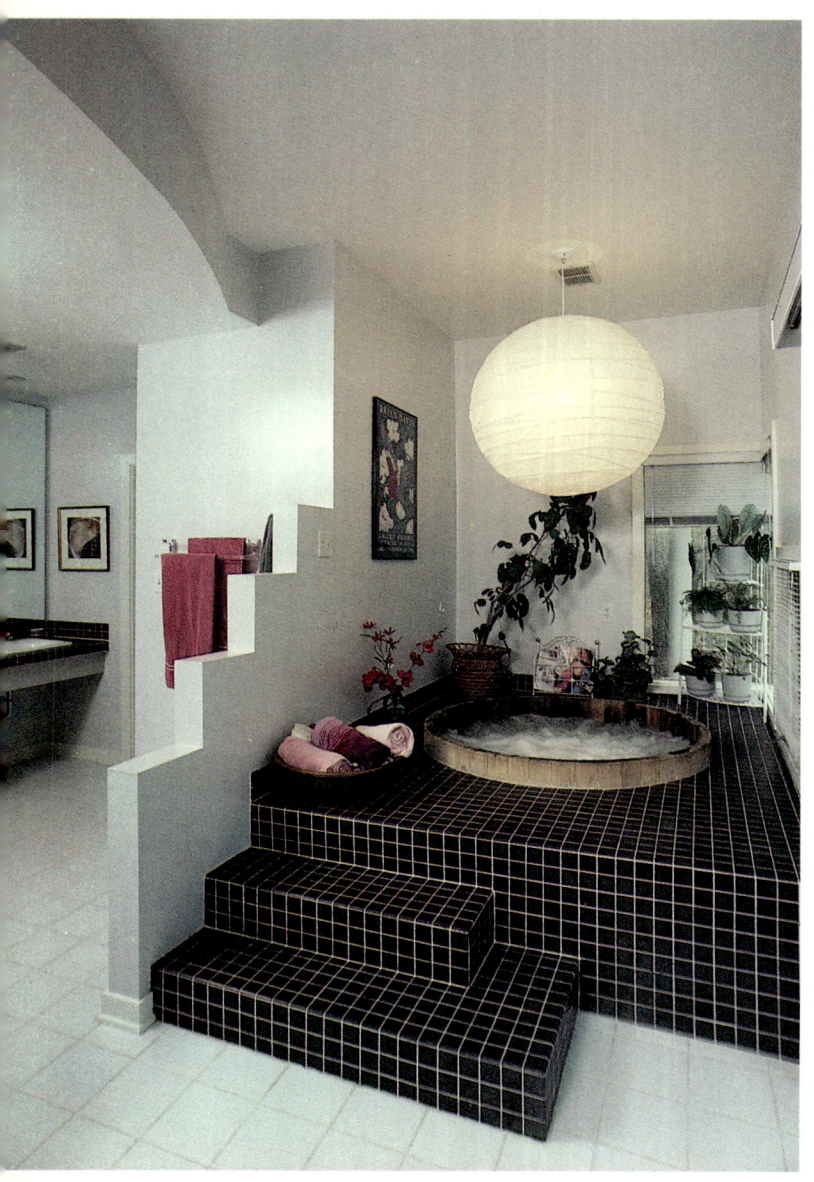

This bath's unique centerpiece is its hot tub, sunken into a ceramic-tile platform. The paper lantern suspended above adds to the tub's mystique.

Dr. Michael Strachan and his wife, Joan, desperately wanted to modernize the master bathroom in their Virginia home. But after examining conditions in their existing bath and considering the renovations they had in mind, they realized a decent remodeling would be impossible. So, they built a brand new house. "The idea to build a house came *after* we had already decided about a new bathroom," Michael says. "We really built the house around the bath."

The master bath in the new Strachan home is a striking combination of simple architectural geometrics, with a decidedly oriental flavor that—surprisingly—the couple did not plan for. Most of the bath, says Michael, "just happened."

The simple yet elegant black-and-white color scheme of the bath was chosen because it was practical. "We knew that we could easily add to those colors," says Michael. In fact, almost everything in the bath was put there for practicality's sake— and it wasn't necessarily planned. The sleek, T-shaped vanity, for instance, was created not for the sake of design but for financial reasons. "At that point we had pretty much run out of money for the project," says Michael, "and we wanted a vanity that would do the job for the least amount of money."

Likewise for the double vanity-to-ceiling mirrors. The price of one huge mirror was more than the Strachans wanted to pay, and so they decided upon two smaller ones instead. To fill the visual space created by the separate mirrors, Joan bought a simple black vase and filled it with silk flowers—the effect is striking. Even the large, white globe suspended above the hot tub was a spontaneous addition. It's made of paper, believe it or not, and was procured from a local gift shop for about $5.

Perhaps the most obvious oriental touch in the room is the redwood hot tub, recessed in a striking black and white tiled platform. But even the tub wasn't planned for traditional Japanese bathing experiences. The Strachans just wanted an indoor hot tub—plain and simple.

Since the water is not drained from the tub after each use, the bath needs good ventilation to prevent moisture buildup and to exhaust vapors given off by chemicals used in the tub. To that end, architect Joseph Boggs employed an innovative air recirculation system. A vent located in the ceiling right above the tub dehumidifies the air and directs it back to the heat pump, where it enters the heating system for reuse. A window near the tub and a sliding glass door provide extra ventilation and pleasing natural light. The glass door opens onto a small backyard deck that overlooks a pretty lake; the same lake view can be enjoyed while soaking in the hot tub.

Planned or not, the separate elements of the Strachans' bath blend to give the room a soothing, oriental look. While much of the bath's design evolved spontaneously, the Strachans made very definite plans for certain practicalities, like the double sinks. The pedestal sink in their previous home, while elegant, did not adequately meet the needs of two working people—who often must use the sink at the same time. The Strachans also installed double shower heads in the extra-large, completely tiled shower and added a walk-in closet for dressing convenience. Heat lamps above the vanity keep the room toasty on chilly mornings.

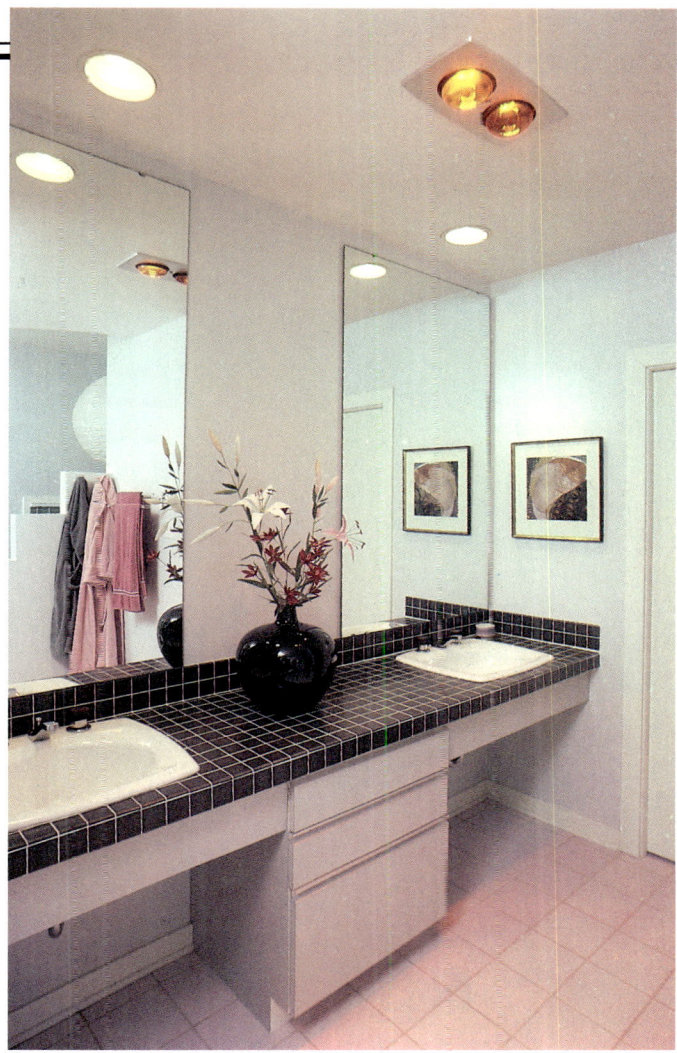

Double sinks in a ceramic-tile countertop provide convenience for two working people.

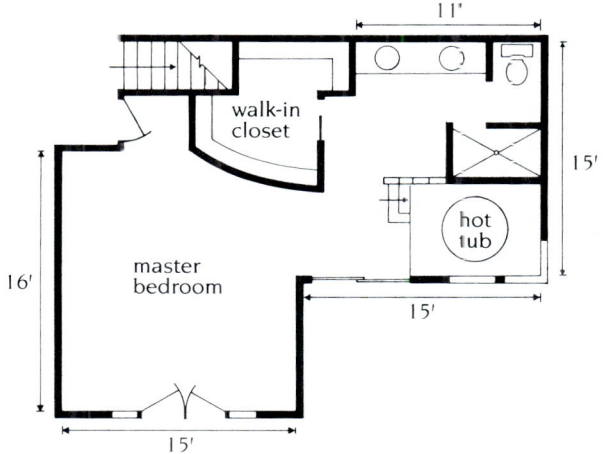

# A Bath in the Woods

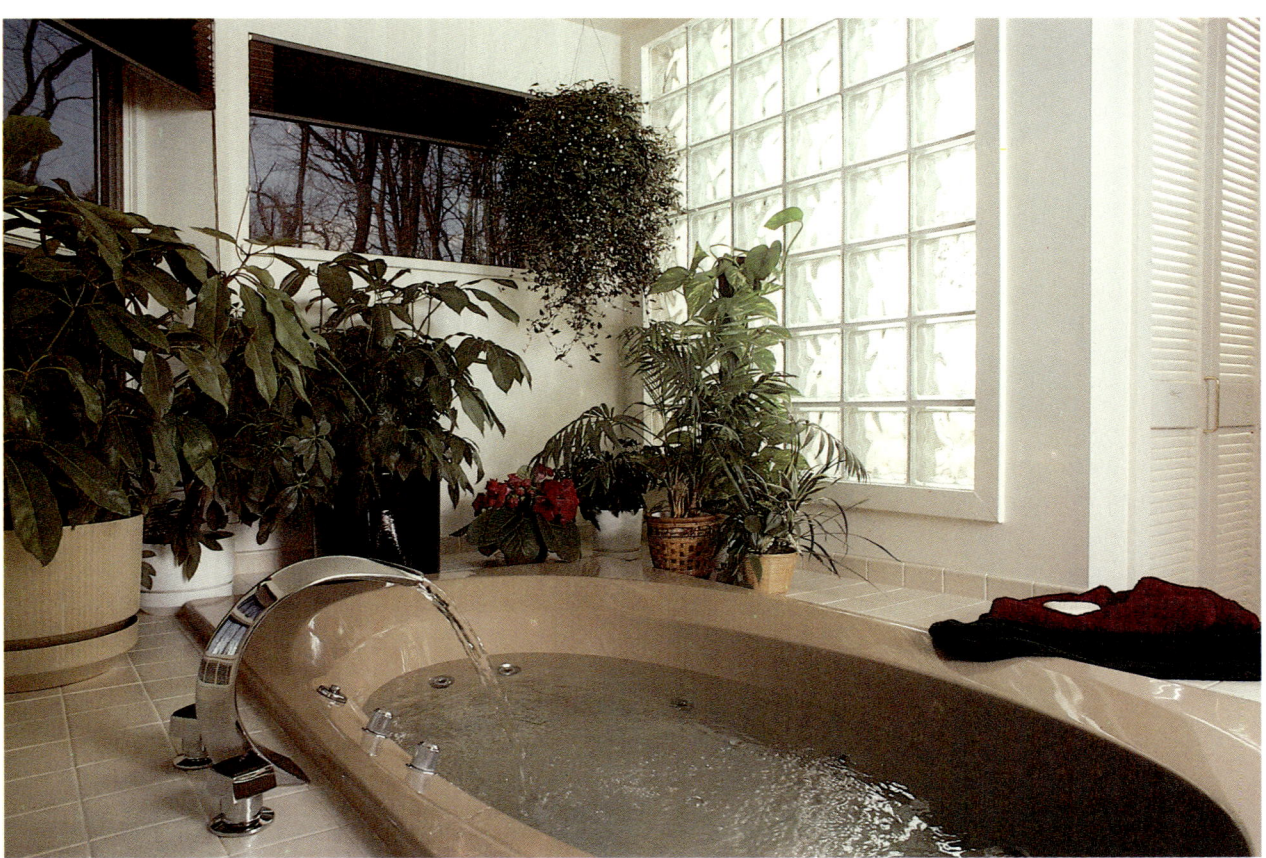

A sleek, European-style faucet gives this whirlpool tub the look of luxury; light filtering through the glass-block wall creates a romantic mood.

When Cecily Laidman and Phil Thorpe found a beautiful piece of property in western New Jersey, they knew that the house they built there would have to be special. The land, a lovely wooded area undisturbed except for the footsteps of an occasional deer and the gurgling of a nearby creek, needed tender loving care. So the couple turned to Princeton Energy Group's Harrison Fraker for a home design that would complement and preserve the land's natural beauty.

Having lived in their new solar house for just over four months, Cecily and Phil are delighted with it. It fulfills all their expectations and blends beautifully into the surrounding landscape. The house features a large, light-filled kitchen and a deck just outside the master bedroom where a hot tub sits. But the couple's favorite room in the house is the master bath. It's huge, measuring 24 feet by 10 feet, and it includes a "room within a room" for the toilet and bidet. "My goal was to be able to have two people use this room at the same time without bumping into one another," Cecily says.

The bath features a European-style laminate vanity and a Corian sink and vanity top, lighted with a strip of theatrical bulbs and mirrored on three sides. The triptych mirror was one of Cecily's clever contributions to the bath's design. "I grew up in a family of four girls," she explains, "and that type of mirror was a wonderful feature in our bathroom."

Since she despises medicine cabinets—"they're unsightly, and when you open them up everything falls out"—Cecily had their bath equipped with a large closet; its plentiful shelves hold bathing needs, toiletries, health aids, and a small supply of towels. The rest of the couple's bath linens are stored in cabinetry just outside the master bedroom.

The pièce de résistance of the bath, however, is the tub. Sunk into a raised, tiled platform, it's a Water Jet whirlpool tub that's 6 feet long, 3½ feet wide, and 21 inches deep—perfect for luxurious double soaks. The bumpout that houses the tub is circled by large windows that afford a peaceful view of the quiet, wooded area outside. "Deer come right up to the window," Cecily adds. Cecily and Phil watch the seasonal changes in their little wooded paradise—from the bathtub vantage point. Earthy neutral colors wash the bath, accentuating the view in the tub area and making it the focal point of the room.

The couple did encounter a problem during the installation of the tub. Because of a federal electrical code that prohibits the placement of overhead light fixtures fewer than 7½ feet above an electrically powered whirlpool tub, the couple could

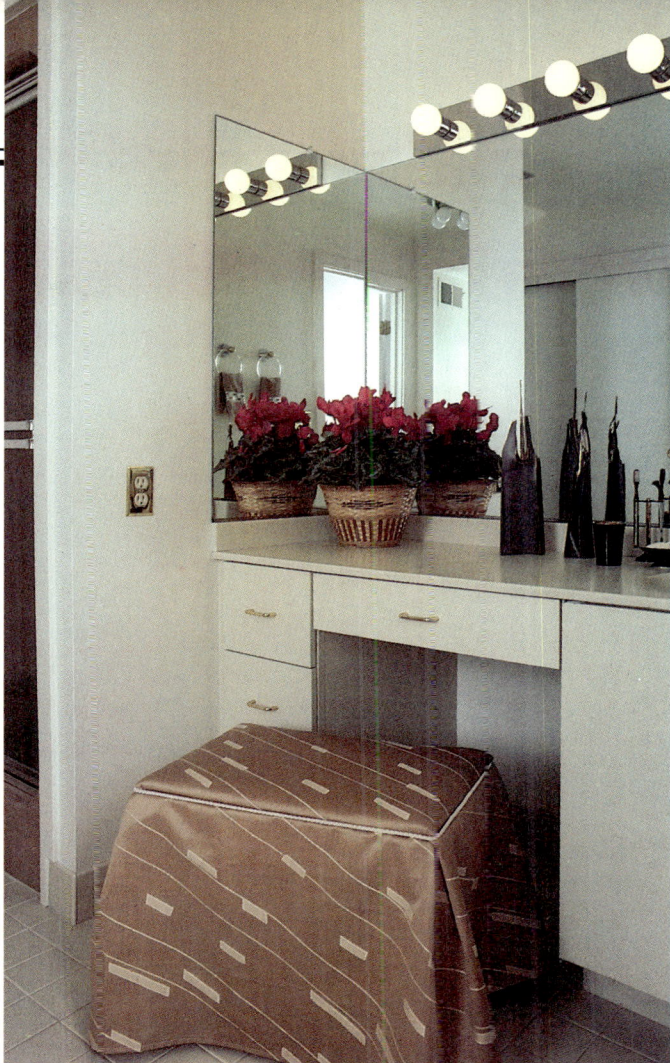

The triptych mirror above the vanity—a feature that Cecily Laidman specifically requested—allows for more flexible use of vanity space.

not use electric lights in that area. But they find that the windows provide plenty of natural light during the day. And at night, the light filtering through the glass-block wall separating the tub and toilet areas sheds a soft glow that is warm and romantic.

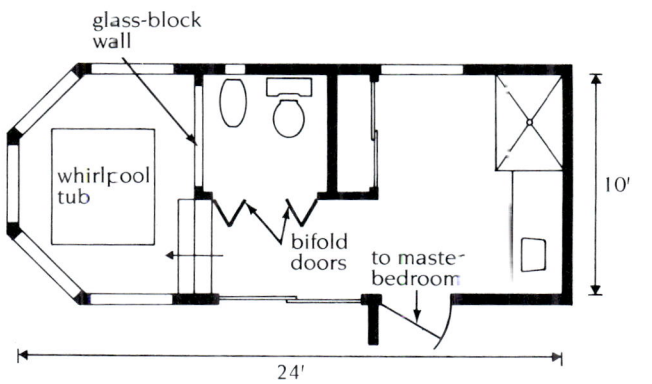

# A Tranquil Retreat

Stephanie and Jack Evanson wanted much more than a master bedroom and bath in their new, custom-built house in Texas. Busy executives who count the few precious hours they can spend at home, the Evansons wanted a retreat, a place where they could escape from the madding crowd to relax and regroup—and from which they could emerge refreshed and completely ready for the day.

This master-suite bath's uncluttered look is largely due to its unique storage systems. The mirrors are actually bifold doors that conceal a vanity and shower.

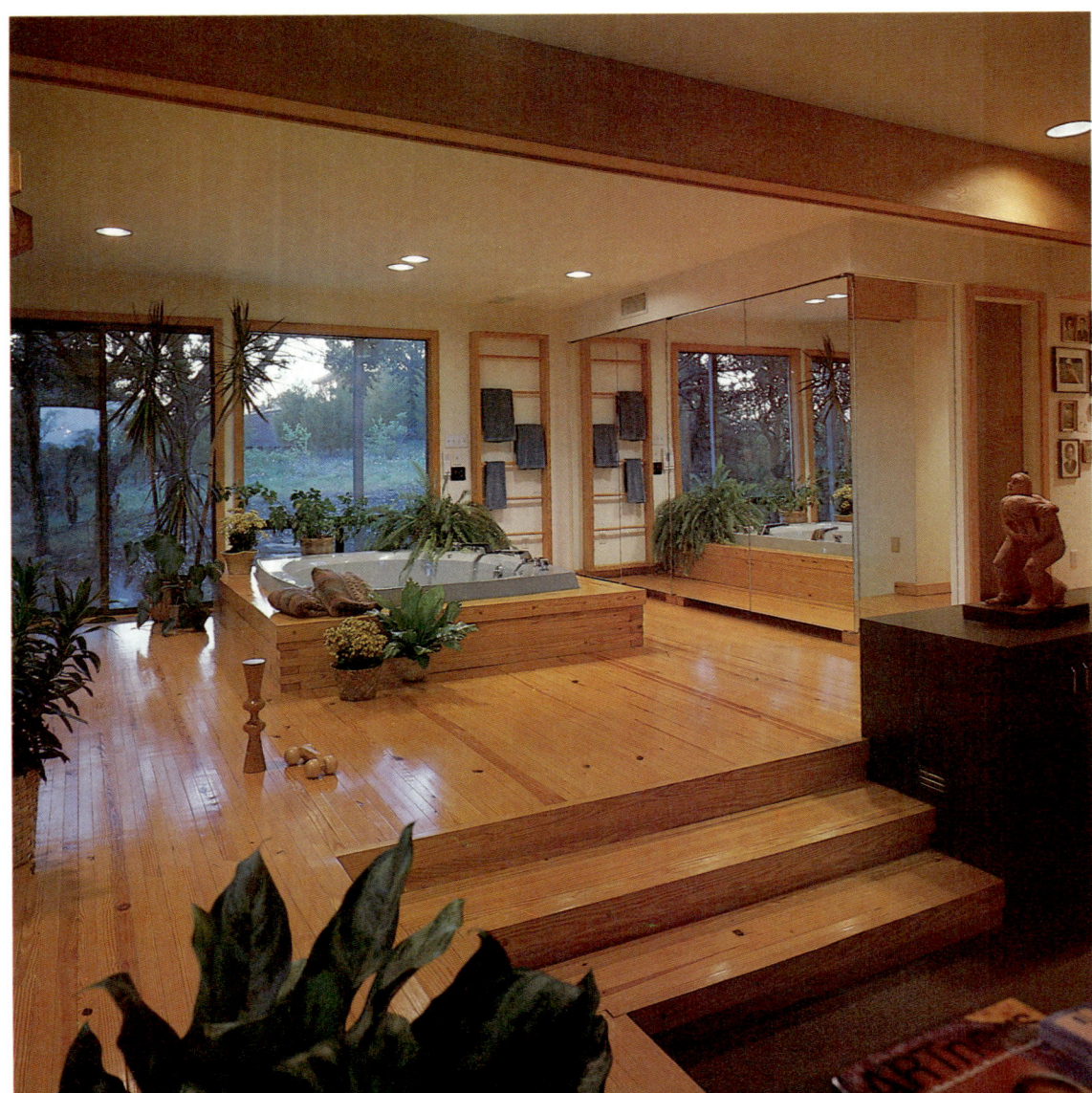

Modern convenience and tranquillity don't always go hand in hand, but architect Alan Taniguchi succeeded in producing a master suite that is as functional as it is beautiful and relaxing. The area is spacious and clean looking, much like the rest of the house Taniguchi designed. A wide expanse of pine flooring marks the bath entrance and warms both rooms, and natural light floods in through surrounding windows. There are no doors in the suite, which contributes to its natural, open feeling.

Yet for all its calming aesthetics, the master suite is practical and self-sufficient. So self-sufficient, says Taniguchi, that the couple practically lives there when they are at home. A giant walk-in closet accommodates the wardrobes of two busy executives. Stephanie had a special vanity installed behind the headboard of the bed to speed her morning routine, and an island/snack bar complete with its own refrigerator and toaster turns the room into a minikitchen. There is even an access door from the master suite to the garage—the couple can get ready for work and rush out the door.

The showpiece of the bath itself is the large, centrally located whirlpool bathtub, which is built into a raised pinewood platform. Sunlight doesn't warm just the room: solar panels on the roof transfer heat to the tub's water supply. The area surrounding the tub serves as exercise space—something the Evansons had requested—and mirrors on two entire walls exaggerate the area's openness and reflect the wild beauty outside. A patio just outside the tub area is a favorite place for lazy weekend breakfasts.

The mirrors on the right side of the bath area serve another purpose: They are actually bifold doors that conceal a double-sink vanity and shower. "They wanted a very uncluttered look," says Taniguchi; to make it even cleaner, the architect installed special out-of-view door hinges. The toilet is also hidden from view, in its own compartment around the corner.

Plants provide the decor for the suite, and they couldn't be more at home in such a natural setting. Neither could the Evansons, who find their tranquil master suite is the perfect retreat after a hectic workday.

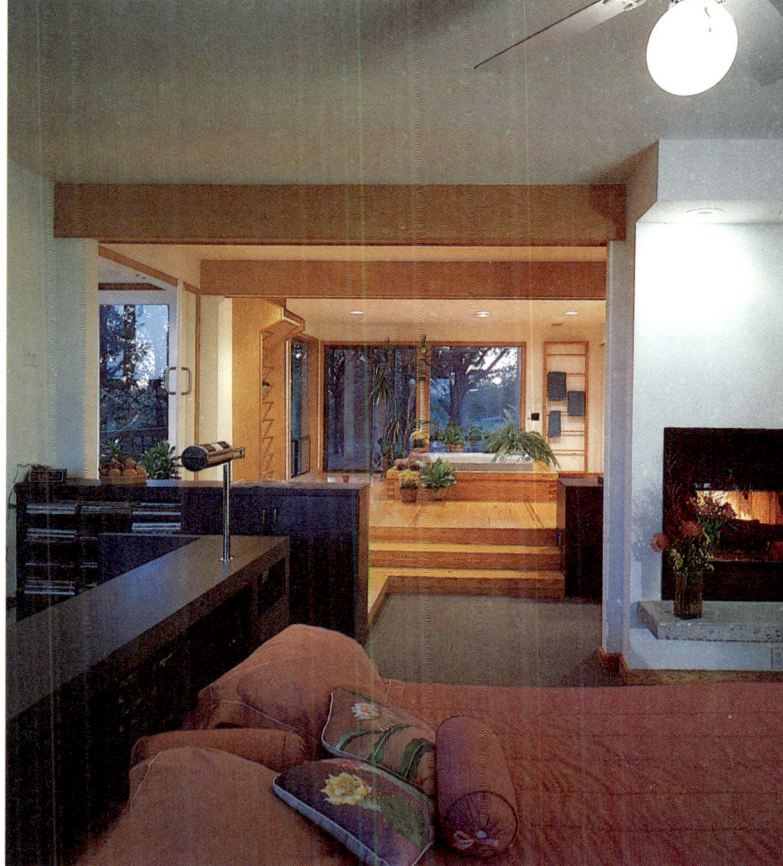

This master-bedroom suite is designed as a retreat from the madding crowd. The bath area also doubles as a gym: A rowing machine, exercise bicycle, chinning bar, and resistance machine often occupy the space next to the tub.

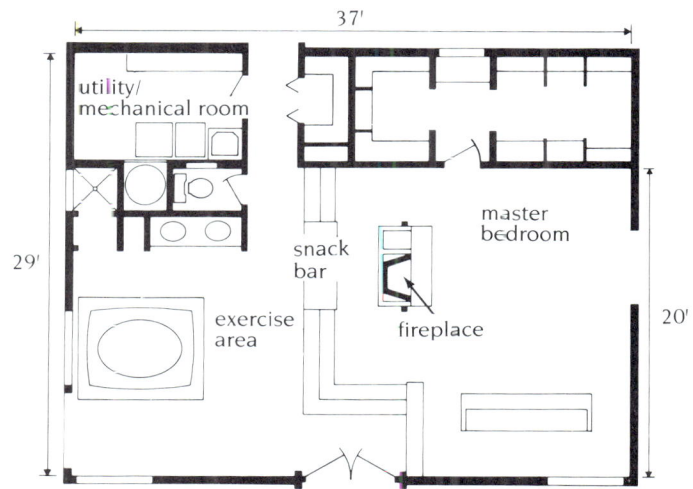

# A Bath of Soft, Soothing Colors

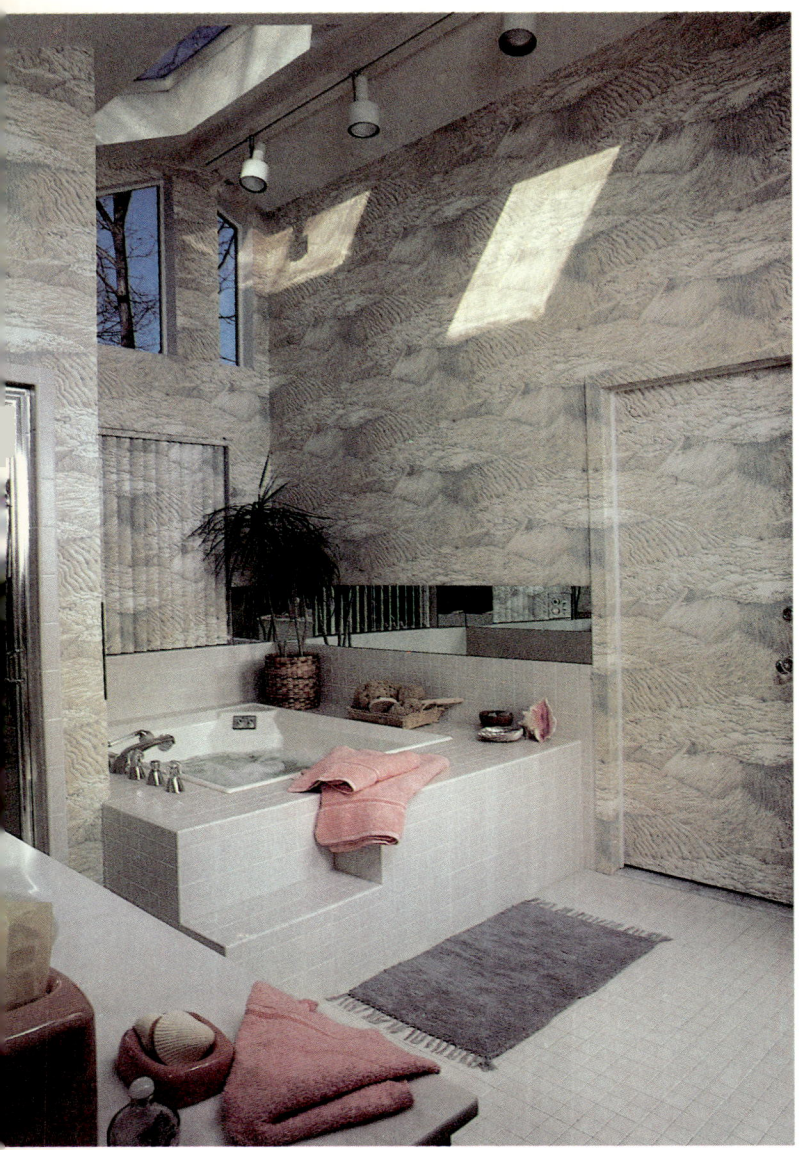

The abundance of tile and window glass in the Sussmans' bath might have made it chilly; but a special radiant heating system in the floor keeps the room toasty.

It was either remodel or sell. And after thinking over the options, Lila and Richard Sussman decided to remodel their 30-year-old home in suburban New Jersey. One of the first projects they undertook was renovation of their master bath.

Because they started their bath remodeling at a time when "super baths" were just emerging, the Sussmans didn't have many resources to draw from. But they did have some very clear-cut ideas about what they wanted. The new bath had to be a pretty space, a relaxing space, done in soft, neutral colors and filled with natural light for an open, airy feeling. Ample closet space in the bath for wardrobe and bath storage was paramount to Lila; and since Richard is owner and president of a company that manufactures residential and commercial steam baths, space had to be designated for their own steam shower. They called on interior designer Rhoda Schuman to turn their ideas into reality.

Rhoda started by expanding the bath out over a porch below to make room for the luxury touches she planned to include. To brighten the room and add a touch of drama, the roof was raised and opened with a series of skylights over the tub area. A creamy ceramic tile on the floors and tub surround, white laminate cabinetry, and a white Corian sink and countertop soften the room even more. But the pièce de résistance of the bath is the wallpaper. Appropriately called "Dunes," it's done in hushed tones that set a quiet mood in the room. "It makes the bath very relaxing," says Lila. The vertical blinds on the window above the tub area are also covered with the paper to match the walls.

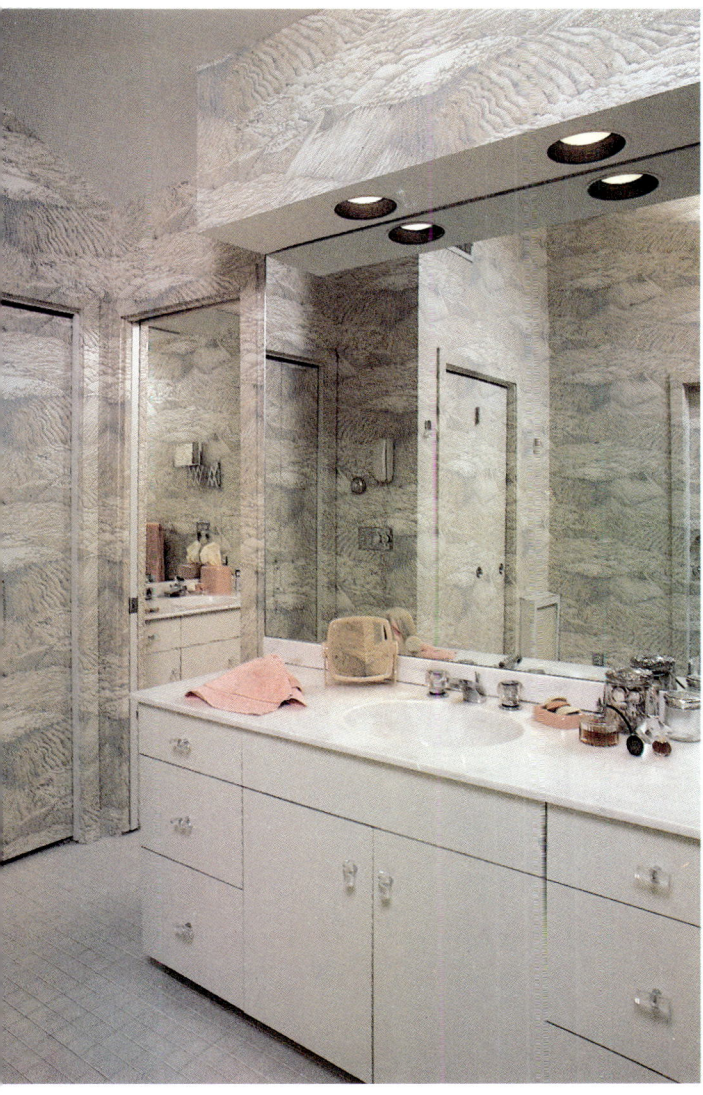

The door to the left of the vanity opens into a huge walk-in closet, something Lila Sussman wouldn't do without in her master bath.

Other luxury touches in the bath include a Mr. Steam steam-generating unit built into the shower; rheostatically controlled lighting for mood setting; heat lamps just outside the shower; and a gigantic walk-in closet. Perhaps the most unique luxury in the bath, though, is a special radiant-heating system installed under the tile floor. It keeps what might otherwise be a chilly bath warm and toasty.

Though it was built before the luxury-bath wave hit this country, the Sussmans' master bath is as luxurious as any. Its soft, soothing colors and relaxing atmosphere will always be in style.

Although she admits the tub is a bit large for everyday use—"My kids once had 13 people in it," she says with a laugh—Lila says it does serve important functions. Since the Sussman family enjoys skiing, the giant-size whirlpool, with its muscle-massaging jets, is a favorite aprés-ski hangout—especially in the evenings, when the skylights afford a peek at a starlit sky. Because of its size, however, the Sussmans did have to beef up the home's water-heating system.

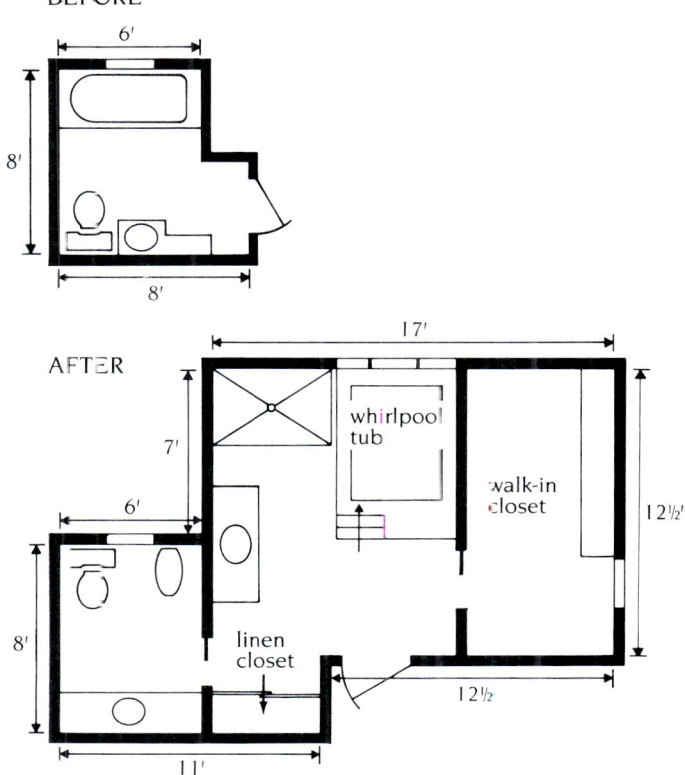

89

# A Bath of Color

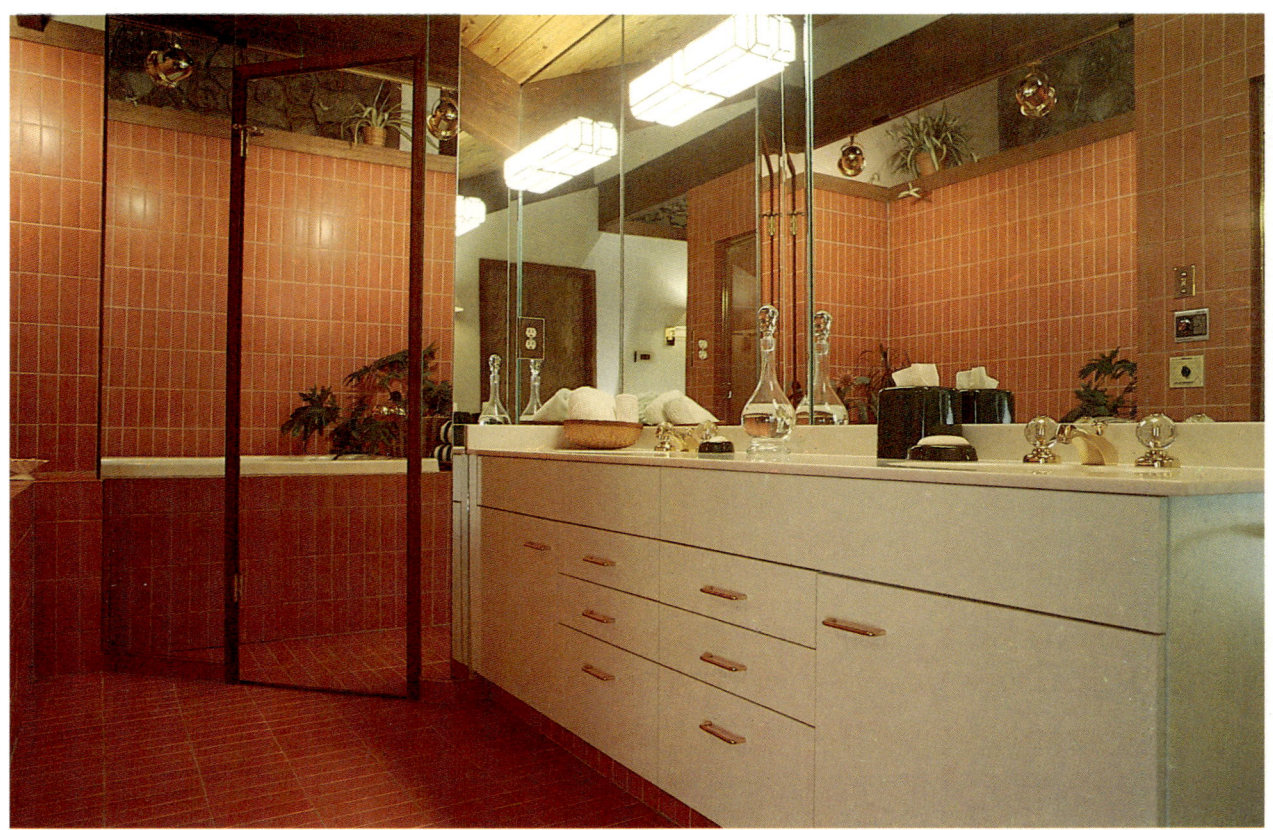

The many mirrors in the Catons' colorful master bath help expand the narrow space. One of the mirrors is actually a door, behind which is the toilet compartment.

It started with a colorful swatch of clearance-house fabric that Cassie Caton found while shopping one day. "I knew even before we built our house that I wanted that color *somewhere*," she says.

Cassie and Michael Caton put the finishing touches on their custom-built Atlanta home in June of 1984. The master bath is where that color ended up, in the form of a striking coral tile by Villeroy & Boch. It's a bright, dynamic color, but warm and elegant just the same. There are three different kinds of lighting in the room, and the coral tile takes on new moods with each light change.

To create more excitement in their bath, the Catons chose bright white for a contrasting color. Custom-designed laminate cabinetry, a Corian countertop with built-in sink, and a whirlpool tub, all in sparkling white, help to create crisp, clean lines. The rectangular pattern of the coral tile accentuates the lines and actually adds height to the room.

Using the vertical pattern on the tile to add dimension to the bath was just one trick Cassie and Mike pulled from their hats to create more space in the room. (They designed the master-suite interior.) It's long but narrow, and a huge walk-in closet consumes the last 11 feet of length. Another way to create the illusion of space, they knew, was to let in lots of natural light. Since the bath itself had no window access, the couple took advantage of north-facing clerestory windows in the master bedroom by only partially enclosing the bath; the wall shared by the master bedroom and the bath stops just short of the ceiling. This allows sunlight into the bath and creates a sense of openness.

They also utilized lots of mirrors—on doors and walls as well as over the vanity—to visually enlarge the room. (The toilet sits in its own compartment behind one of those mirror-clad doors.) The shower/steam unit is enclosed with brass and clear glass to maintain the bath's open feeling.

Both Cassie and Mike had wanted a whirlpool tub for evening relaxing. But an oversize tub would have taken up too much space, so the Catons opted for a standard-size, extra-deep model—an economical use of space *and* a comfy soak. The brass fixtures above the tub are fitted with soft-pink bulbs that emit a warm, romantic glow, making a soak even more relaxing.

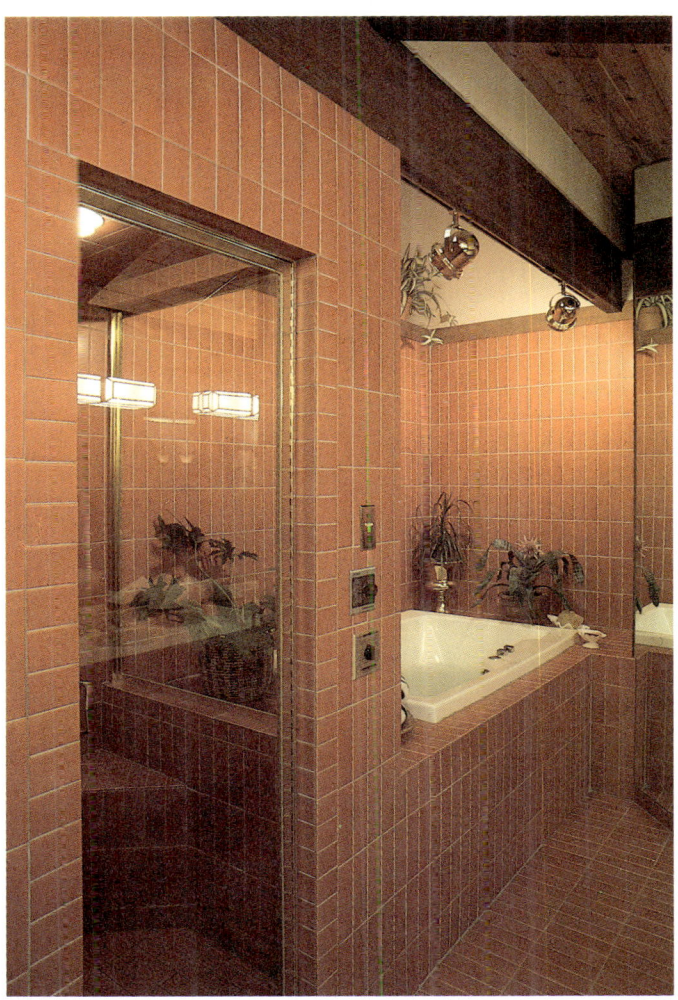

The Catons wanted a whirlpool tub separate from the shower; they chose an extra-deep model that requires less length and width than most soaking tubs.

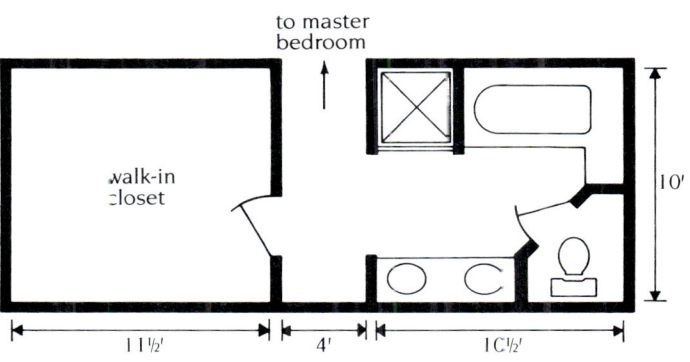

# A Garden Bath

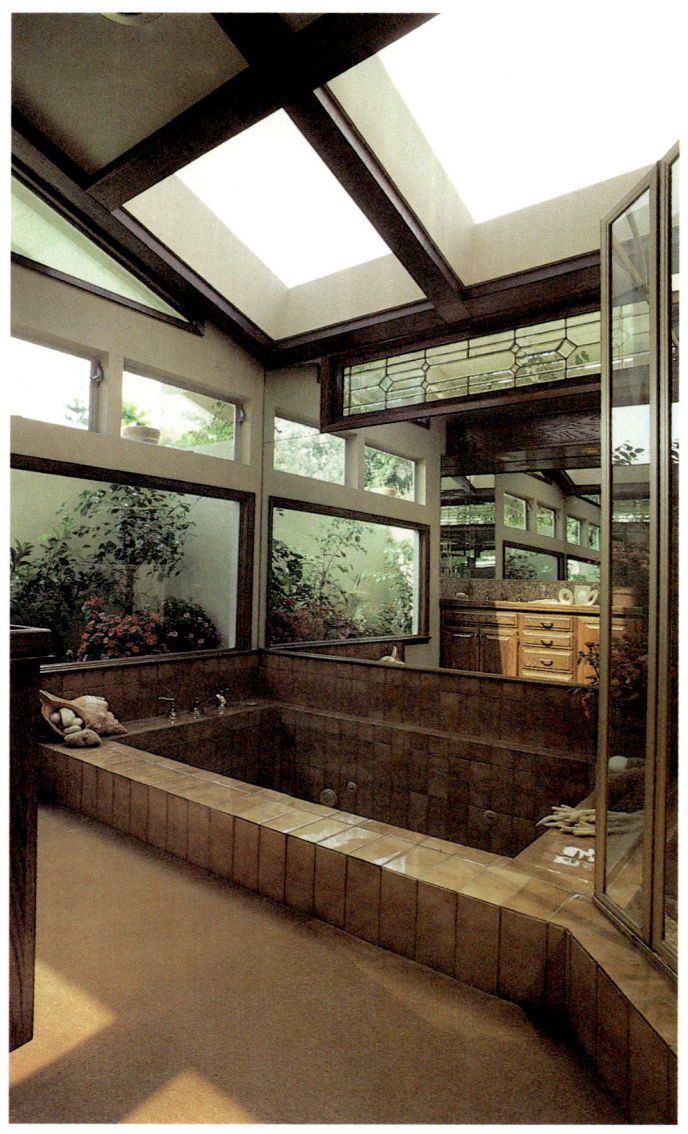

The small patio outside the Hahnes' bath is just big enough for a small garden and to house the whirlpool equipment for the custom-built tub.

Linda and Wally Hahne's 30-year-old home on the Southern California coast was nice enough. But many of the rooms were beginning to look dated, and the bathroom just wasn't measuring up. There wasn't enough space in their existing 5-by-8-foot bath for stretching out and moving around comfortably.

So when architect Brion S. Jeannette of Newport Beach, California, was contracted to design a new bathroom for the Hahnes, his first order of business was to create a space that was as roomy as it was aesthetically appealing. "I wanted it to feel large even though it's not a big space," he says. Knocking out some walls helped, as did lifting the bathroom ceiling—the highest point is now about 15 feet. But rather than borrow all of the necessary space for the bathroom from existing rooms in the house, the architect chose to expand into the Hahnes' large backyard.

To keep the bath private, Jeannette constructed a 7-foot fence around the addition and created a secluded garden patio just outside. The effect is remarkable. Not only does the garden visually expand the space in the bath but the natural beauty of the garden greenery enhances the look of the entire room. The natural light that floods in from three large skylights and several windows adds to the garden's appeal and creates an almost outdoor atmosphere in the bath. Mirrors make it possible to view the garden from almost anywhere in the room.

The tiny patio garden is the inspiration for the bath's decor. Natural earthtones warm the new fixtures, carpeted floor, and imported ceramic tile on the countertops, tub, and shower surround. Cabinetry for the "his" and "her" vanities (Wally's is conveniently

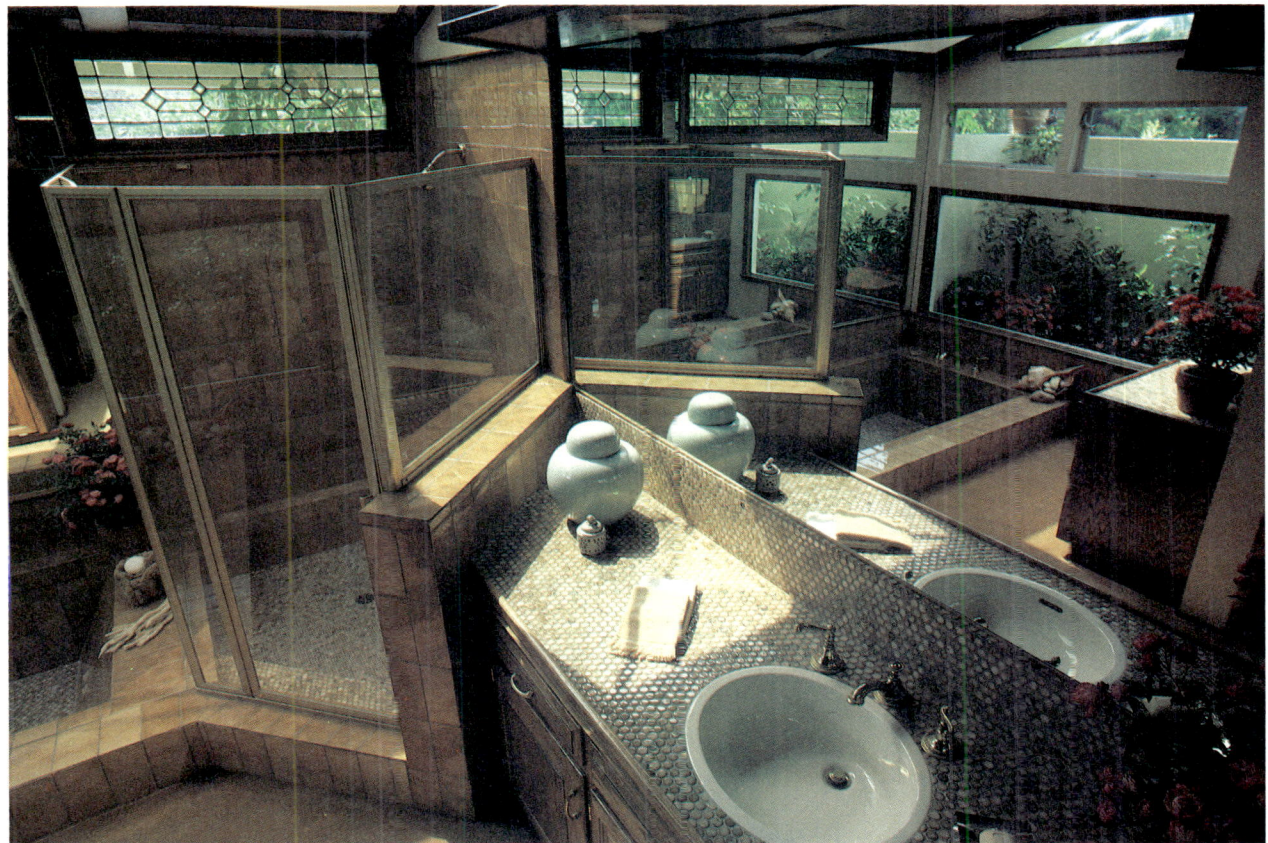

Imported ceramic tile on the countertops, shower stall, and tub surround and the abundance of natural light give this bath an earthy feel.

close to his extra-large shower, and Linda's is across from her sunken whirlpool tub) is handcrafted from a rich, stained oak. Glowing brass faucets and shower hardware work as elegant accents.

The toilet and bidet are located in their own separate compartment, which also has a window to the garden. To make the bath an even more restful place, Jeannette ingeniously located the whirlpool pump machinery, which can get noisy, outside on the patio. To assure maximum comfort, windows and skylights in the room are east-facing to take full advantage of the warm morning sunlight.

The Hahnes' bath is now a wonderfully relaxing place to spend time after a long day. And the mild, Southern California climate keeps their little patio garden fresh and lovely year-round.

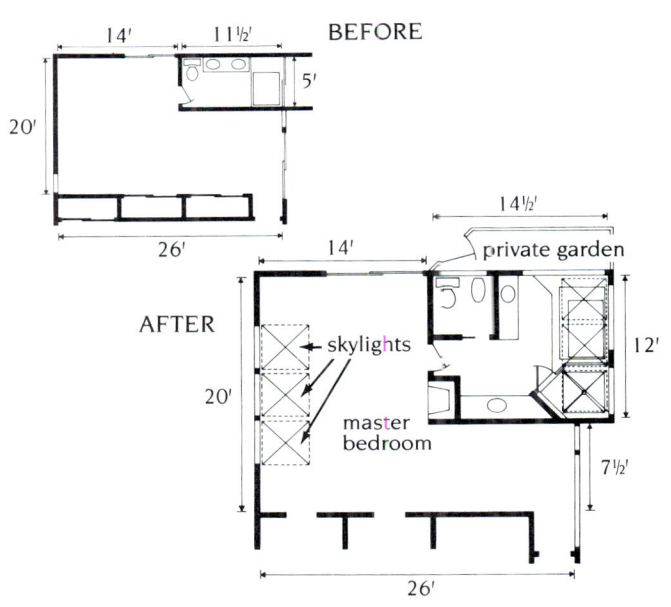

# An Octagonal Bath

Claire and Ted Jarek loved their octagonal house in coastal Maine. But their octagonal bath needed a face-lift. Located right in the center of the house—with no windows at all—the bath was small, dark, and oppressive. It needed a few rays of sunshine to cheer it up. And interior designer Philippe Favet's job was to bring in that sunshine.

That wasn't going to be easy. Since the bath's location wouldn't be changing, Favet still had to deal with the fact that the room had no windows. Somehow, he had to brighten the room without relying on direct, natural light. To accomplish his goal, he employed natural color, reflection, and lots of theatrical lights.

The resulting bath is so bright and warm that you'd never guess how dismal it had been before. Part of that warmth is due to Favet's liberal use of wood in the Jareks' bath. The light pine of the ceiling and the rosy maple of the cabinetry are trimmed with rich mahogany for an unusual yet beautiful combination. Mahogany trim also runs from the floor to the ceiling at each of the

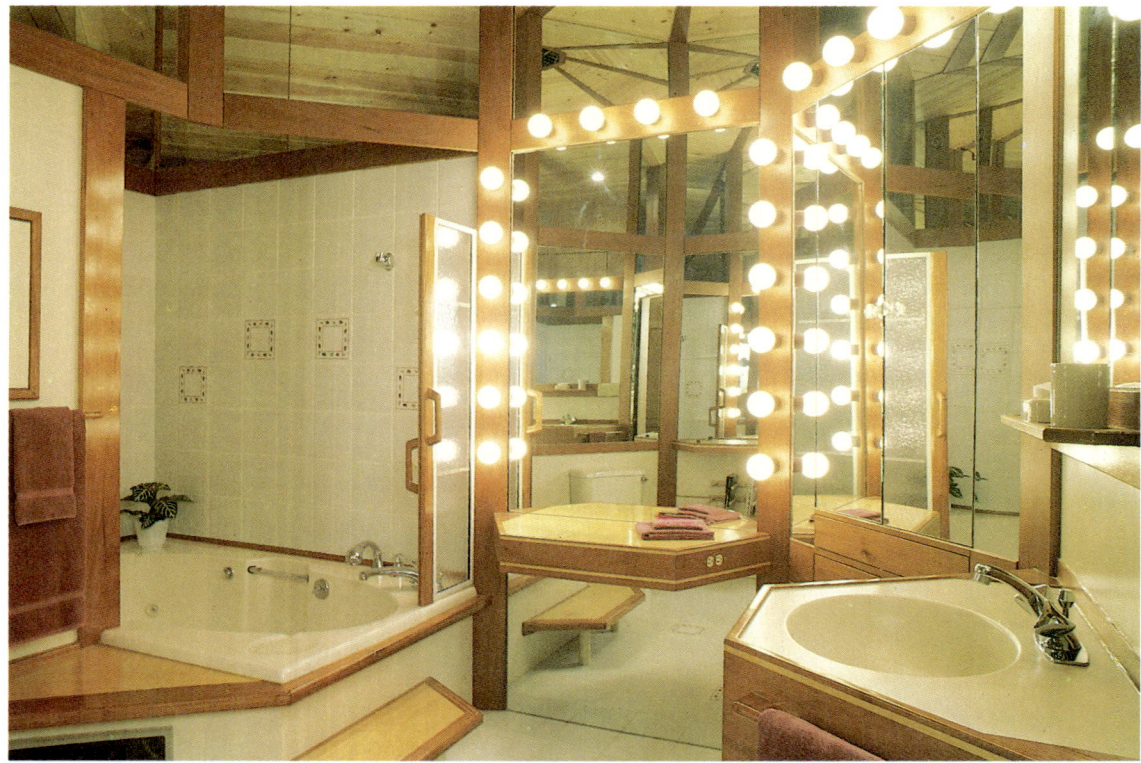

A bumpout in one wall of this octagonal bath allows just enough space for a large whirlpool tub and shower.

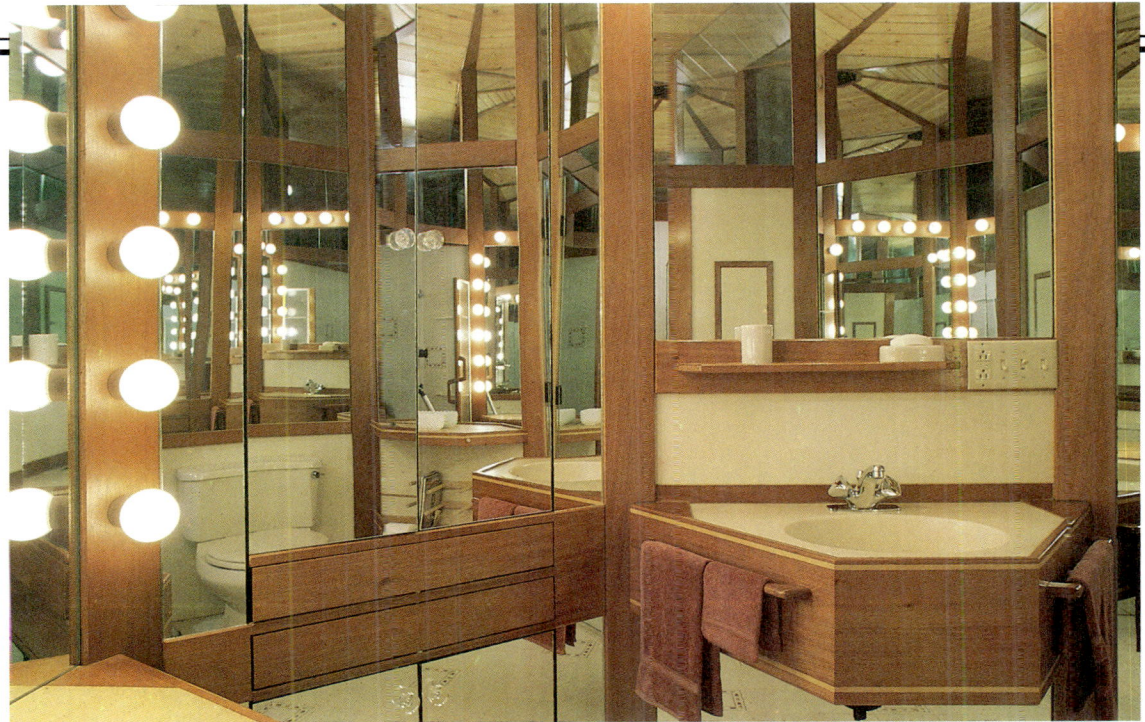

Although the Jareks' bath has no windows, the theatrical lighting and its reflection off the mirrored walls provide plenty of illumination.

eight corners of the octagonal room.

The rich wood trim serves to define the eight walls of the bath, each of which are 3 feet wide. Floor-to-ceiling mirrors on those walls create the illusion of space and make the bath look much bigger than it is. Another space stretcher is the bath's high ceiling: The height from the floor to the top of the bath's cupola above is 20 feet.

To add color and life to the bath, the Jareks had a stained-glass dome custom-designed and fitted into the top of the cupola. Eight small mirrors on the interior surface of the cupola reflect the bright red, blue, and amber throughout the bath, creating constantly changing patterns of color and light.

The 24 theatrical lights in the bath provide plenty of warm light. And to give the feeling of windows in the bath, Favet glassed the top half of two walls shared with the living room. This allows natural light from the windows in the rest of the house into the bath.

The bath's amenities, like its unusual lighting, complement its unique shape. The custom-designed sink vanity, makeup vanity, and tub/shower enclosure repeat the bath's geometric motif, as do a number of innovative storage ideas and design elements—like two pivoting drawers recessed into one wall, and the handcrafted wood bench in the tub area. The wood cabinetry and several mirror-clad cabinets recessed into the walls provide plenty of bath storage, making the Jareks' octagonal bath as functional as it is warm and beautiful.

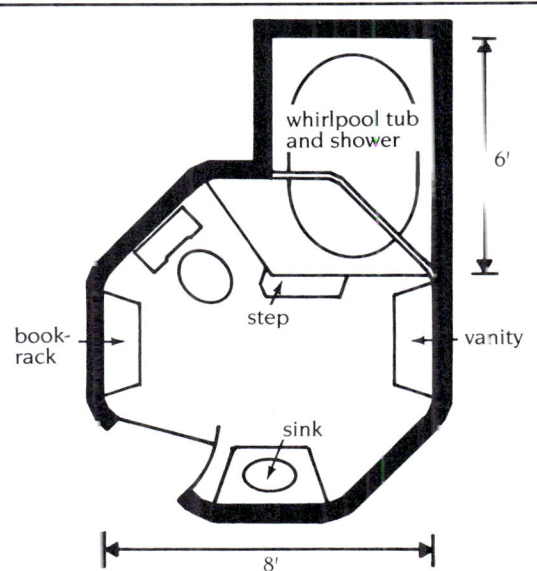

# A Bath of Simply Stated Luxury

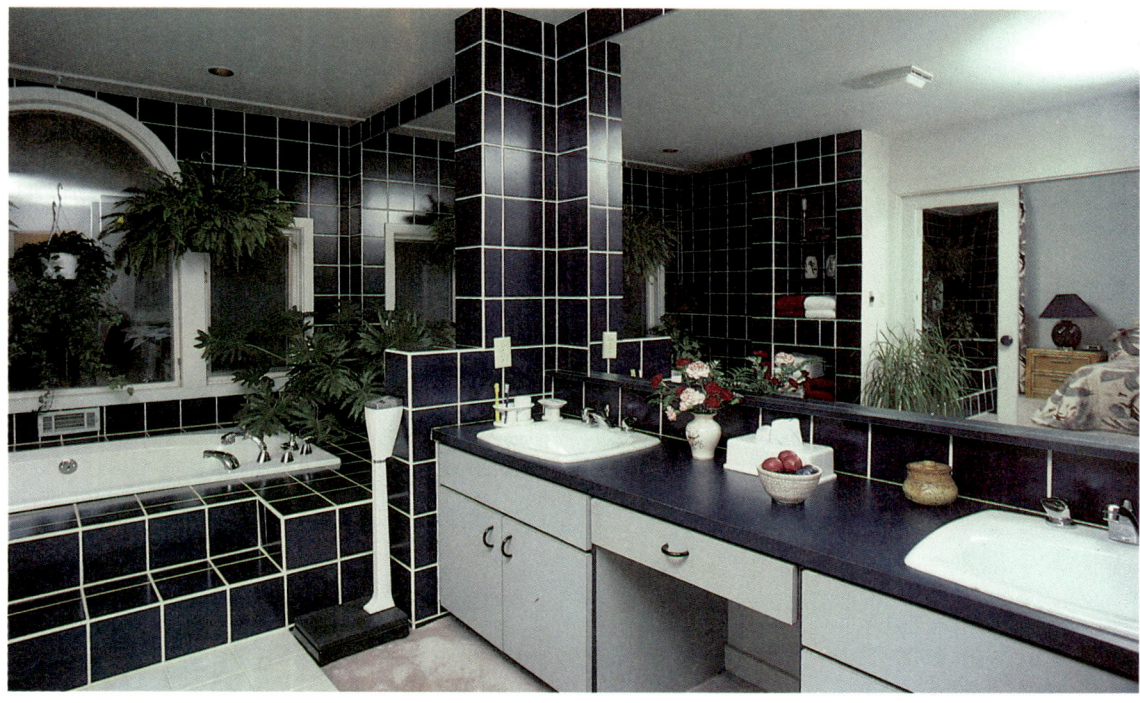

Who says plain white is boring? In this bath, the white tub, cabinetry, and sinks look dazzling against the blue tile background.

You won't find many decorative embellishments in this master-suite bath. Yet the room exudes elegance, as well as luxury—proof that a simple, almost understated, approach can be a powerful statement.

The request communicated to Karel Pruner, AIA, the architect, by Edward Karlin, M.D., the homeowner, was for a practical, easy to maintain, spacious bath. Karlin, a physician by profession, an entertainer at heart, and a bachelor at the time, wanted a bathroom design that would be compatible with his casual life-style. Karlin left most of the detail work up to Pruner.

The resulting bath is right in tune with the rest of the house Pruner designed: simple, spacious, and unencumbered, yet luxurious at the same time. Striking cobalt blue ceramic tile with white grout covers the walls, shower, and tub surround. The style is simple and bold, while the rich colors lend a look of understated elegance to the bath.

To offset the blue of the walls and to provide continuity of colors with the adjoining bedroom, Pruner chose a neutral-colored tile for the floor; plush carpeting around the vanity offers extra comfort on cold morn-

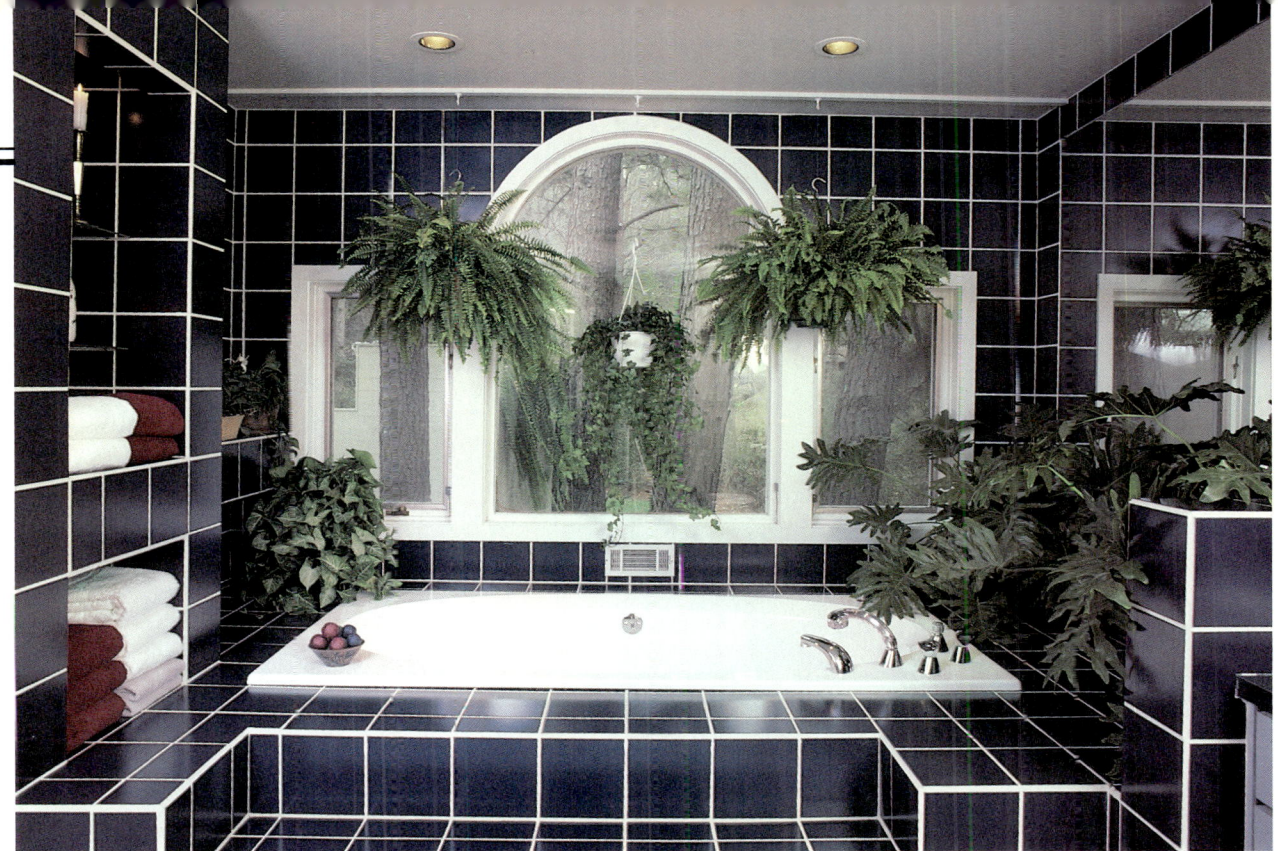

A quiet backyard view, visible through a custom-designed window, creates a picturesque setting for the large whirlpool tub in this master bath.

ings. Tile niches in the wall provide a unique storage system for bath linens. Accent lighting above glass shelves filters through to showcase a few treasures.

Mirrors on several walls and on the door to the master bedroom make the space even larger and lend to the bath's overall excitement. Clean-white fixtures and smooth laminates on the countertop and vanity cabinetry also add to the sense of openness in the room.

While he had few requests, Karlin did want his "toys," as Pruner calls them. A giant whirlpool tub sits on a platform just below an exquisitely shaped window, which lets in lots of light and affords bathers a peaceful backyard view. A stepped wall outside assures privacy, and the many green plants in the tub area help to bring the outdoors in. The extra-large shower, equipped with a built-in bench, converts to a steam bath with the press of a button. All lighting is controlled by dimmer switches—for creating just the right mood.

Expensive bath toys aside, the style of the room is straightforward and simple—just what the doctor ordered. Yet it's that simplicity that makes this bath so luxurious and inviting.

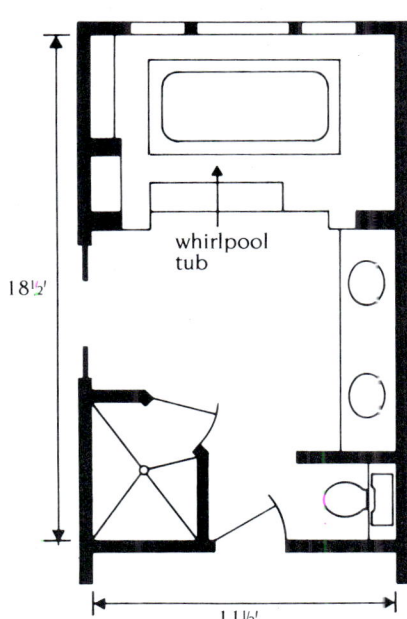

# The Best of Both Worlds

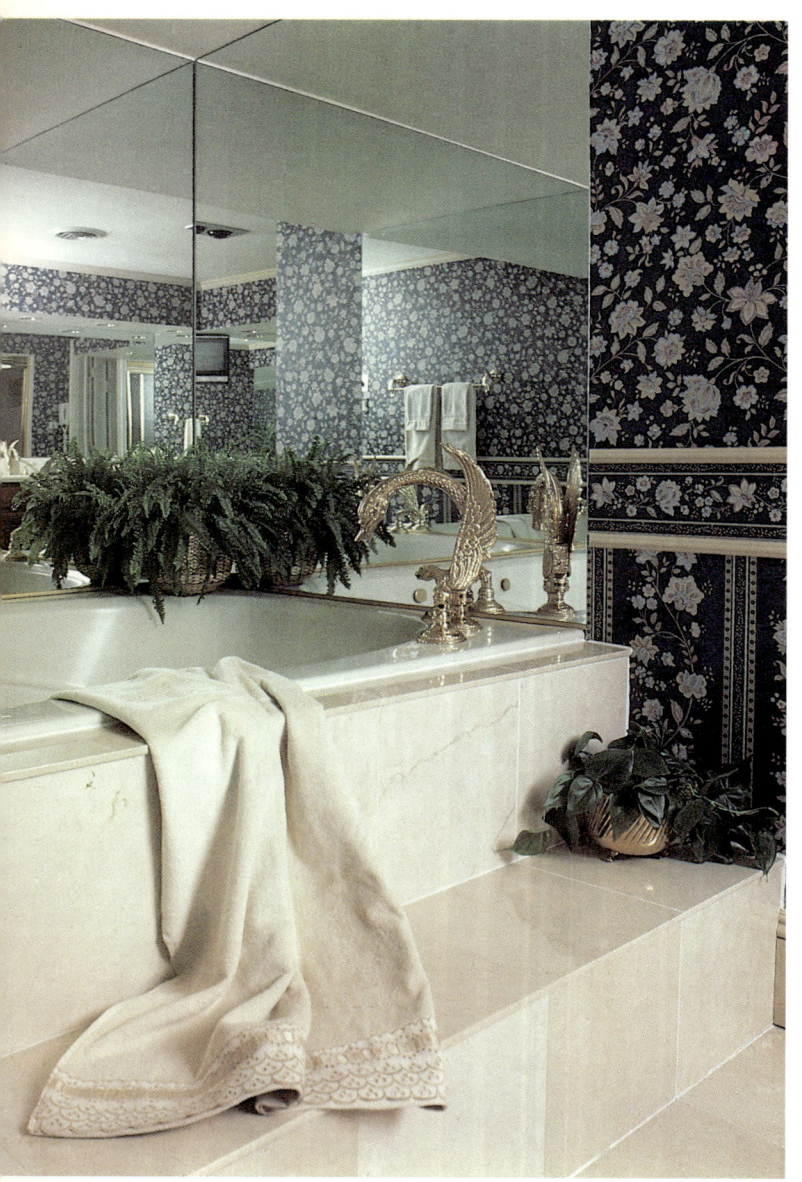

A swan-shaped, solid-brass faucet and a marble-tile surround add touches of elegance to the whirlpool tub in the Bollingers' master bath.

Barbara and David Bollinger had wanted a stone farmhouse for as long as they could remember. But they couldn't find a genuine article with room enough for all the modern conveniences they wanted to include. So they built their own, designing and decorating it just like the stone farmhouses of old—with thick, fieldstone walls, three fireplaces, a large, comfy kitchen, and plenty of country furniture.

With its old-fashioned floral wallpaper and colonial-style wood cabinetry, the bath also has an old-world flavor. But luxury is the first word that rushes to mind. The room is huge—about 270 square feet—and its large mirrors make it look even bigger. Creamy marble graces the floor and makes a regal setting for an elegant whirlpool tub. Stunning brass tub fillers shaped like swans match the sink faucets and towel hangers in the room. "The swans," says Barbara, "were bought during a moment of madness. We had been looking for something much simpler."

The cabinetry, custom-built and corner-fitted, is crafted of a rich cherry wood and accented with the same brass hardware that appears on the furniture in the master bedroom. The cream-colored Corian countertop has double sinks; vanity lighting is recessed into a soffit above and, like the lighting in the rest of the bath, is controlled by dimmer switches.

The extra-large shower is custom-built with marble and ceramic tile and contains three separate shower heads; one is mounted fairly low on the wall "so I can shower without getting my hair wet," Barbara explains. Also extra large is the walk-in closet, which provides storage for the Bollingers' wardrobes as well as bath linens and other sup-

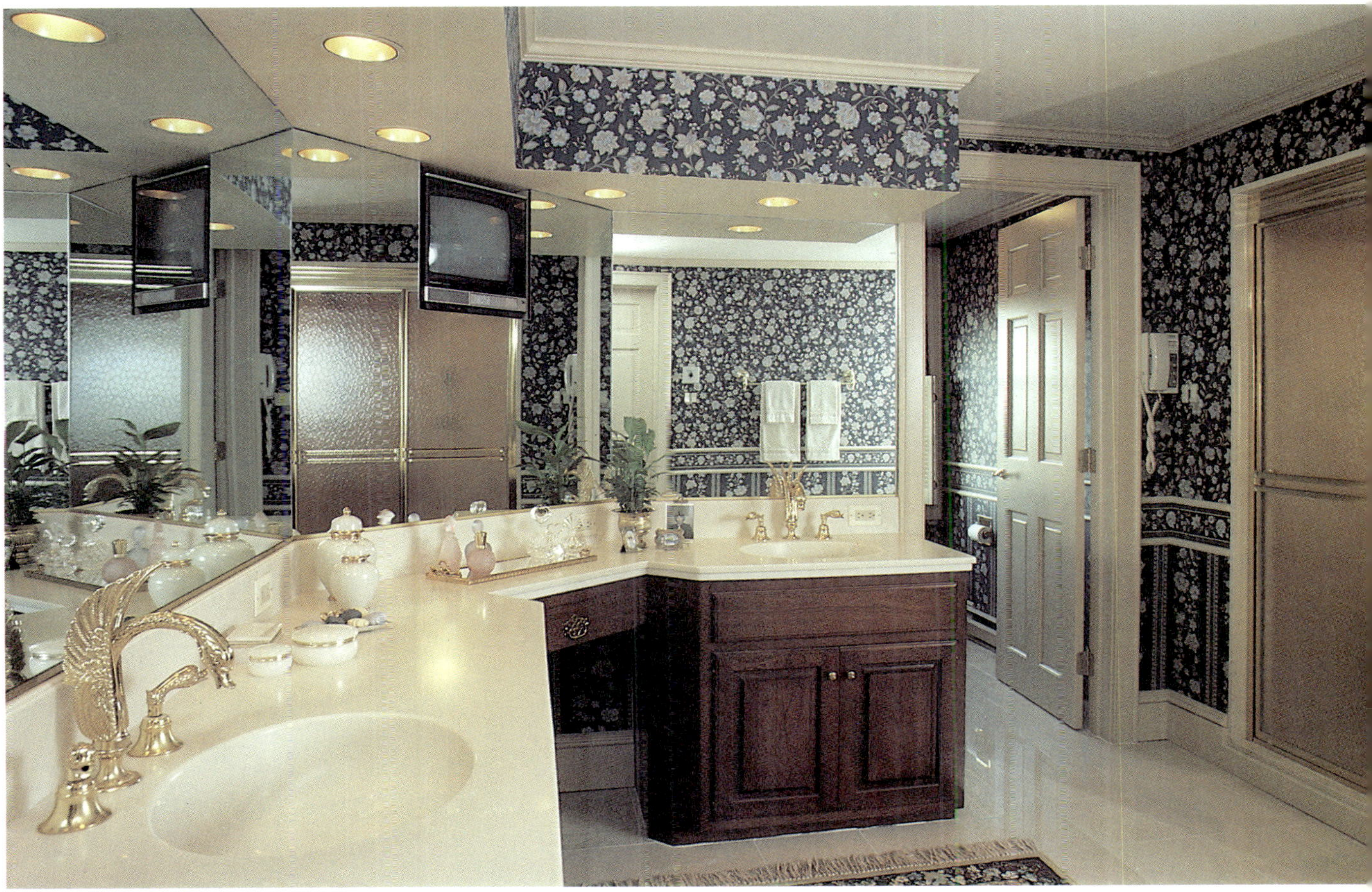

Cherry-wood cabinetry and country-style wallpaper lend a traditional look. But the room isn't lacking in any modern conveniences, as evidenced by the TV recessed into the mirror.

plies. To create more space, a separate compartment was built for the toilet.

Like the rest of the Bollinger house, the master bath contains all the modern conveniences—and a few electronic luxuries. The television set is recessed into a niche in the vanity mirror. An intercom allows the Bollingers to answer the door without leaving the bath. And the telephone, with its extra-long cord, can be conveniently answered from anywhere in the room.

But for all its electronic gadgetry, the Bollingers' master bath still exudes a warm feeling, the same feeling you get walking through the rest of their cozy, country-style, Pennsylvania home. Modern convenience and traditional style give this bath the best of both worlds.

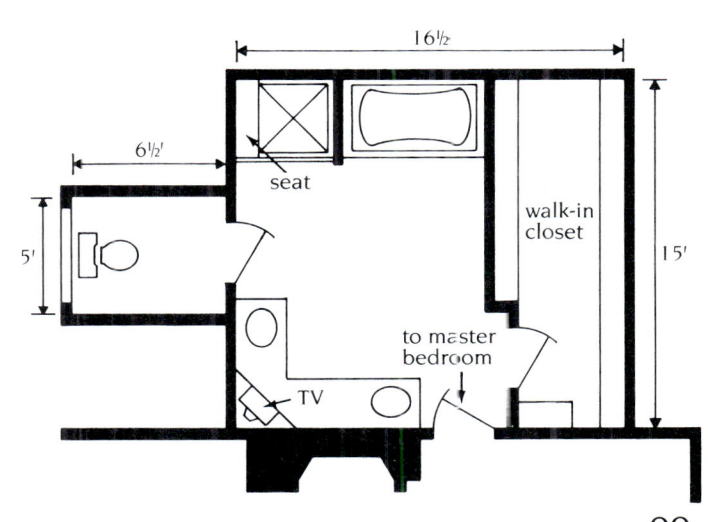

# A Bath of European Elegance

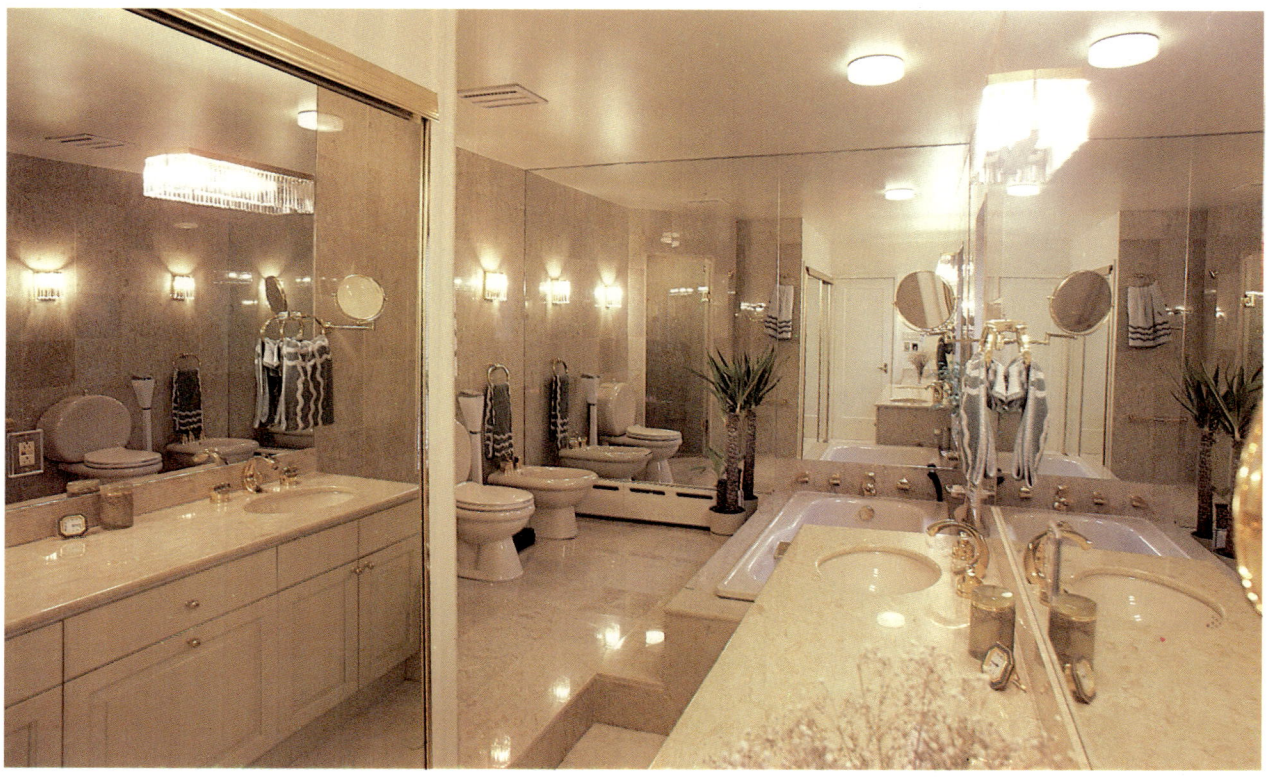

Although this bath is narrow, the designer was successfully able to include all the luxuries—even a large shower (around the corner from the mirrored closet).

When it came to redesigning the master bath in their Canadian home, Heather and Allen Scott asked for a formal, elegant atmosphere with all the luxury amenities, which was compatible with the style of their home. Creating a formal atmosphere was one thing, but "making" enough space was tough. The existing room that designer Barbara Munn had to work with was not large, and fitting everything in—which included a large whirlpool tub, a shower, a bidet, a double-sink vanity, and a large clothes closet—looked impossible. "We really put her through the wringer," Heather admits.

But they say it's the seemingly impossible task that stimulates the greatest amount of creativity, and Munn rose to the occasion, finally producing a floor plan to accommodate all the luxuries *and* with space to move around. A surprisingly large shower

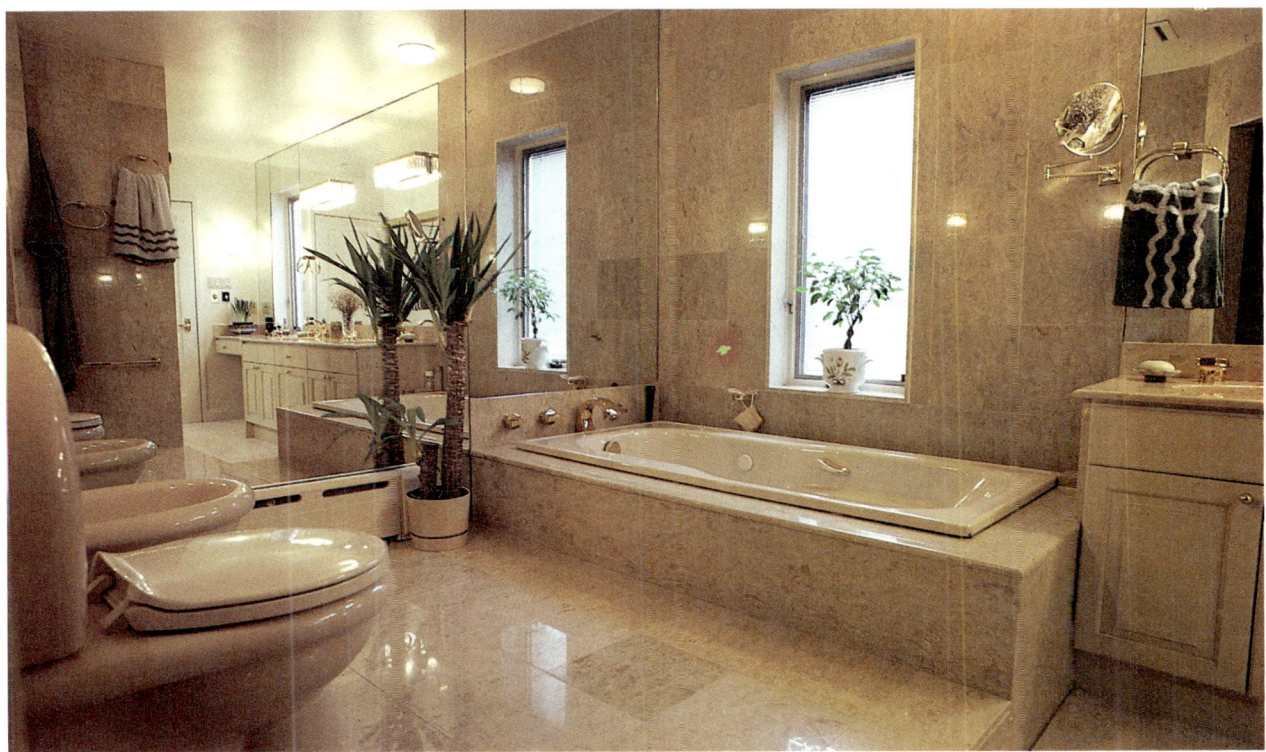

To give the bath an elegant look, the Scotts used marble on walls, floors, and tub surround.

is tucked into a space behind the closet, and the toilet and bidet are tastefully positioned around the corner and out of direct view.

Heather and Allen chose soft, light colors and used lots of floor-to-ceiling mirrors to visually expand the space in the bath. Marble on the walls, floors, tub surround, and vanity countertop gives the bath the elegance they wanted. Light from the cut-crystal lamps Heather chose for the bath enhances the marble even more.

The imported European fixtures the Scotts selected blend nicely with the marble tiles and add a special style to the room. The tub is from Spain; the other fixtures are Italian. The tub is extra long and deep with built-in armrests and handgrips; the two sinks, as well as the tub, are equipped with solid-brass, gold-plated faucets. But it's probably the toilet, with its uniquely shaped tank, that attracts the most attention.

The closet, concealed behind mirror-clad doors, is Heather's closet. (Allen's closet is in the bedroom.) The extra-long vanity is constructed with white laminate and accented with brass door and drawer pulls. Knee space is built into the cabinetry for close-up work at the vanity mirror.

Thanks to a creative designer and the Scotts' active participation in the design of their bath, this master bath has everything they could want. And the use of a few simple finishing materials and stylish European fixtures gives it elegant beauty.

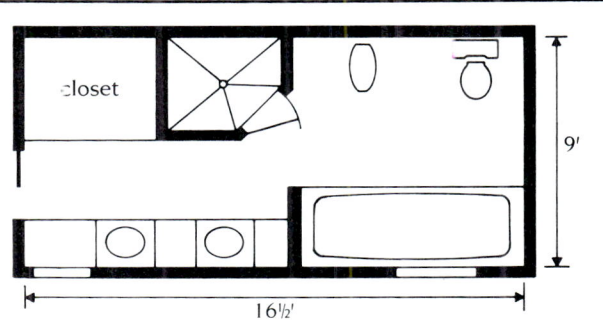

# A Split-level Country Bath

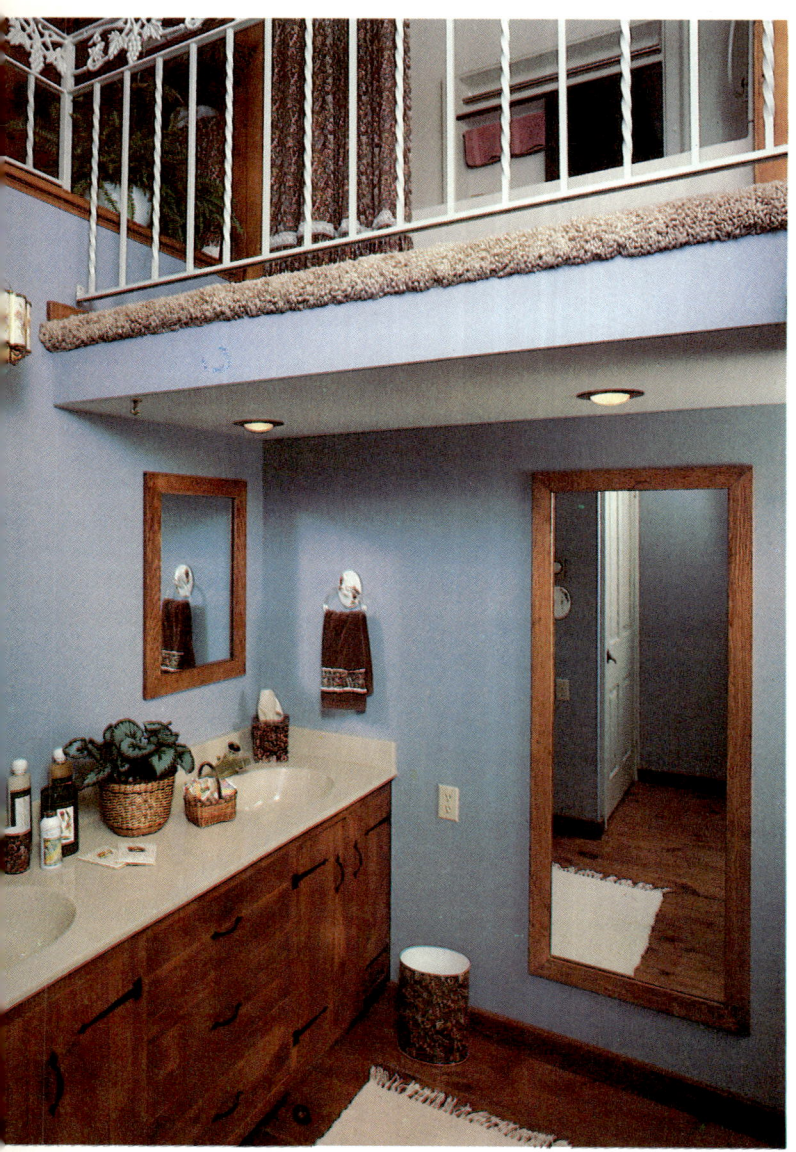

The cabinetry in this split-level bath was crafted from original knotty-pine floorboards in the Landises' nineteenth-century farmhouse.

Robin and Sam Landis were delighted when they found their wonderful old stone farmhouse in eastern Pennsylvania. Built in the nineteenth century, the house is cozy and charming. But for all its charm, it had one major flaw: no serviceable family bathroom. A small bath downstairs provided a shower, but barely enough room to move around. And the upstairs bath, equipped only with a sink and toilet, could hardly have been called a family bath.

So they decided to convert a spare upstairs bedroom into a bath big enough for a nice-size tub and double-sink vanity. To Sam, a contractor and president of A. P. Houser, a contracting company, the job seemed easy. But those plans soon fell through: No matter how Sam laid it out, the room just couldn't accommodate all the fixtures and accessories the couple wanted to include. That's when Sam decided to put the tub in the attic.

Unbelievable as it might sound, the Landis family now has a two-story bath—and the tub is on the second level. The original winding staircase from the spare bedroom to the attic is what inspired the owner/builder to create it. Two steel beams provide added reinforcement for the combination tub/shower, and a landing, created by removing part of the attic floor, opens up the space. With the tub in its attic niche, the spare bedroom below was left free for the double-sink vanity. The tiny original bath became a toilet compartment.

While most stone farmhouses don't sport split-level baths, this bath has all the charm you'd expect to find in an old country home. This is a direct result of Robin's

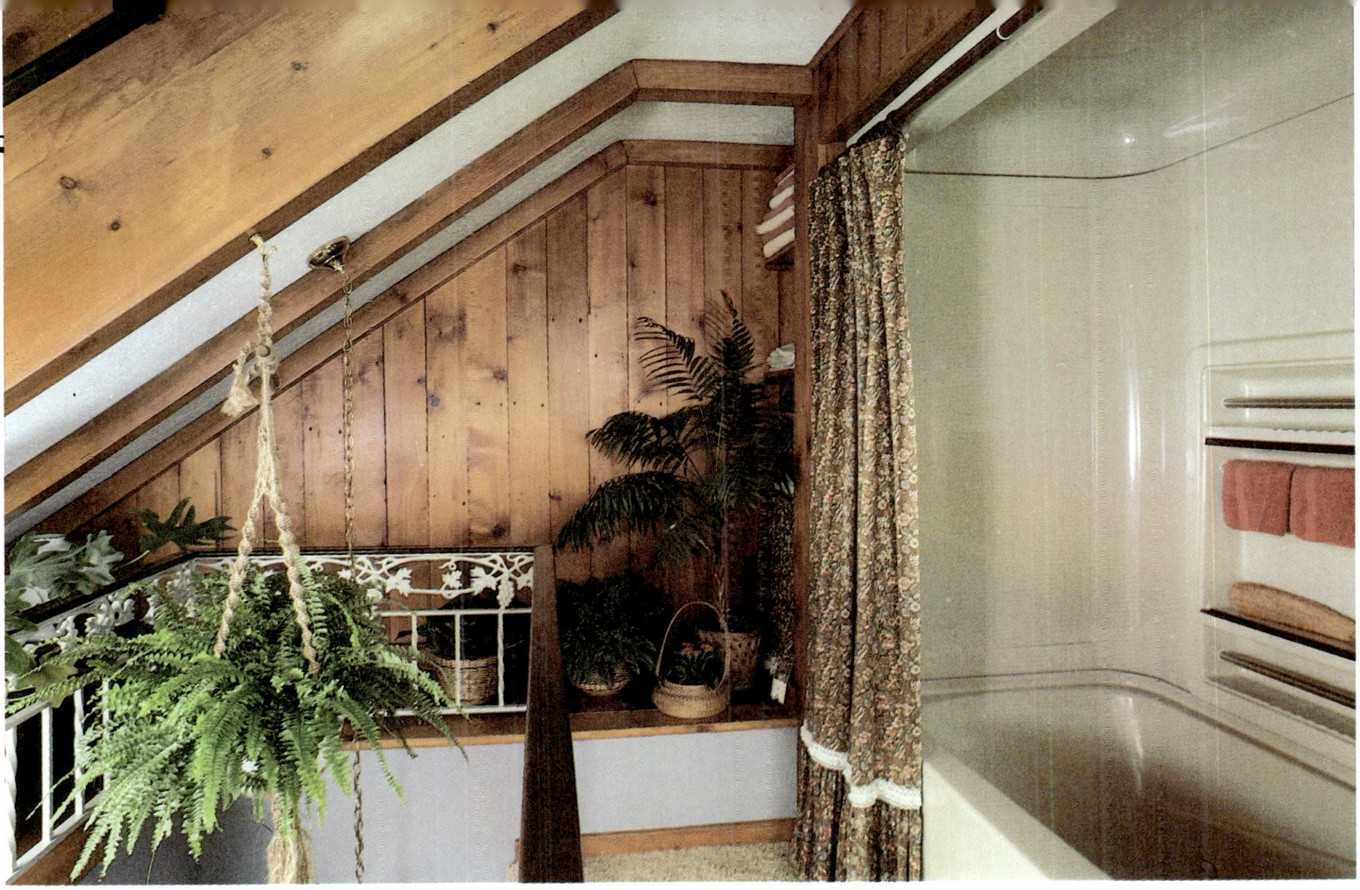

To support the weight of a combination tub/shower, the attic floor had to be reinforced with two steel beams.

good taste in decorating the bath. The original knotty-pine flooring in the vanity area is polished and glowing; the cabinetry, with its old-fashioned hardware, is handcrafted of the same old wood. A country-style, wrought-iron railing wraps around the staircase and landing upstairs, and more knotty pine covers the stairwell and upstairs walls.

The bath is filled with other homey touches, like the hand-stitched, floral-print shower curtain and matching towels, the macramé hangers and wicker baskets filled with green plants, and the pretty Victorian light fixtures. The room is bright, warm, and cheerful; it's a cozy, country farmhouse bath. And, Robin and Sam are sure, the only two-story bath in town.

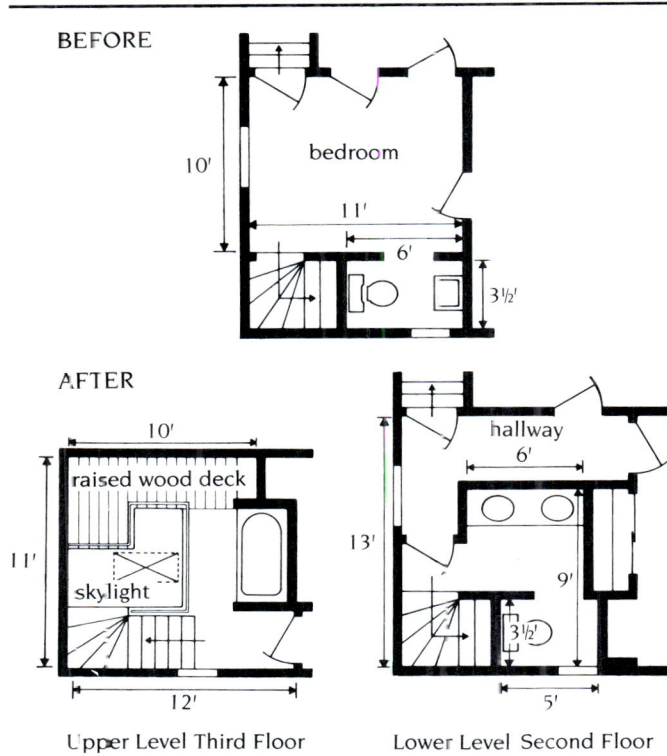

Upper Level Third Floor     Lower Level Second Floor

# A Body and Soul Room

Think about the bath of your wildest dreams, about what it might look like and all the wonderful things you'd find in it. If our guess is correct, the bath we call a body and soul room has all those wonderful things—and some you might never have imagined.

Created by Eric Bernard Designs of New York, this bath is one of the very first "bodyrooms"—if not the first—constructed in the United States. Bernard doesn't like to refer to it as a bathroom. "It's much more than that," he says.

That's obvious. This is an escape room. It's a place to spend time on a rainy afternoon—it's so sumptuous that you might be tempted to retreat there even on a gorgeous, sunny day. And the room is as functional as it is sinfully luxurious. "It's

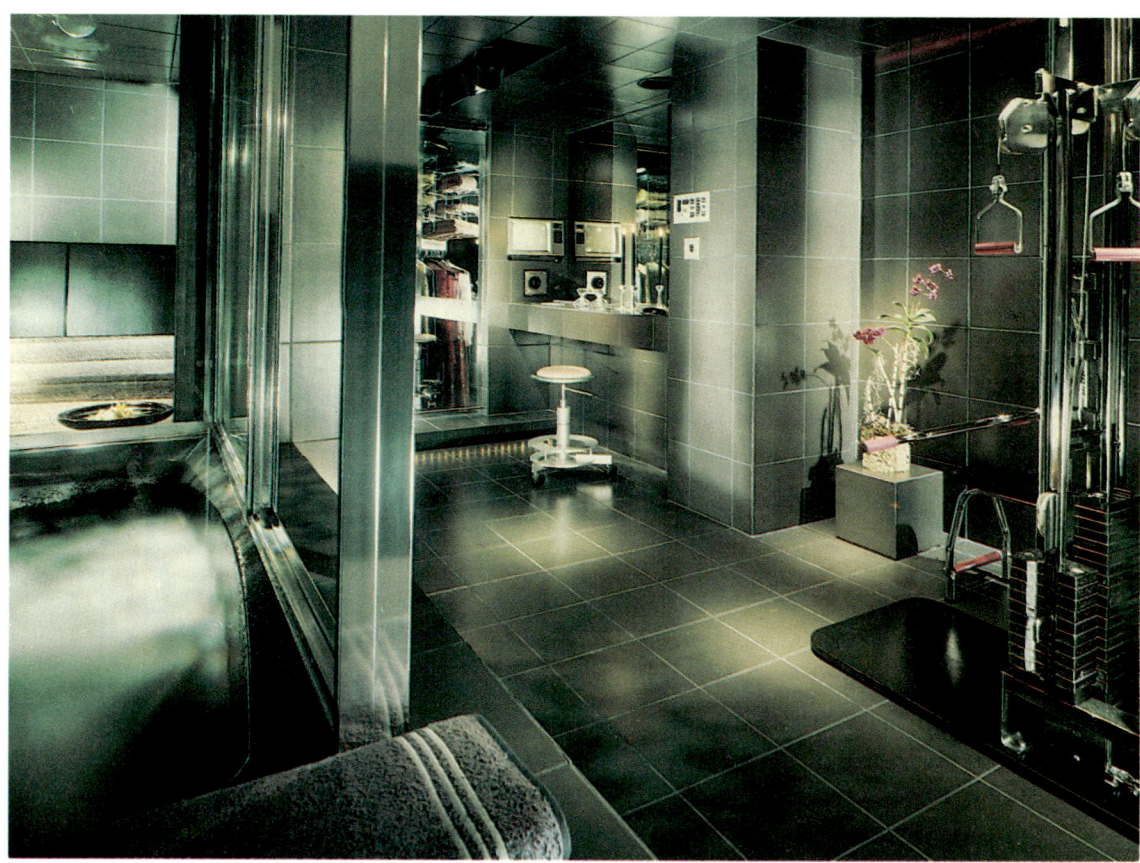

With its automatic garment organizer, computer-controlled lighting and whirlpool, and gym equipment, this bodyroom could be the shape of things to come.

all-purpose," says Bernard. "If you need to take a whirlpool bath, balance your checkbook, get in a quick workout, take a catnap, put on makeup, get dressed—you can do it all, right in this room."

Who wouldn't want to do it all in a room like this? The fabulous amenities make it almost irresistible. The tub, for instance, is no ordinary tub. The enclosure houses not just a jetted whirlpool, but a shower and steam bath as well. Vaporproof speakers in the walls pipe in stereo sound, and two projectors situated above the enclosure's two-way-mirrored ceiling shoot images of falling leaves into the steam as you soak—relaxation at its most extraordinary.

The chaise lounge just behind the tub is also extraordinary. Exclusively manufactured and upholstered with a handwoven silk chenille, the lounge is made of separate "rolls" that at the push of a button move up or down independently to elevate head, neck, knees, or feet. Another button activates a stimulating massage in each roll, and another controls a soothing heat. A rest on this lounge might be the perfect way to cap a workout.

The closet, too, is one of a kind. Desiring a better use of space than typical walk-in closets afford, Bernard employed a Railex automatic garment organizer, the kind used in the dry-cleaning industry. Everything is compartmentalized—shoes, scarves, hats, stockings, handbags, dresses, blouses, slacks, and coats. A computer screen shows you exactly what's there; the automatic system brings your selection right to your fingertips.

The computer performs additional functions. All the lighting in the bath can be preprogrammed: to light one area of the bathroom only, to simulate various lighting environments at the vanity mirror, to create almost any mood desired. The computer also operates the remote-control stereo system, telephone, and temperature/humidity controls. If you want to check your calendar or work on your personal finances, you can do it at this computer; it will even help you coordinate your makeup with your wardrobe!

Such an abundance of mirrors and chrome would scream high-tech anywhere else. But this room is surprisingly soft-looking and sensuous. The innovative lighting helps

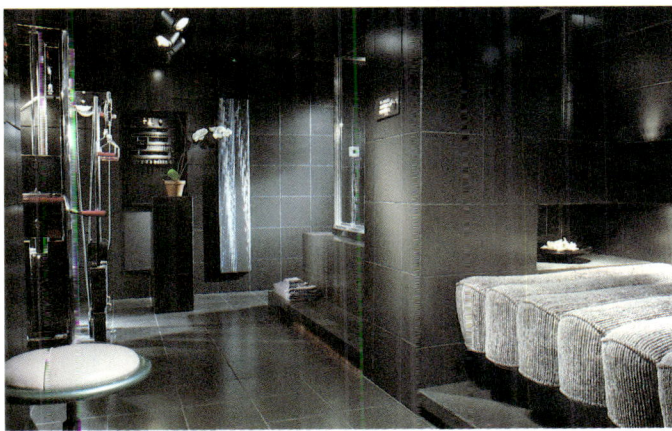

The bath's custom-built, electrically powered chaise lounge provides soothing heat and massaging action—great after a workout.

to create this softness, as does the dove-colored Italian tile on the walls and floors. The tile looks so much like kid leather that it might prompt you to run a hand over it—just to make sure it's really tile.

The soft, comforting atmosphere and the accessibility and convenience of the accessories make this a room for nurturing both body and soul, the basic philosophy behind the bodyroom concept. "It zeroes in on comfort," Bernard says of the bodyroom, "and makes all those things you have to do each day a lot easier. There's so much technology at work in today's homes—why have it at all if we can't use it to enhance our personal well-being?"

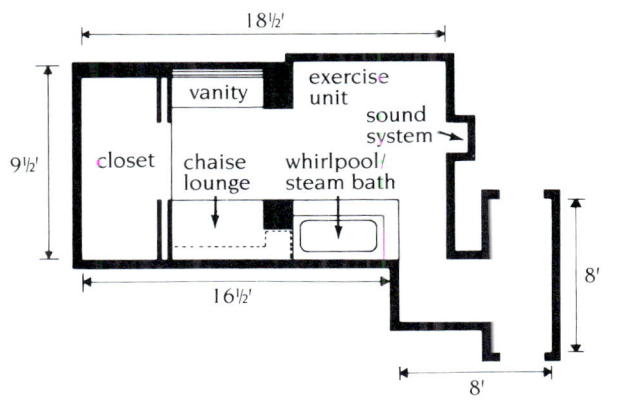

# A Terrarium Bath

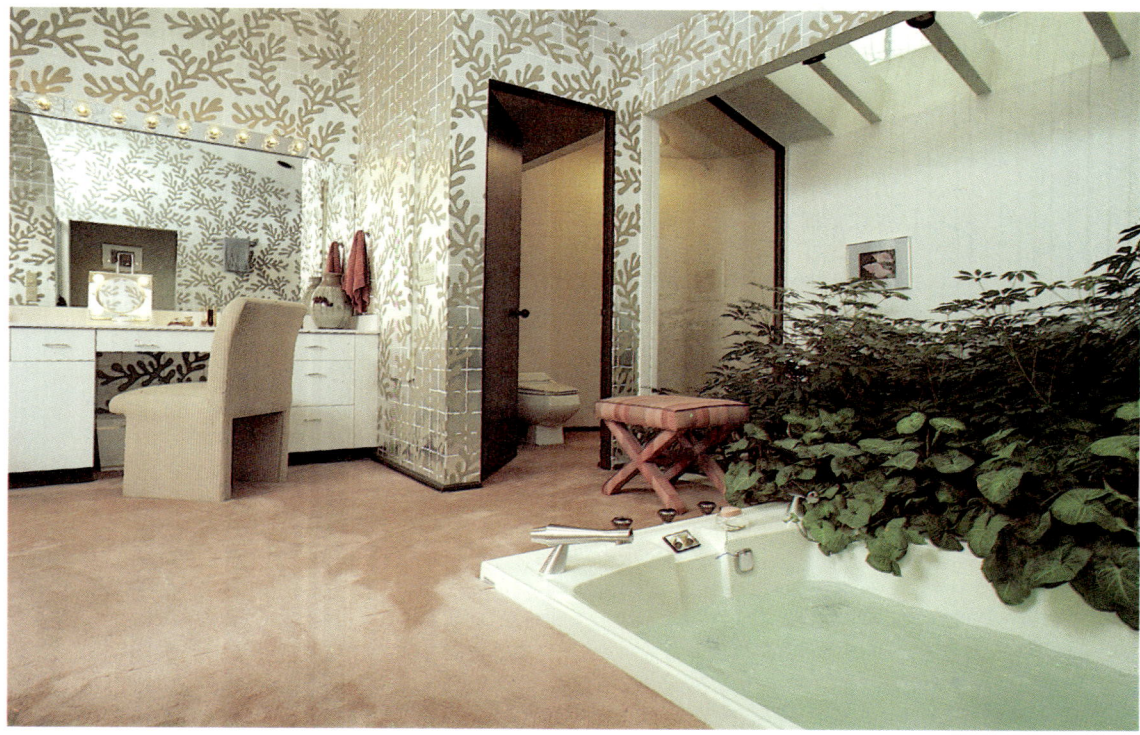

The Dornbushes' master bath is large and luxurious; the whirlpool tub, sunken into the carpeted floor, adds a dramatic touch.

Diane Butler loves plants—so much, in fact, that she has five indoor gardens throughout her custom-built Atlanta home. And one of those lush, green gardens is in her master bath.

The garden is the first thing you see when you walk into the bath. You feel as though you're in the middle of a tropical terrarium: The plants have all but overtaken one corner of the room, their vines climbing up the walls toward the skylights and trailing into the tub. Apparently, the plants find the bath's steamy atmosphere to their liking—they grow so fast that Diane can hardly keep them under control!

While the garden is the biggest attention-grabber in this master bath, its large whirlpool tub runs a close second. Sunken directly into a plushly carpeted floor and equipped with sleek, European-style faucets, the tub lends a dramatic touch to the room—although Diane admits that since she and her husband, Robert, are both runners, the shower is a more popular fixture.

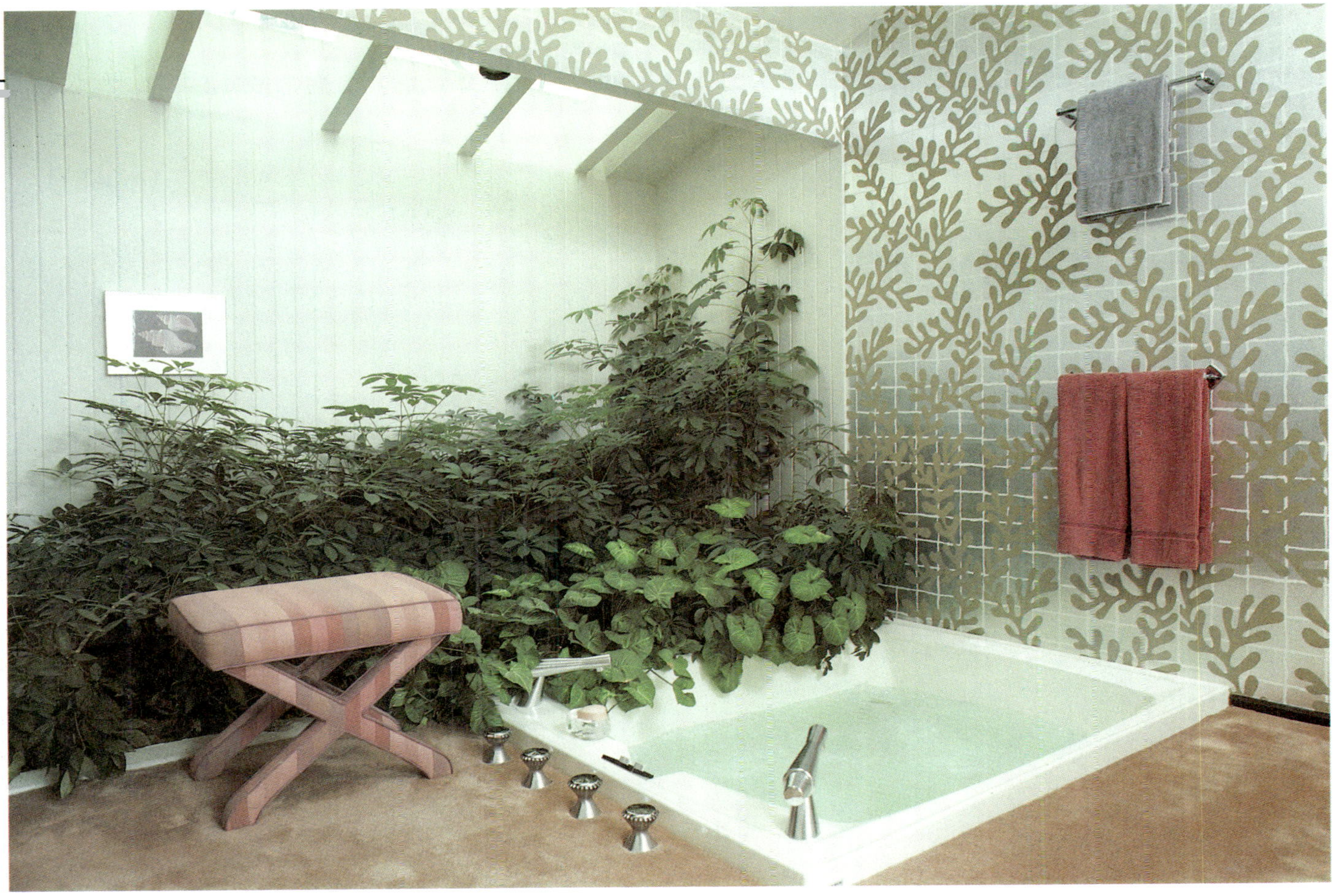

The humidity from tub and shower use and the abundance of natural light in the bath create a lush garden.

The white laminate cabinetry in the bath is fitted with a Corian countertop and built-in sink; theatrical lighting and a cushioned seat make closeup work at the vanity easier. A unique cosmetic storage cabinet is built flush with the wall and covered with wallpaper for a low profile. Electrical outlets in the vanity mirror are disguised with mirror-clad plastic when not in use.

The room is large, comfortable, and luxurious, echoing the light, open feeling throughout the house. The bath is open to the master bedroom and has access to an adjacent walk-in closet and dressing area. Skylights fill the bath with light—another reason the garden looks so fresh—and the metallic wallpaper helps to reflect the light even more.

The Butlers were at first leery of installing wall-to-wall carpeting in their bath. But they now find that the luxurious, soft feel of carpet underfoot is well worth the extra upkeep. And its earthy color is the perfect complement for the garden's greenery. The wallpaper, with its unique botanical pattern, is the perfect wall covering for this terrarium bath.

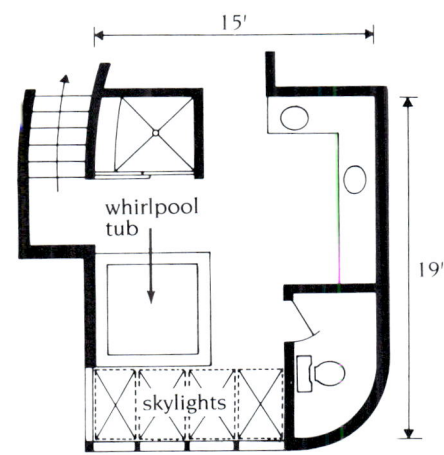

# A Bath of Wide Open Spaces

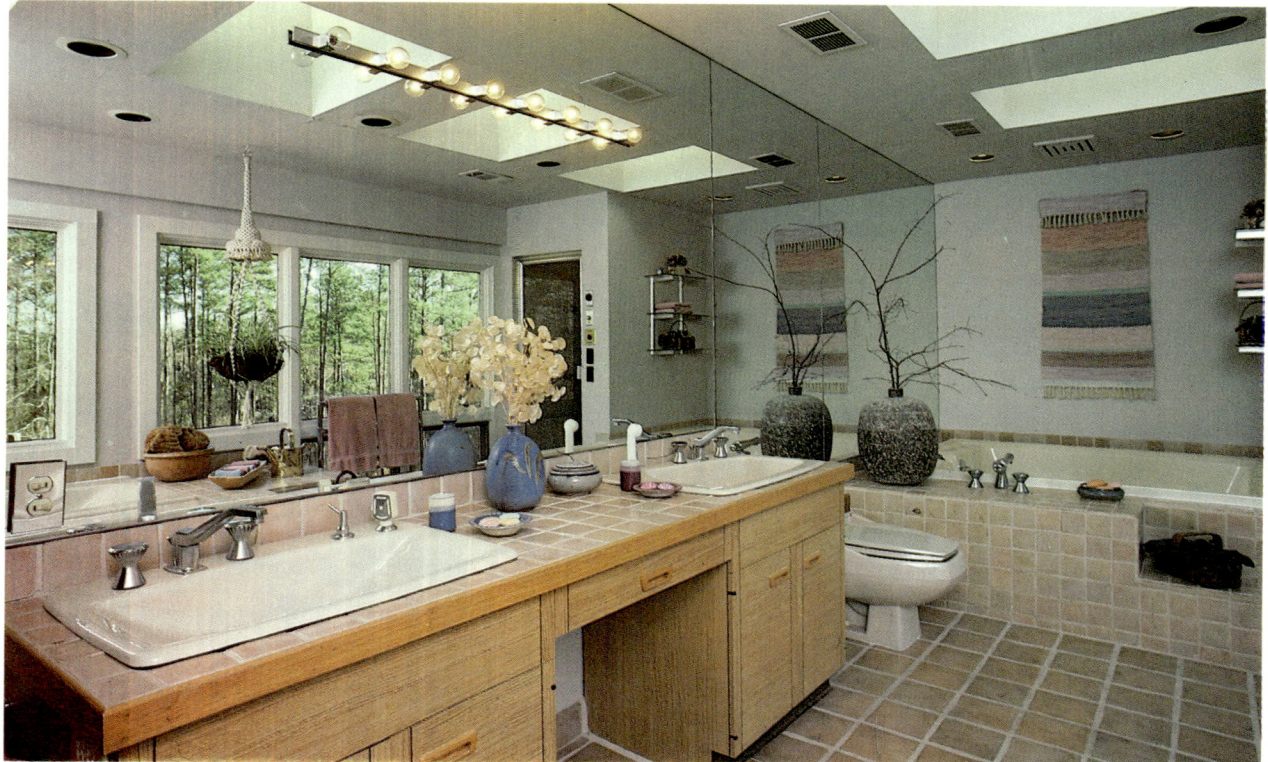

The use of light colors and floor-to-ceiling mirrors on several walls of this master bath create the illusion of endless space.

When Tommy Caswell's Atlanta clients decided to remodel the master bath in their 15-year-old house, they wanted to splurge on all the luxuries: a double-sink vanity; a separate, extra-large shower; and *two* oversize tubs. Squeezing them all into a room that measured just 9 feet square would not be easy. So Caswell bumped out some walls and used lots of mirrors and glass to create a bath of seemingly endless space.

Floor-to-ceiling mirrors cover two entire walls of the new master bath, which gained an extra 10½ feet of length from two enclosed porches on either side of it. The effect is startling: Not only do the mirrors make the bath look gigantic but they reflect the beautiful backyard and forest view from the north-facing wall of windows throughout the room. Four large skylights brighten and expand it even more.

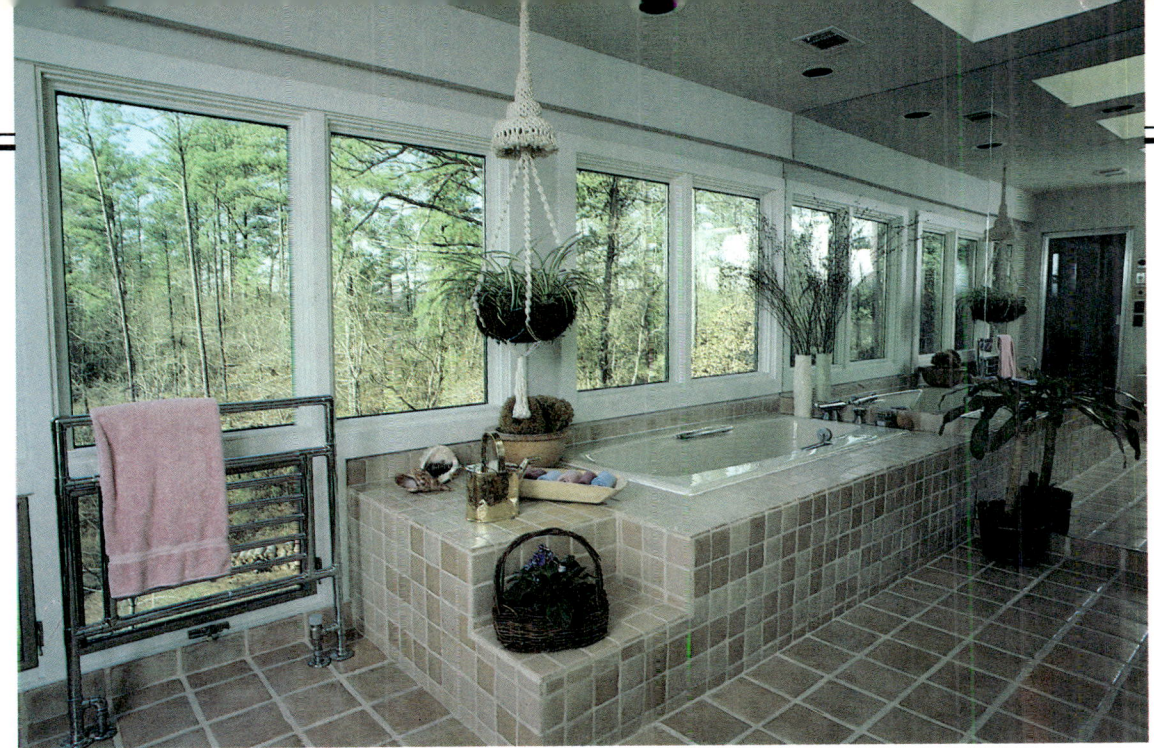

A European-style towel warmer adds a unique touch. Hot water for the tub flows first through the warmer; towels are kept toasty for bathers.

The abundance of light and space in this bath inspired its natural decor. Sand-colored Mexican tile and matching fixtures, woodgrain laminate cabinets, and a distinctive collection of tapestries and ceramics give the bath a warm, south-of-the-border feel.

But the space itself was created to make room for the amenities—not the least of which were two tubs. One is a 5-foot bathtub for regular bathing, the other a giant-size whirlpool for more leisurely soaks; both are recessed into raised, tiled platforms. A European-style towel warmer, heated by hot water, services the tub near the windows.

The separate shower features six shower heads and a built-in steam machine. Since there were so many potential sources of humidity in the bath—like the steam shower and the whirlpool—designer Caswell installed a heavy-duty ventilation system necessary for a bath with so much glass. The excess humidity also prompted the use of laminate for the vanity rather than wood.

The vanity is equipped with a few luxury touches as well. The two sinks have extra-large bowls; a hand-held spray attachment makes one sink perfect for hair washing. Special dispensers for soap and lotion provide added convenience, and a row of theatrical bulbs light up the vanity.

But for all its luxury details, it's the spaciousness of this master bath that really captures the eye and the imagination. And with its many mirrors, it's a pleasure to see reality end and illusion begin.

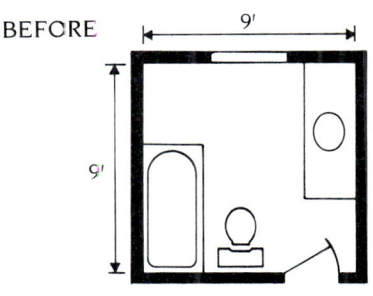

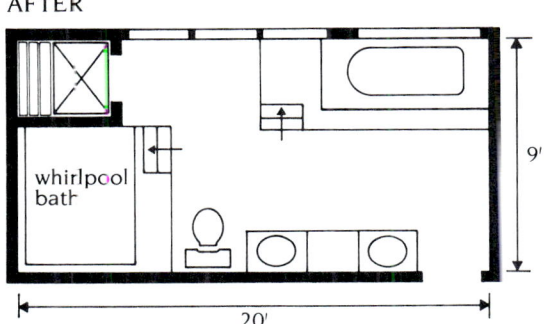

# City Sophistication

Designing an aesthetically pleasing room requires a lot of creative energy. But architect Heidi Kleinman's job was even more taxing: to create an open, spacious master suite in an apartment in a New York City high-rise.

Juanita and Frank Witt landed a treasure when they found their Manhattan apartment, but the existing interior wouldn't have garnered rave reviews—especially the master bedroom and bath. Cramped and "indistinguishable," according to Kleinman of Morpurgo Architects, Saddle River, New Jersey, both rooms were completely gutted to

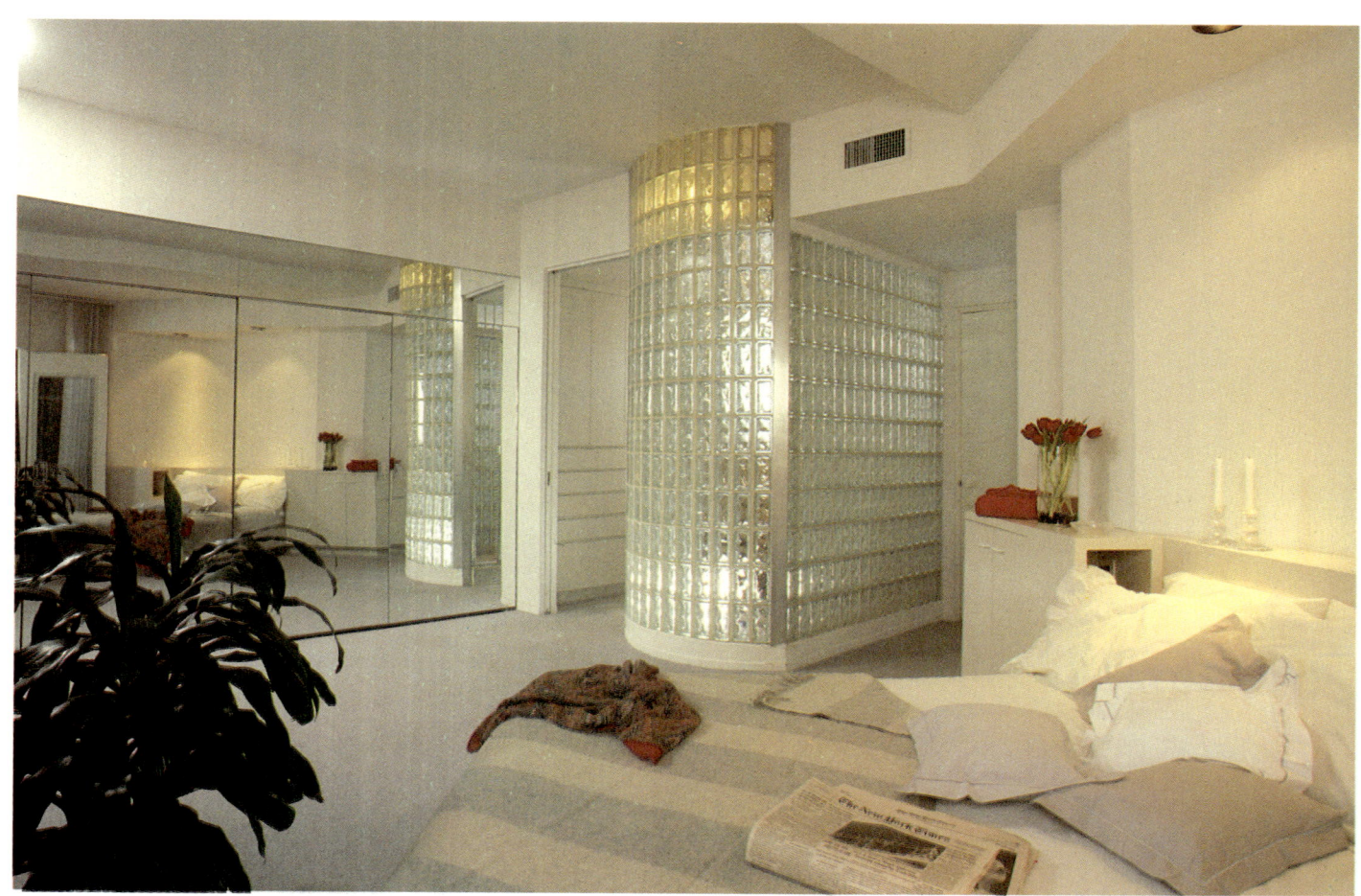

The stunning glass-block shower enclosure is the showpiece of the Witts' sophisticated master suite.

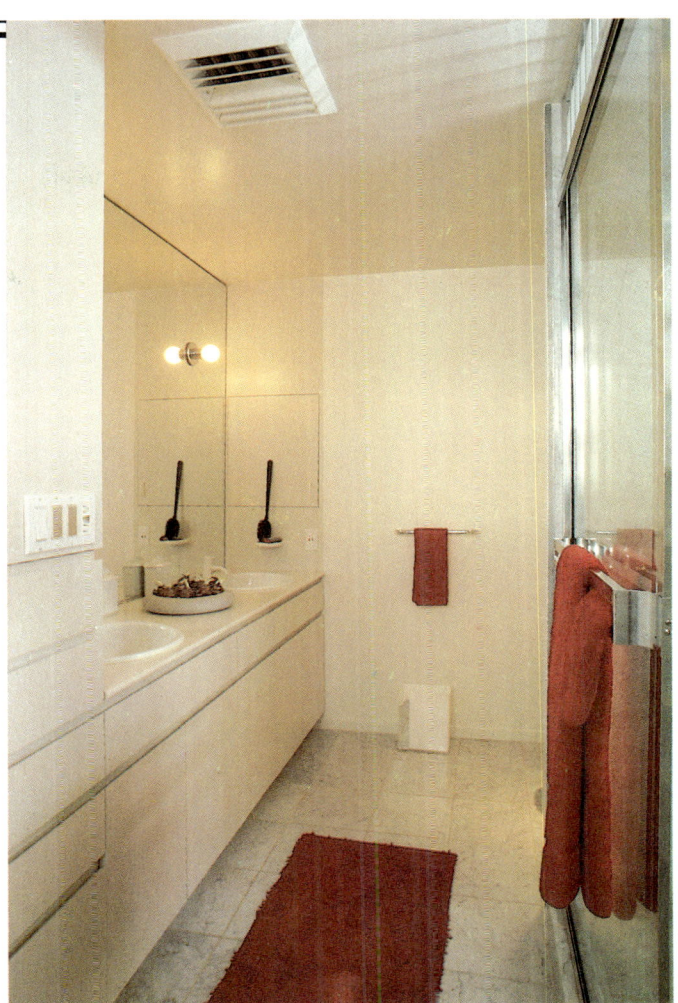

pave the way for a new master suite.

Space proved to be a precious commodity, and the architect had limited options from which to choose. But with the help of very open-minded and design-oriented clients, Kleinman succeeded in creating a master suite more than worthy of its sophisticated urban surroundings. The "barely there" gray on the walls makes the room look open and spacious, and the simple, curvilinear design of the suite gives it a cosmopolitan feel.

And, like a New York City art gallery, the suite has its showpiece: a striking glass-block structure that houses a marble-tiled shower and separates the bath from the rest of the room. The cool tint of the glass is reflected in floor-to-ceiling mirrors that conceal a large closet; a light above the shower compartment filters through the glass block, creating a lantern effect and setting a sensuous mood in the room. This unique shower enclosure is a tribute to the Witts' open-mindedness, says Kleinman. "They were willing to take chances on some innovative concepts that others might have balked at."

The bath itself, like the rest of the suite, is simple in design and decor. The cabinetry is made of bright white ColorCore; all hardware is disguised for a clean, unencumbered look. European faucets add a touch of class to double sinks, dropped into a white Corian countertop. The floor, like the shower, is tiled with marble. Because of limited space, the Witts have a whirlpool tub in another bath.

This master suite is unmistakably luxurious, but in a very untraditional way. It's not colorful, or terribly large, or filled with extensive embellishments. But like a sophisticated gallery exhibit, it gets glowing reviews.

To make the look cleaner, the designer used smooth marble tile and European-style laminate cabinetry in the bath.

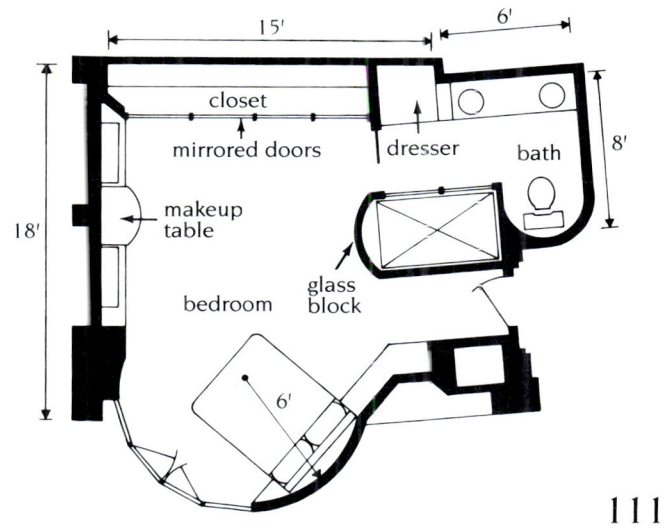

# A Victorian Bath

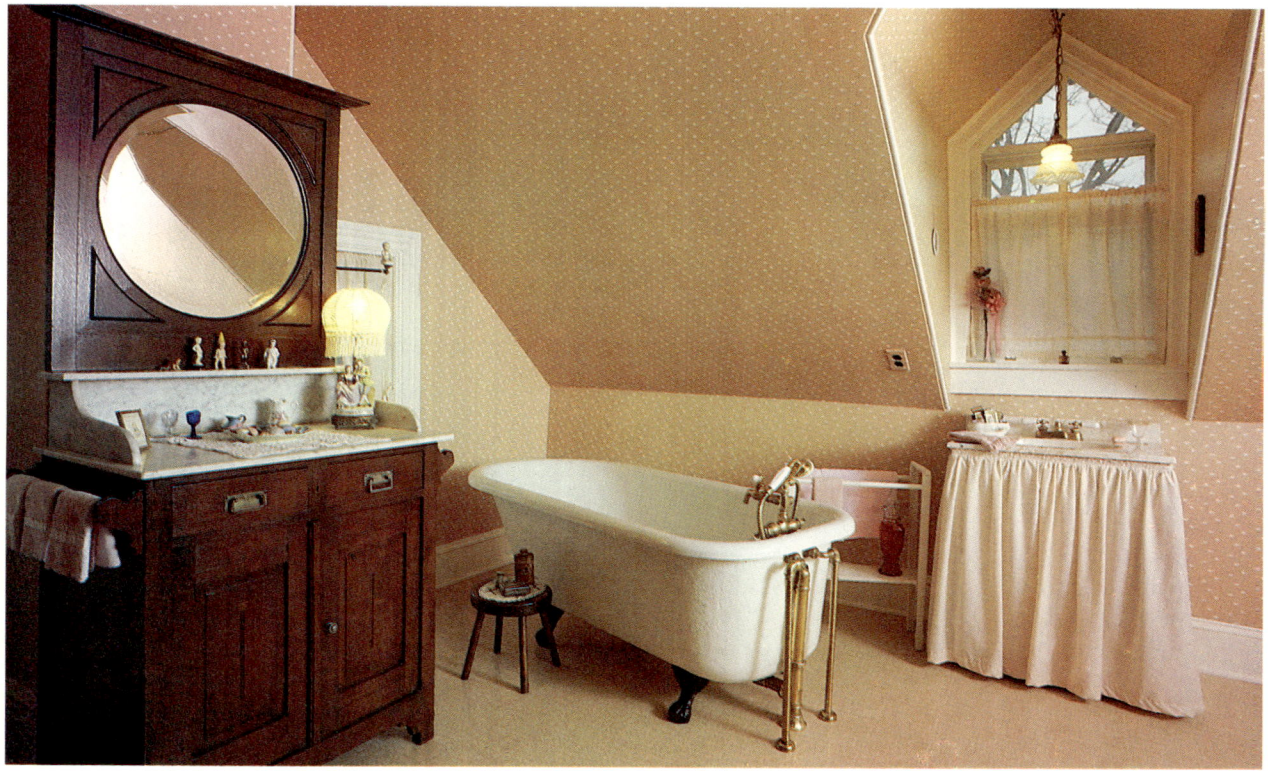

The sloping ceiling and the dormer window in this third-floor attic bath add to its cozy and inviting decor.

Walking through the seashore town of Cape May, New Jersey, is like walking into the past. Located far from the glamour and glitz of Atlantic City, Cape May recaptures yesteryear with its tree-lined streets and Victorian bed-and-breakfast inns and houses. Joyce and Spurgeon Smith are the proud proprietors of one of these Victorian homes.

The Smiths purchased their little cottage in June of 1984, but charming seaside home it was not. Built in 1883, the house had served as a summer home for many years before the Smiths bought it, and it was not in the best of shape. As with many old houses, its problems had been masked under layers of plywood paneling, gypsum board, and stucco. So the Smiths stripped the house to its bare bones and started over, with an eye toward comfort and nostalgia.

What emerged was White Dove Cottage, a home restored with lots of love and care—and elbow grease. Spurgeon drew

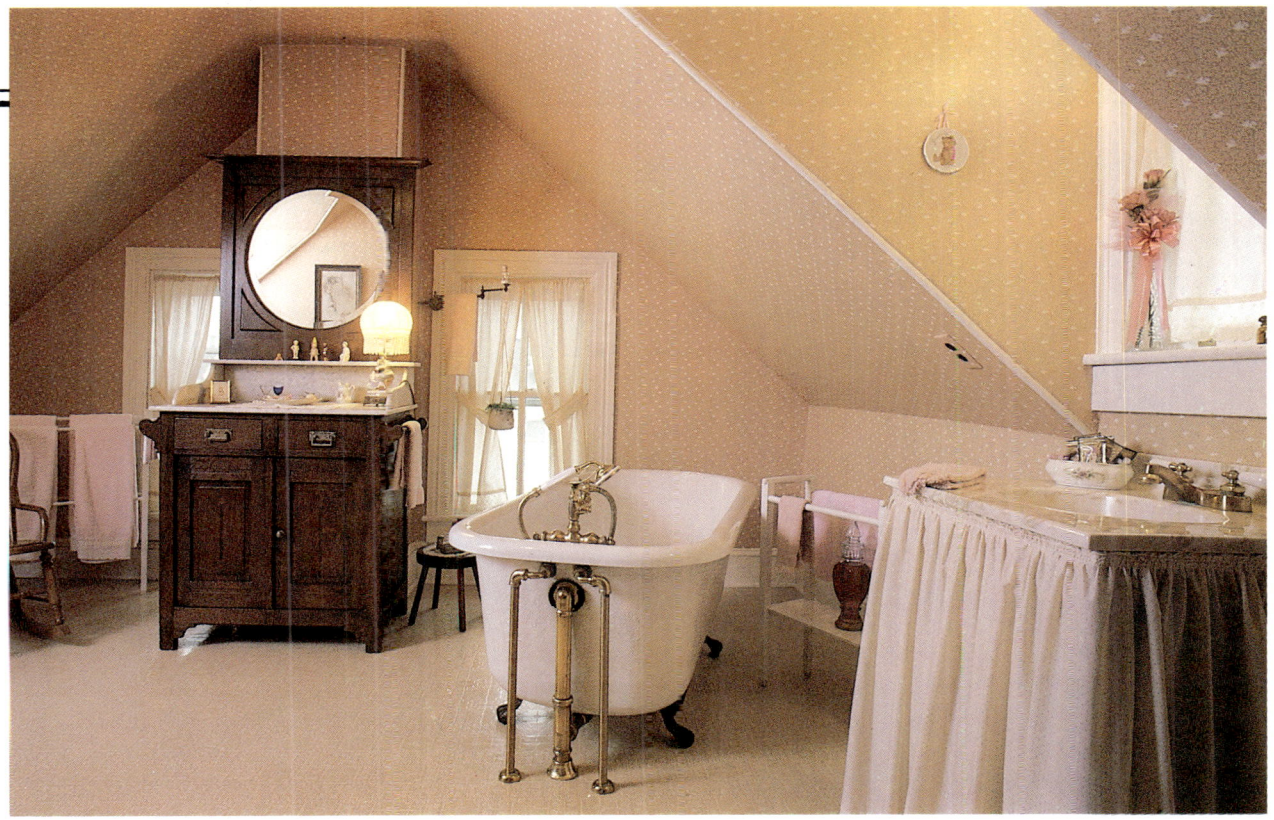

Although this bath has an old-fashioned look, almost everything is new—even the claw-foot tub.

the floor plans for every room and did most of the construction work himself, while Joyce lent her artful eye to interior decorating. The guest suite in their home is comprised of a bedroom, sitting room, and bath. It was the bath that caught our eye.

Located in what had been the third-floor attic of the cottage, the bath is cozy and charming, a vestige of the past. But although it looks truly authentic, most everything in the room is new. Even the fixtures—including the wonderful claw-foot tub—are reproductions. "We wanted the old-time look," Spurgeon says, "but the old cast-iron fixtures would have been too heavy for the old attic floor." The sink vanity, in fact, was a damaged model the couple found at a plumbing-supply store; Joyce's hand-sewn fabric skirt dressed it up and gave it a new lease on life.

Placement of the fixtures in the bath was pretty much dictated by the room's configuration—more specifically by the sloping attic roof. The tub sits in the middle of the room because if it were anywhere else, a person would certainly "conk his head on the ceiling," Spurgeon explains. Yet the Smiths like the tub's dramatic, center-stage presence in the room. The sink and toilet are located underneath the attic's two Gothic dormer windows to compensate for the sloping ceiling.

Special decorative touches like pretty pastel wallpaper, an old-fashioned washstand with an antique mirror and a marble top, lacy curtains, and an assortment of treasures make the bath homey and inviting—just as it might have been in 1883.

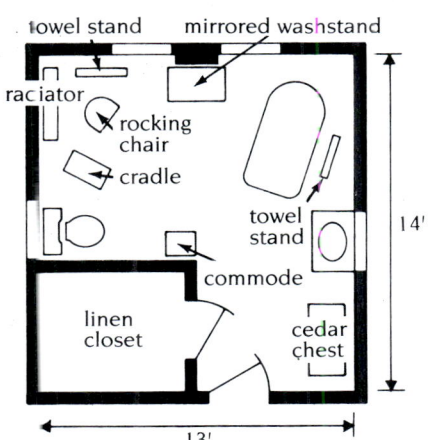

# A Spa with a View of Pikes Peak

The site that Susan and Tom Tucker chose a few years ago for their home was nothing short of breathtaking. It's a natural balcony in the mountains of Colorado with a spectacular view of Pikes Peak to the south and extensive pine forests to the north and east.

In keeping with the grandeur of the site, architect Dominique Gettliffe and builder Lee Cerioni of Terra-Sol, designed an equally spectacular house. The 3,300-square-foot structure is completely solar-heated, and its windows command incredible views of the alpine scenery. But the 12-foot waterfall that cascades from the great room into a light-filled spa room below is its most striking feature.

The waterfall is the realization of one of Tom Tucker's lifelong dreams. While growing up, Tom often visited with an aunt and uncle whose mountain home had an indoor waterfall. And he always dreamed of one day having his own mountain home with its own waterfall.

The spectacular Pikes Peak view from the Tuckers' sunspace makes a soak in the spa all the more relaxing.

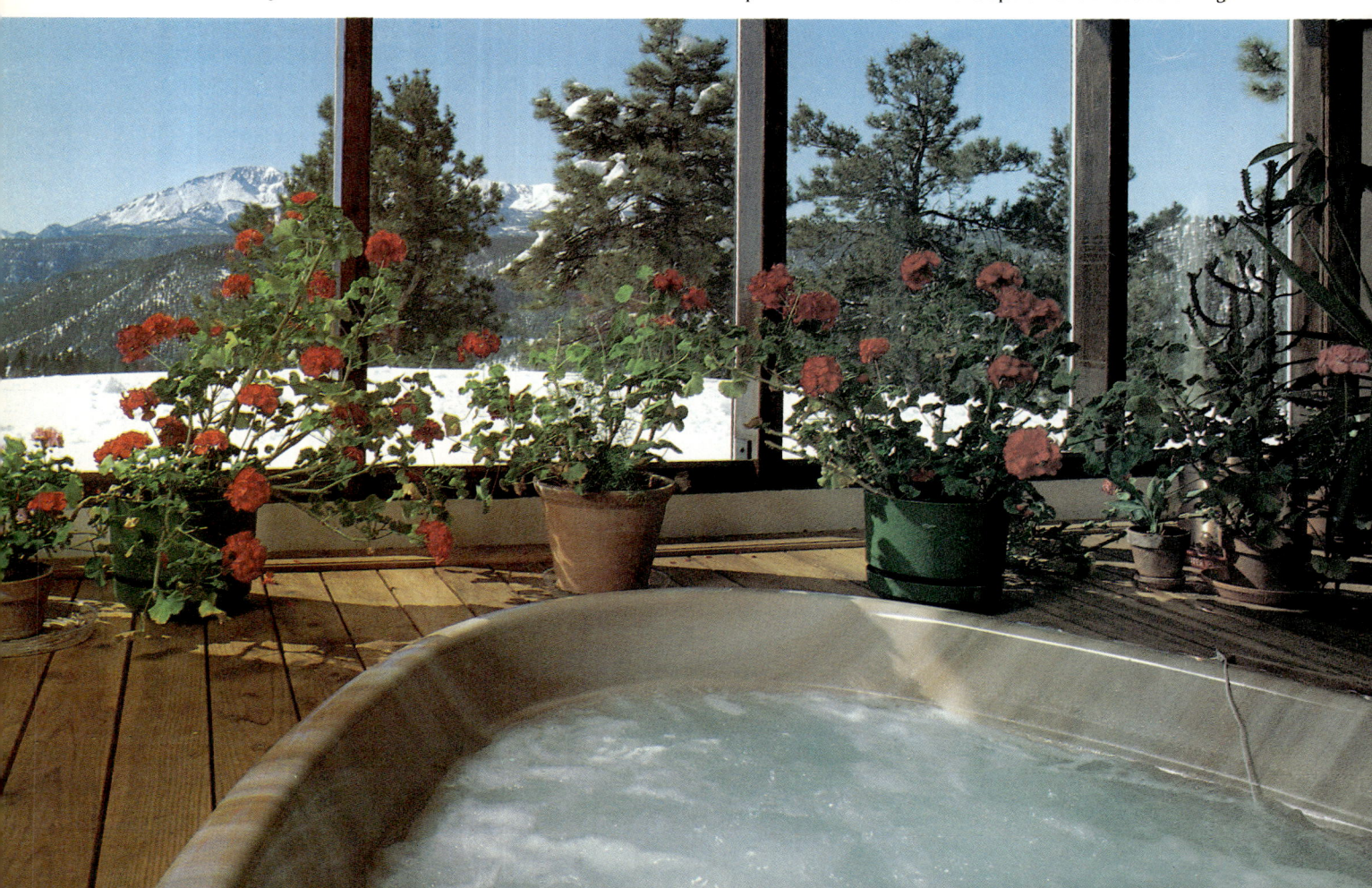

This waterfall, however, is more than just a pretty sight. Built of masonry, it receives direct sunlight from a summer room and skylights directly above the spa room. With its 50,000 pounds of concrete mass and the 120 gallons of water contained in its pools, the waterfall is a solar collector that provides a substantial amount of heat for the house.

The spa room itself is comfortably cool in the summer and warm in the winter, as the sun—lower in the sky during this time of year—streams in through the room's many windows almost all day long. Ventilation is not a problem. Excess heat and moisture generated by the waterfall and spa rise to the summer room above, where large fans distribute it to colder areas of the house during the winter. In the summertime, the excess heat is vented outside the house.

Besides being a marvelous feat of solar engineering, the waterfall provides aesthetic benefits as well. Its tumbling and gurgling create a soothing atmosphere in the room and make a soak in the large spa even more relaxing. "It's a getaway room," Susan Tucker says of the spa room. "We go down there to get away from the kids for a while, and they go down there to get away from us!" A dressing room is situated just off the spa room for convenience. Stereo sound, piped in through several strategically placed speakers, makes spending time there even more enjoyable.

The room's environment is ideally suited to its natural outdoor surroundings. It is simply decorated, with lots of Susan's plants and a few well-chosen landscape prints.

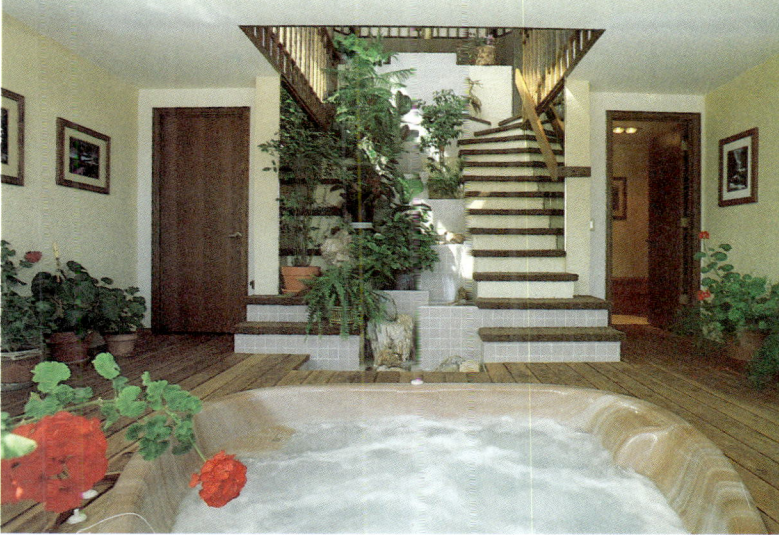

The masonry waterfall built into the staircase provides aesthetics as well as humidity for the house and thermal mass for solar collection. Susan Tucker's tropical plants thrive in the spa room's humid atmosphere.

Earthy redwood floors, ceiling beams, and landing and stair railings work to bring the forest inside. Some accent and night lighting is provided by hanging fixtures, but most of the room's illumination comes from sunlight that streams in through six skylights above and the floor-to-ceiling picture windows on the room's south wall—which provide a breathtaking, bird's-eye view of Pikes Peak.

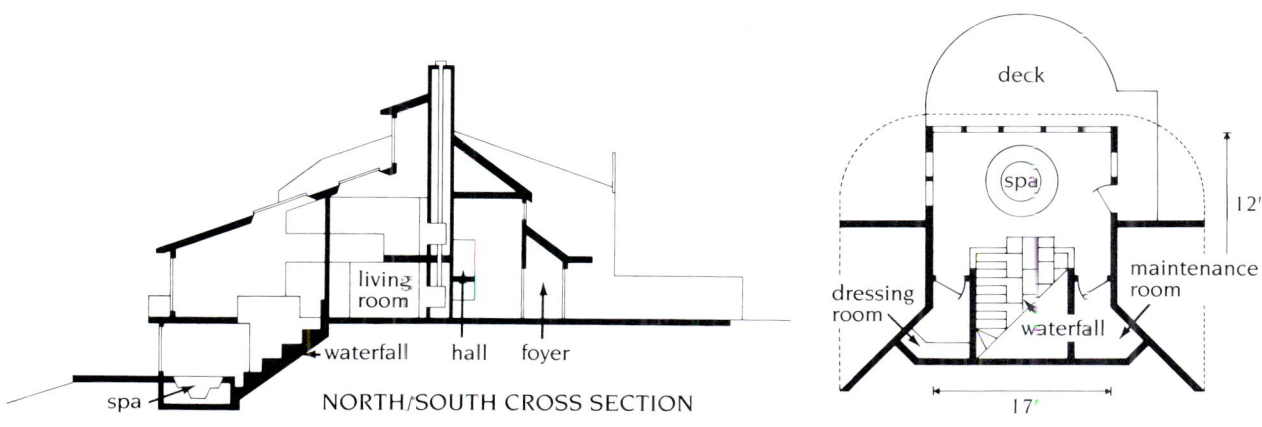

# An Atrium Spa—Underground

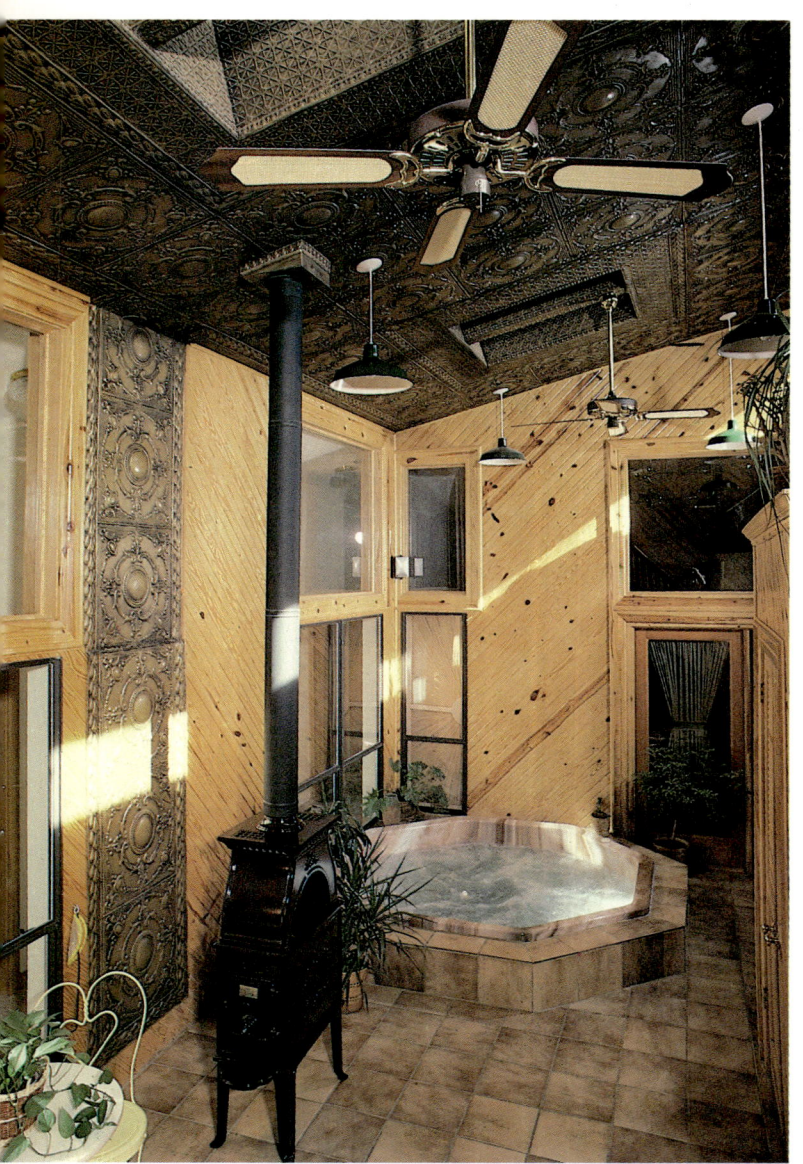

The first thing to catch your eye in the Greers' atrium is its beautiful ceiling, made of hand-pressed, hand-stained tin.

The spa room in the Oklahoma home of Marsha and Scott Greer is beautiful, but when you realize it's an atrium in an underground home, it becomes even more fantastic.

Only about one-fourth of the home's total surface area (3,584 square feet) is visible from the outside world. Gradually sloping ceilings start at 18 feet in the atrium and decrease to a height of just 7½ feet at the rear of the structure. Scott drew up the floor plans for the house; Joe Hylton, an architect and the author of Earth Sheltered and Solar Homes: A Book of Plans (Norman, Oklahoma: Joe Hylton Publishing Company, 1984) helped him to refine those plans and put them into action.

The atrium is more than just a pretty entryway for the Greers' home; in fact, it is probably the most important area of the house. Clerestory windows above the wall between the atrium and the living room and two skylights flood the room with natural light during the day. Since it is the only room in the house with windows above ground, the rooms surrounding the atrium have access to daylight through windows in the atrium's walls. Put simply, virtually all the natural light for the house comes from this room—it's a sunspace in the truest sense of that word. Utility lamps suspended from the lofty ceiling provide soft, incandescent light at night.

The atrium provides warmth as well as light. A woodstove located next to the spa is a major source of heat in the house (along with a solar greenhouse on the south-facing living room wall). Since it can get bitterly cold in central Oklahoma during the winter, this room performs a vital function for the family.

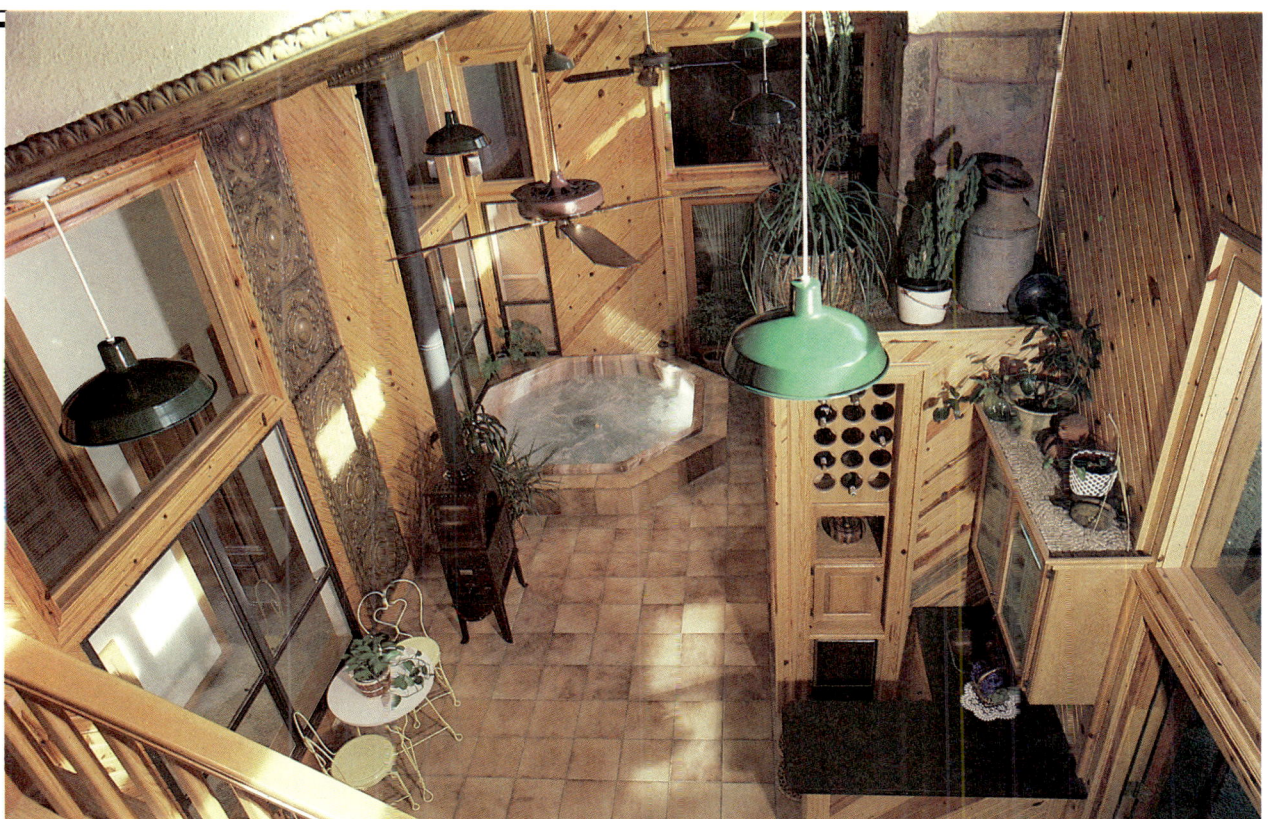

The atrium not only serves as a spa room but also provides a majority of the light and heat for the Greers' underground home.

Besides serving basic needs, though, the atrium is cozy and inviting and sets the tone for decor in the rest of the house. Warm, yellow pine graces the walls, door trims, and window sashes, and the floor and tub surround are covered with sand-colored ceramic tile. "We really like earthy colors," says Scott. The imported Danish woodstove complements the room's elegantly rustic design, and a built-in wine rack and wet bar make it an entertainment center for the Greers.

By far the most eye-catching attraction of the sunspace is its ceiling. Truly a work of art, it is constructed of tin and was hand-painted and stained by craftsmen at Structural Antiques in Edmond, Oklahoma, to produce its desired, well-seasoned complexion. ("We're antique collectors," Scott explains.) Casablanca fans heighten the effect. Although the ceiling is brand new, its history, as well as its paint job, gives it a wonderful, old-time feel. The ceiling, made in a factory in Missouri that recently reopened after a 50-year dormancy, was hand-pressed with the same equipment used there during the 1920s.

The Greers have four small children, and the couple has often talked about putting another spa outdoors. "With all the kids it gets to be a real splashing production," Scott says. But the couple knows that children grow up, and they will soon learn to appreciate the beauty and warmth of this unique room.

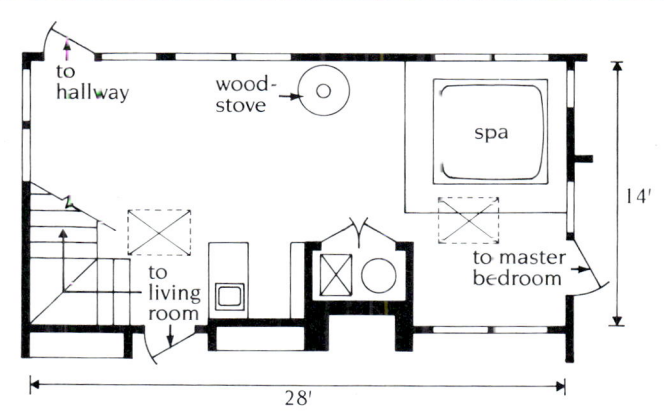

# Small Baths

The baths that follow share a unique quality. They look great while they are also clever uses of very small spaces. For example, it is possible to have a full bath in a space that is just 5 by 7½ feet, as in the Heinemeyer bath. Creative floor plans and special fixtures are just two ways that allow small spaces to give big results. In this section you'll see other ways to "make" space.

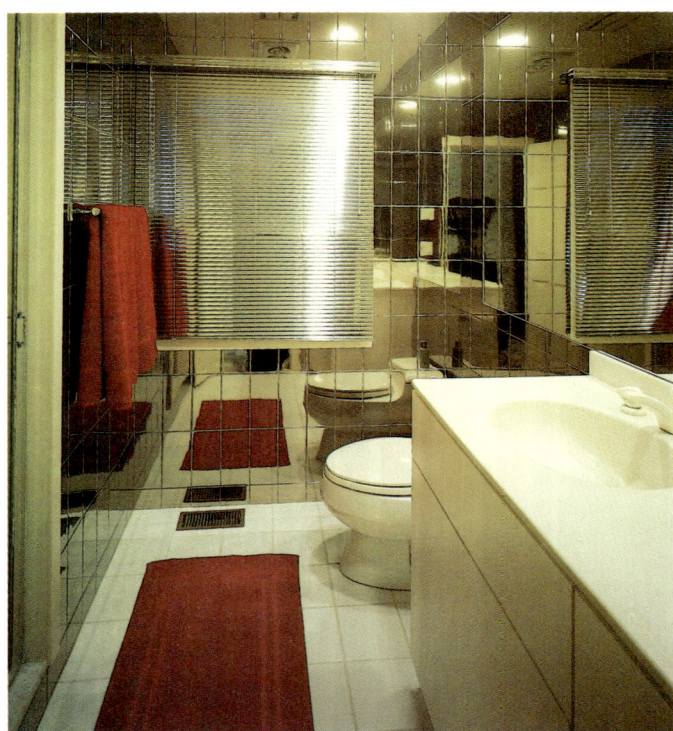

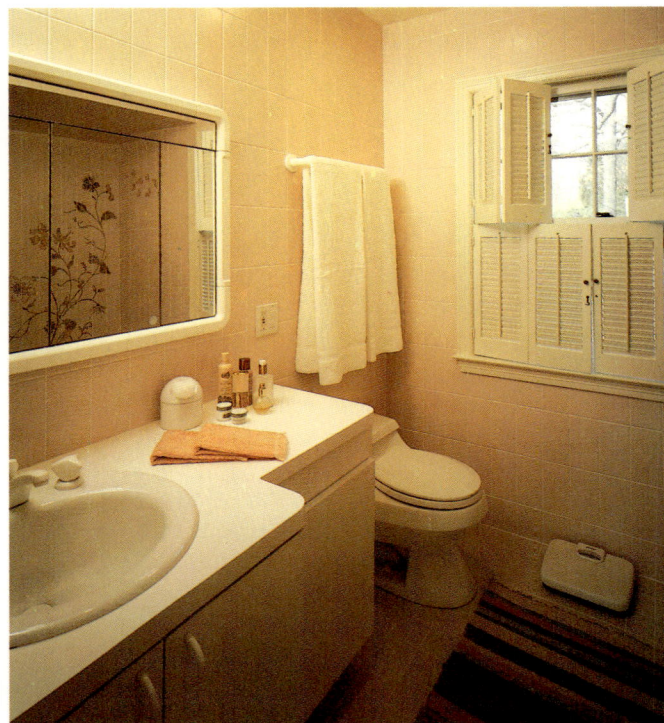

**His and Hers:** Many couples think that a master bath should be one gigantic room. Not Heidi and Gregory Bathon. Busy executives who have different styles, schedules, and needs, they wanted their own separate spaces for bathing and grooming. So instead of creating one big master bath, designer Janine Newlin, CKD, ISID, divided the available space in half to produce double baths. Each serves the needs of the person it was designed for. Heidi, for instance, wanted a pretty atmosphere and a deep steeping tub, while husband Gregory preferred a more functional look and a large shower with several body sprays. The two baths share a common plumbing wall, which made layout and installation of fixtures fairly easy.

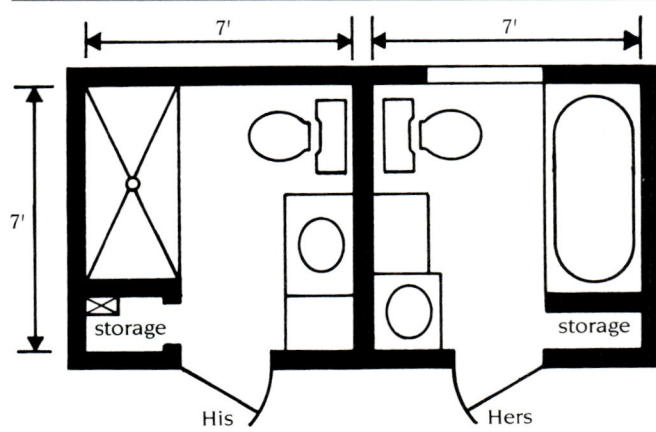

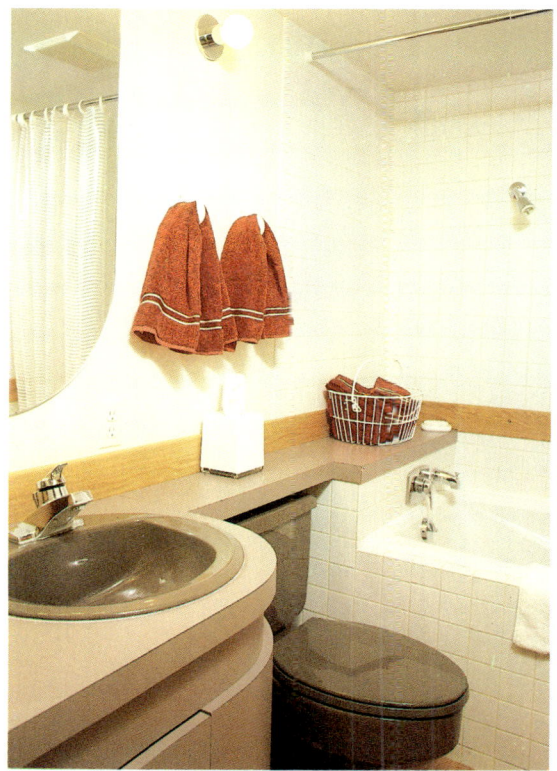

**Fitting It All In:** The guest bath in Diana and Richard Heinemeyer's house is a perfect example of how smart design can turn a tiny space into a livable one. An architect by profession, Richard didn't have much space to work with—just 5 by 7½ feet. Yet he wanted a whirlpool tub, a shower, and a respectable amount of storage space. The tub presented the biggest problem. To solve it, Heinemeyer chose an extra-deep model; it's shorter than a standard-size tub, but the added depth provides plenty of soaking room. To create the illusion of more space, Heinemeyer rounded the corners of the vanity and extended the laminate countertop from wall to wall to provide extra storage. The room has everything you might want in a bath—in half the space.

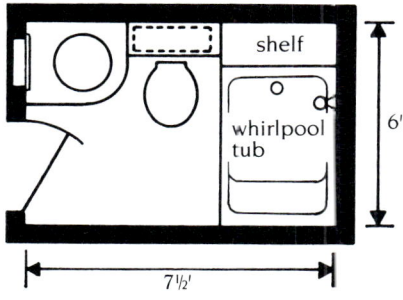

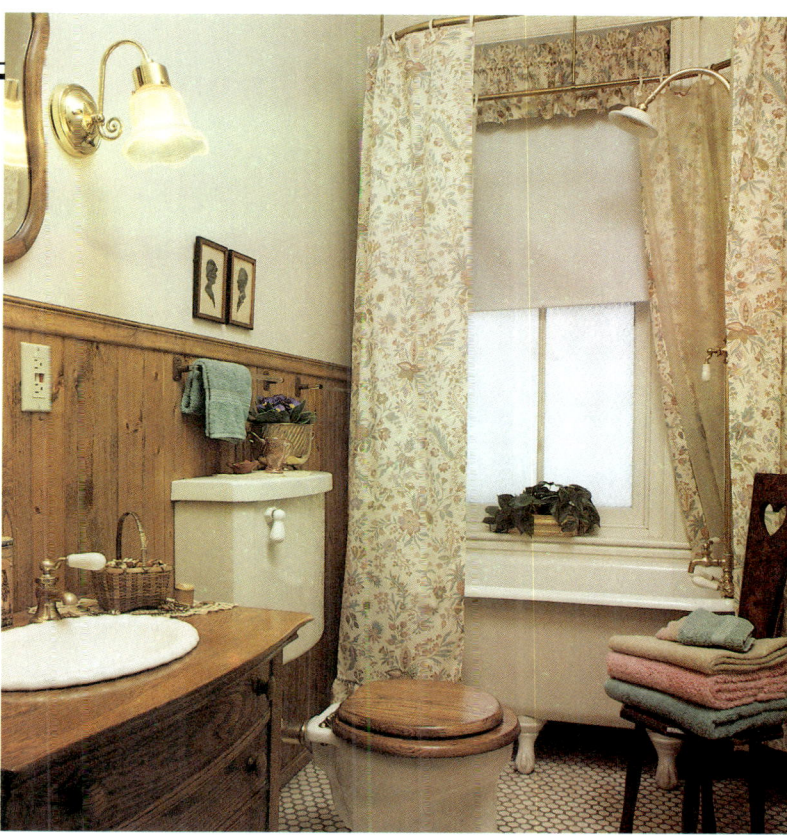

**Victorian Charm:** The original bath in Susan Weaver's turn-of-the-century townhouse was, in her own words, "absolutely unlivable." There was a hole in the floor, the fixtures were unattractive, and their awkward placement had resulted in an atrocious use of space. "The radiator was the centerpiece of the bath," she says. When she began the inevitable remodeling, the fixtures were the first things to go. Since space was limited, Susan chose a 4-foot antique tub and had it professionally refinished; new brass hardware and a floral-print shower curtain dress it up nicely. The toilet, too, is salvaged. Susan refinished the antique washstand and beveled-mirror frame as well as the new pine wainscoting; all are polyurethaned to prevent water spotting. The fixtures and special nostalgic touches give this bath the charm of years gone by.

BEFORE    AFTER

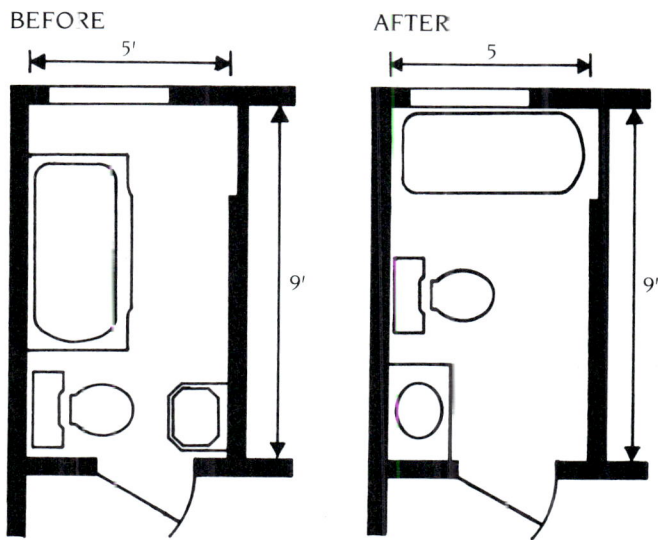

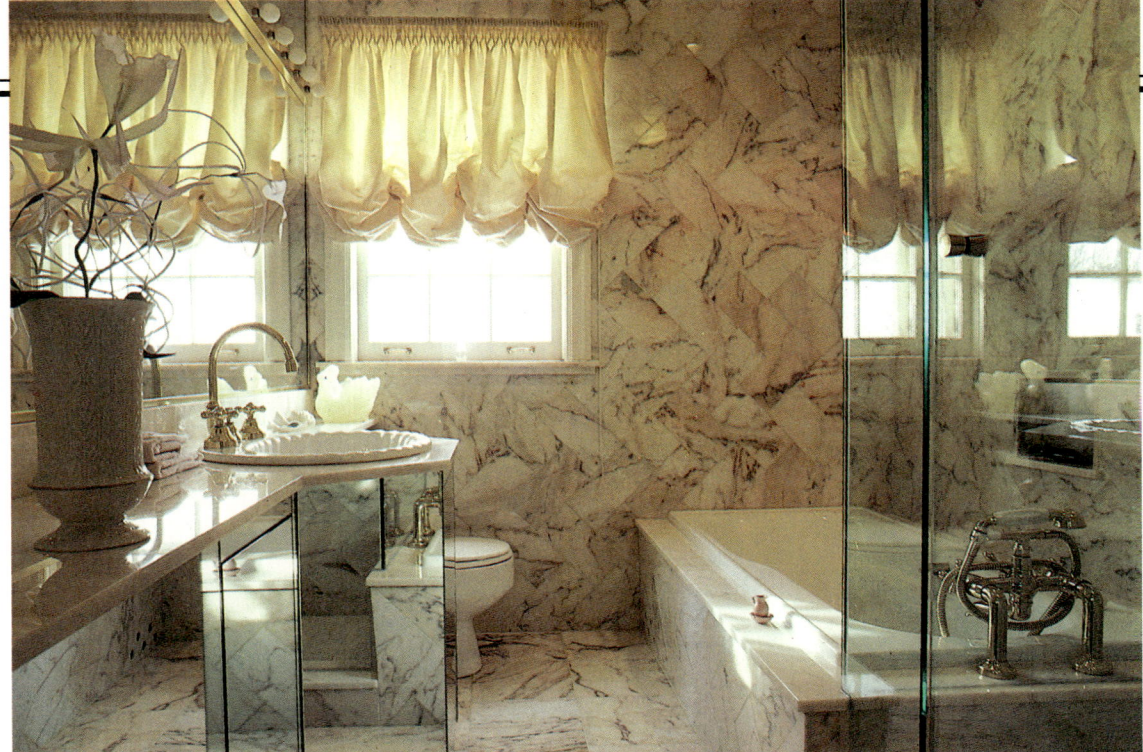

**Pretty and Feminine:** With its cotton-candy-colored walls and floors, balloon shade, and pretty European fixtures and faucets, this bath is a young girl's dream. But besides being a lovely place to spend time, this second-floor bath in Joan Silver's house is also a study in space-making design. It was a narrow room to start with, not more than 5½ feet wide. Yet Joan wanted a vanity big enough for storage, a *separate* shower stall and tub, and plenty of space for walking around. For the shower stall, Karen Nelson of Ginger's Bathrooms installed a double-paneled, tempered-glass enclosure just behind the tub and used a deck-mounted tub filler with a cradle for a hand-held sprayer. The glass opens the space and keeps the bath from looking cramped. Mirrored cabinetry that is tailored around the sink allows sufficient storage and more room for moving around. And the pretty marble tile gives the bath a soft, feminine look—perfect for a girl of any age.

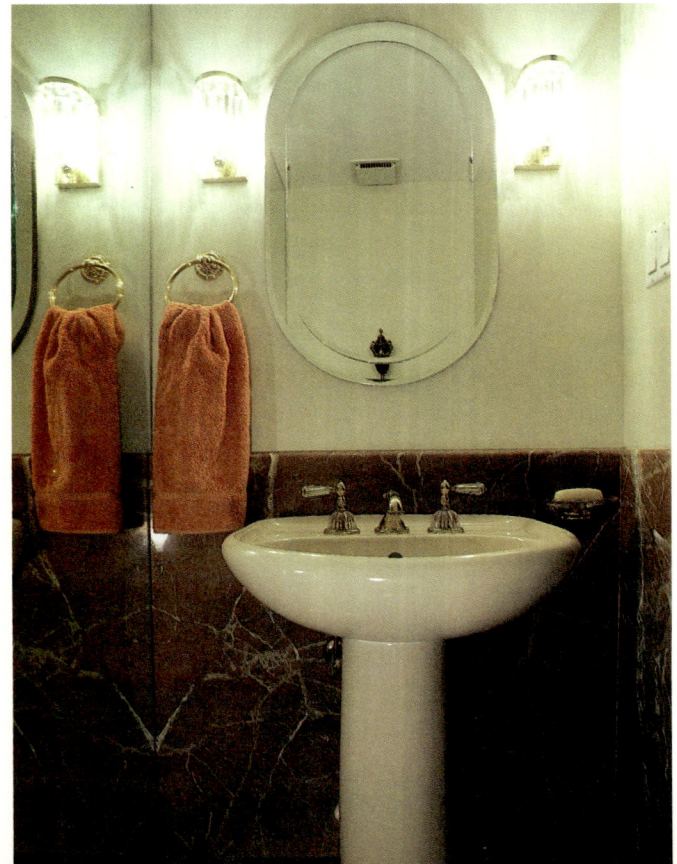

**A Bath in a Closet:** Heather and Allen Scott didn't like the idea of having guests trudge upstairs to use the children's bath. So they decided to create a main-floor powder room—in a coat closet. Designer Barbara Munn borrowed extra space from the kitchen and tapped into kitchen pipes to provide plumbing facilities for a sink and toilet. A mirrored wall helps to open and brighten what would have been a tiny and very dark space. Since the bath is small, the Scotts were able to splurge on some luxurious features—like marble slabs on the floor and walls; an antique, beveled mirror; and lead-crystal light fixtures. The result is a luxurious little guest bath—which goes to show that you never know what you might find in your closet.

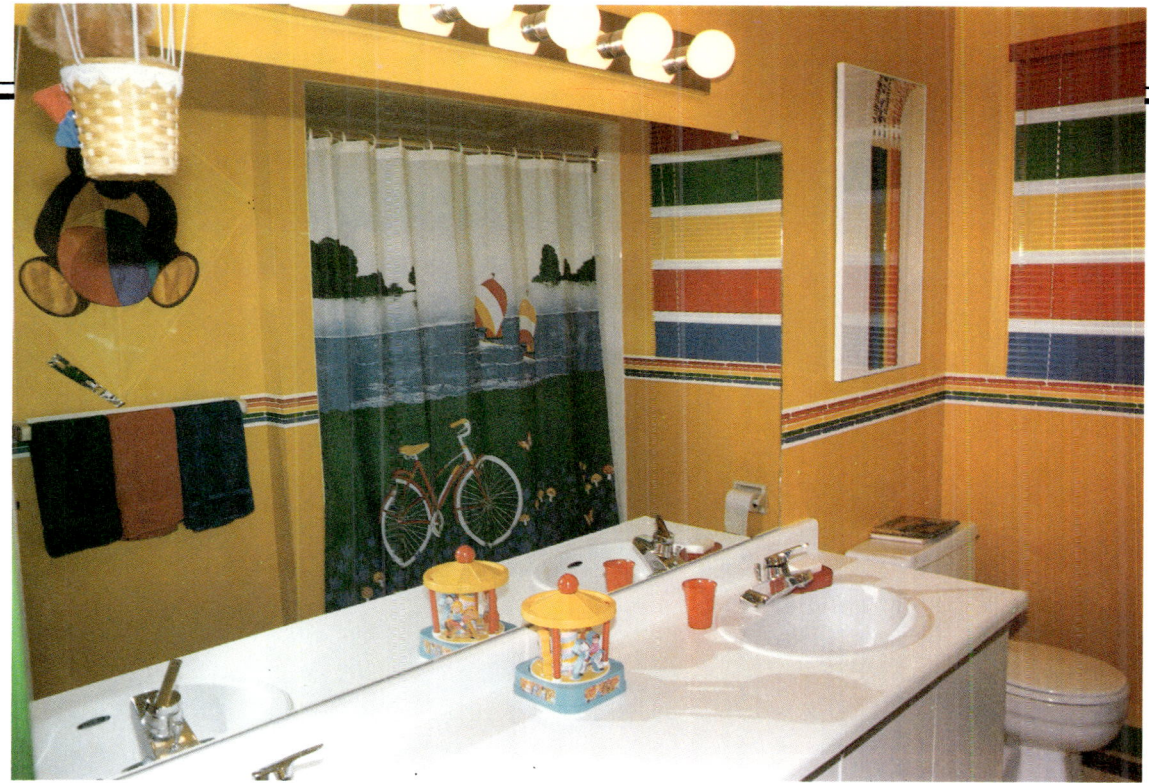

**Making Bath Time Playtime:** With its nondescript fixtures and finishes, the second-floor bath in Fern and Mitchell Larry's home didn't excite anyone—least of all the children for whom it was intended. So when the Larrys decided to remodel the bath, they called on Ann Louise of Children's Design Centre in Toronto, who in turn called on Brandon, Jonathan, and Erica, ages 7 to 2, to help her. Louise likes to involve children as much as possible in choosing colors and accoutrements for their bathrooms. And this bath is testimony to the success of her strategy. Filled with wonderful shapes and lots of bright colors, chosen by the children and woven together by Louise, the bath is a child's delight. Says Fern Larry: "The kids who visit our house just go wild when they see it."

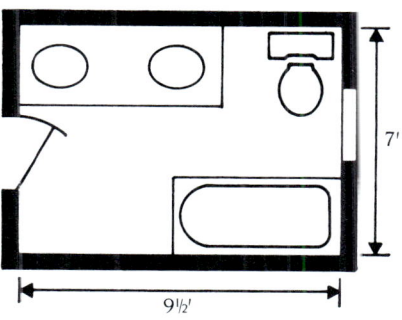

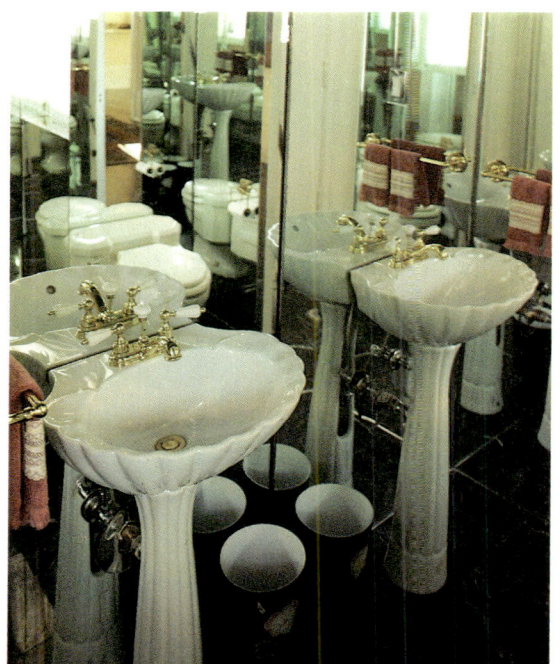

**Mirror, Mirror on the Wall:** They're on every wall in this little powder room in Joan Silver's home, and for good reason. The original bath had been a terribly dismal and tiny space—just 5 feet by about 30 inches! While Karen Nelson of Ginger's Bathrooms could easily turn ugly into beautiful, she could not create any more actual space in the bath. So she relied on space-stretchers—like the mirrors. They run floor to ceiling in the bath, and the room literally grows to twice its size because of them. Nelson also chose tiny fixtures for the bath: The basin of the imported Portuguese pedestal sink is just 19 inches in diameter, and the one-piece, low-profile Kohler toilet is one of the smallest available. Solid brass imported faucets and a marble floor add touches of luxury to a bath you'd never guess was so tiny.

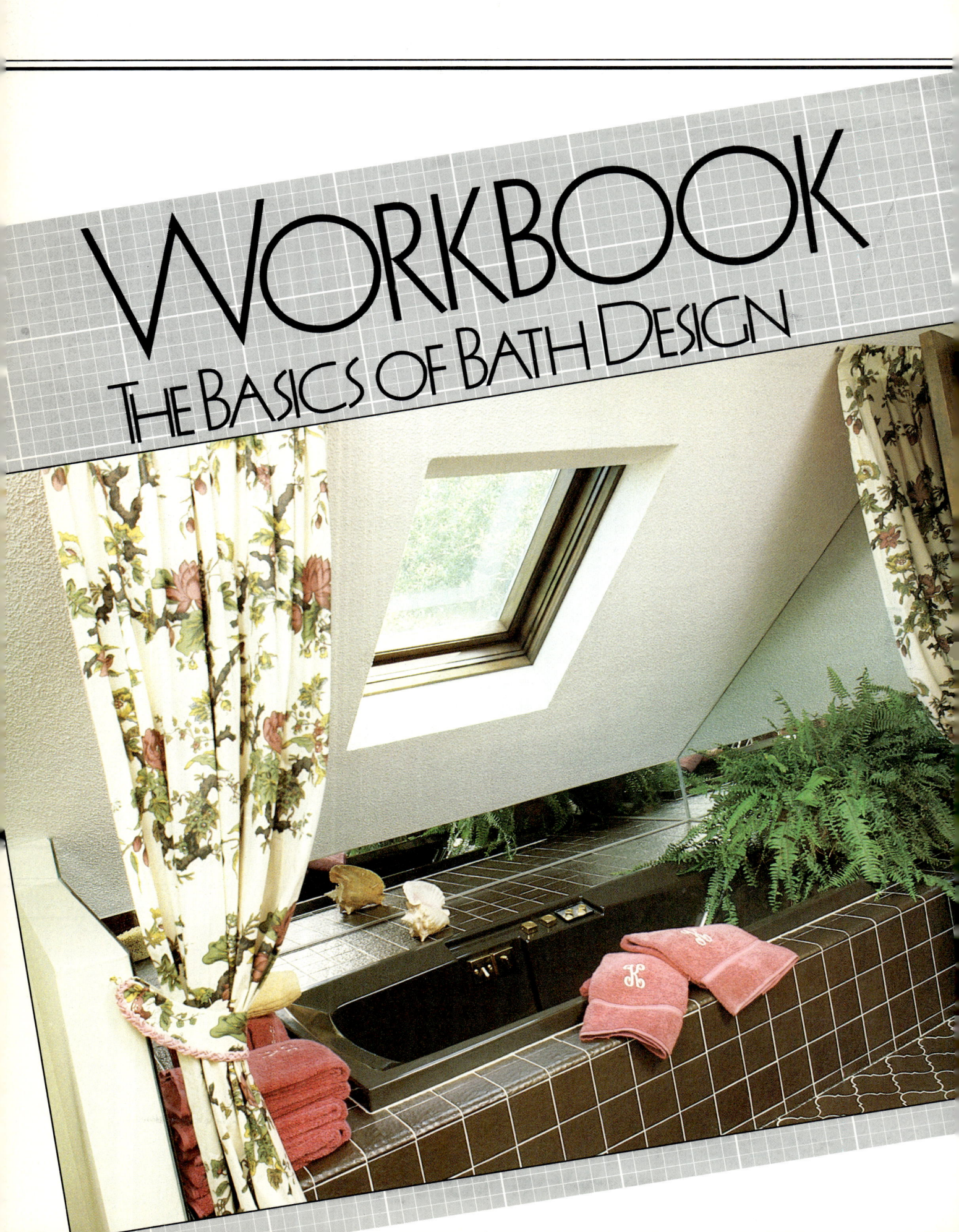

# WORKBOOK
## THE BASICS OF BATH DESIGN

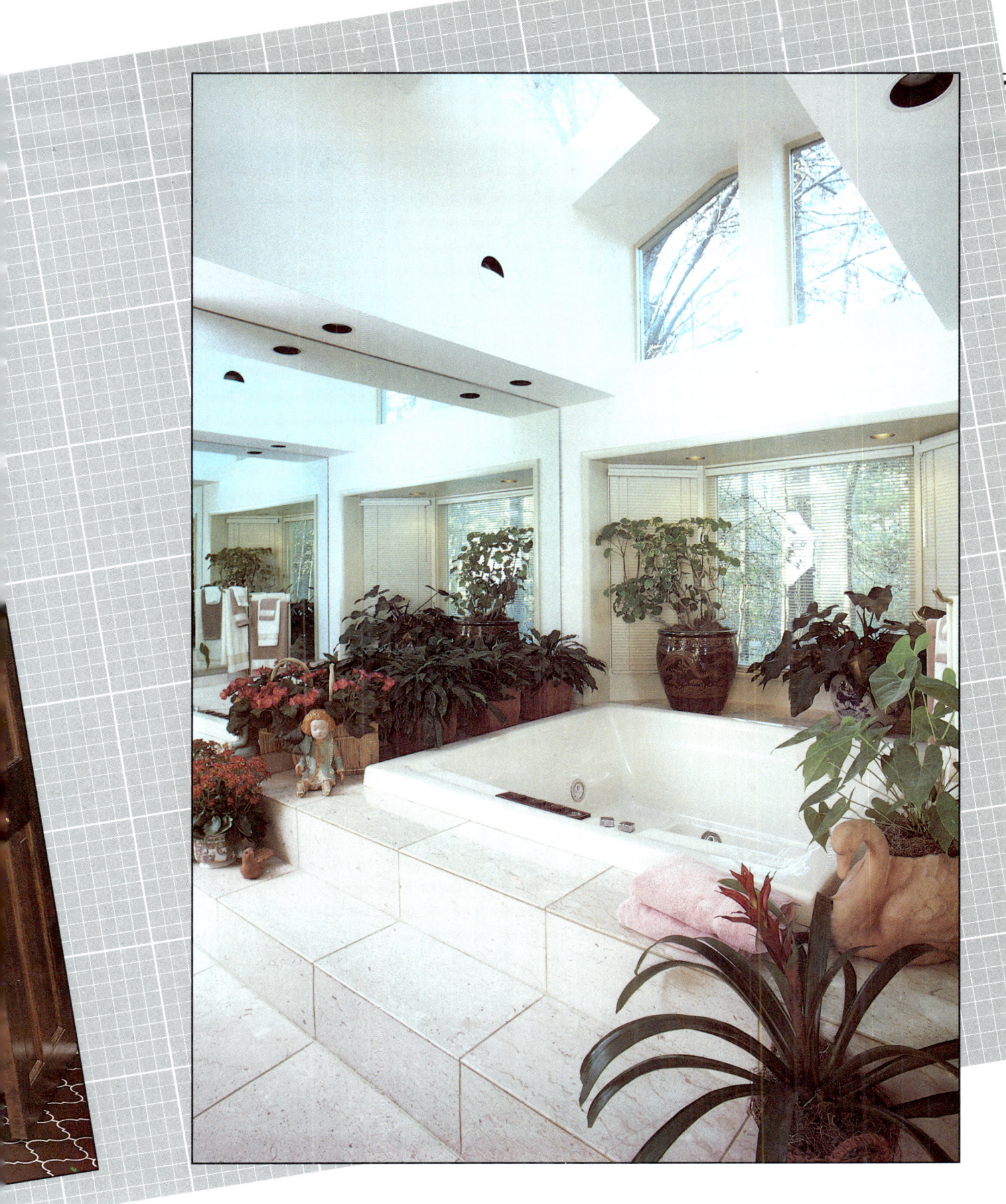

# Designing Your New Bath

How many times have you heard about homeowners who have spent thousands of dollars on a remodeling project—only to be completely dissatisfied with it when it was finished? In many cases, the cause of dissatisfaction can be traced back to a lack of adequate planning. Without enough attention paid to decision making, details slip through the cracks, and unforeseen problems crop up.

The lesson to be learned of course, is that the more time you spend planning your bath, the less chance there will be of your ending up with a room you don't like. You'll know exactly what you want in your bath, and exactly what it takes to get what you want. Planning and detailed decision making are what this workbook is all about.

The first five chapters of this book are devoted to ideas and concepts, laying before you all the possibilities in bath design. The workbook will help you dig in and put these ideas to work. It will help you to make choices based on your needs and your budget and guide you in turning your dream bath into a reality.

It discusses details, like drawing up a floor plan for your bath and making a budget. Even if you plan to hire an architect or designer for the entire project, you will still need to supply that professional with a clear, concise idea of what you want your bath to look like. By planning ahead, you'll be able to communicate your needs more distinctly.

The information in the workbook will help you to establish a good working relationship with the designers, builders, crafts people, and other contractors who will be working on your bathroom. It's important to state your requirements in the very beginning, before any contracts are drawn up. Contracts should serve as sources of mutual understanding and clarification, not confusion, and the information here will help you to attend to this important, but often neglected, detail. Remember to have all contracts reviewed by a lawyer.

"Keep Your Bath Bright" (see page 142) gives lots of hints on how to maintain the beauty of your new bath for years to come.

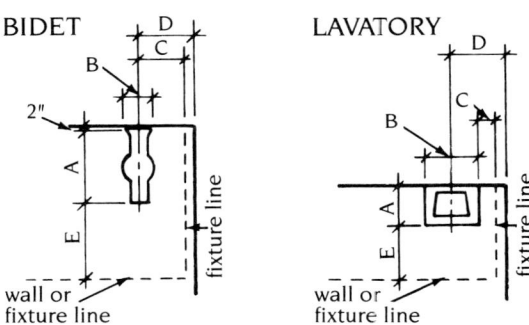

## Fixture Sizes and Clearances

| Dimension | Bidet | | Lavatory | |
|---|---|---|---|---|
| | Minimum (inches) | Liberal (inches) | Minimum (inches) | Liberal (inches) |
| A | 25 | 27 | 16 | 21 |
| B | 14 | 14 | 18 | 30 |
| C | 12 | 18 | 2 | 6 |
| D | 15 | 22 | 14 | 22 |
| E | Wall—18 Fixture—18 | Wall—36 Fixture—34 | 18 | 30 |

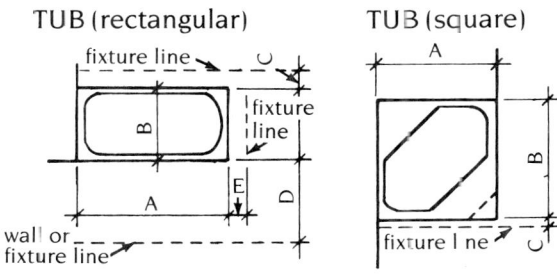

"Helpful Addresses," which begins on page 144, is a list of manufacturers of bath and related products that we have included for your convenience. Always compare prices, performance reports, and warranty terms before you purchase fixtures or other materials. Your bathroom is an investment; choose its components wisely.

## Drawing a Floor Plan

Before you even think about discussing your new bath with a designer, get a plan in mind. It's best to have a definite idea of what you want before calling in an expert. Only *you* know your family's habits and needs, and a beautiful bathroom is not necessarily an efficient bathroom.

The best thing to do is to sit down with paper and pencil and start exploring the possibilities. Ask yourself some questions: How many fixtures will you need in your bath? How big should they be? How many people will use the bath? Where will traffic be the heaviest? Will you compartmentalize? Will the bath have windows? How many doors will it need? You will also need to consider fixture sizes and clearances.

As you consider your own needs, take a look at the examples of the fixture sizes and clearances and bathroom floor plans provided here.[1] They should give you an idea of at least a few of the options you have. Be thorough, but have fun!

### Fixture Sizes and Clearances

|  | Tub (rectangle) | | Tub (square) | |
|---|---|---|---|---|
| Dimension | Minimum (inches) | Liberal (inches) | Minimum (inches) | Liberal (inches) |
| A | 60 standard | 72 | 38 | — |
| B | 30 standard | 42 | 39 | — |
| C | 2 | 8 | 2 | 4 |
| D | Wall—20 Fixture—18 | Wall—34 Fixture—30 | — | — |
| E | 2 | 8 | — | — |

### Fixture Sizes and Clearances

|  | Shower | | Toilet | |
|---|---|---|---|---|
| Dimension | Minimum (inches) | Liberal (inches) | Minimum (inches) | Liberal (inches) |
| A | 32 | 36 | 27 | 31 |
| B | 34 | 36 | 19 | 21 |
| C | 2 | 8 | 12 | 18 |
| D | 18 | 34 | 15 | 22 |
| E | — | — | Wall—18 Fixture—18 | Wall—36 Fixture—34 |

[1]. The illustrations on pages 124-25 and 126 (top) are reprinted, by permission of John Wiley & Sons, from *Architectural Graphic Standards*, 7th ed., Robert T. Packard, ed., copyright © 1981 by John Wiley & Sons.

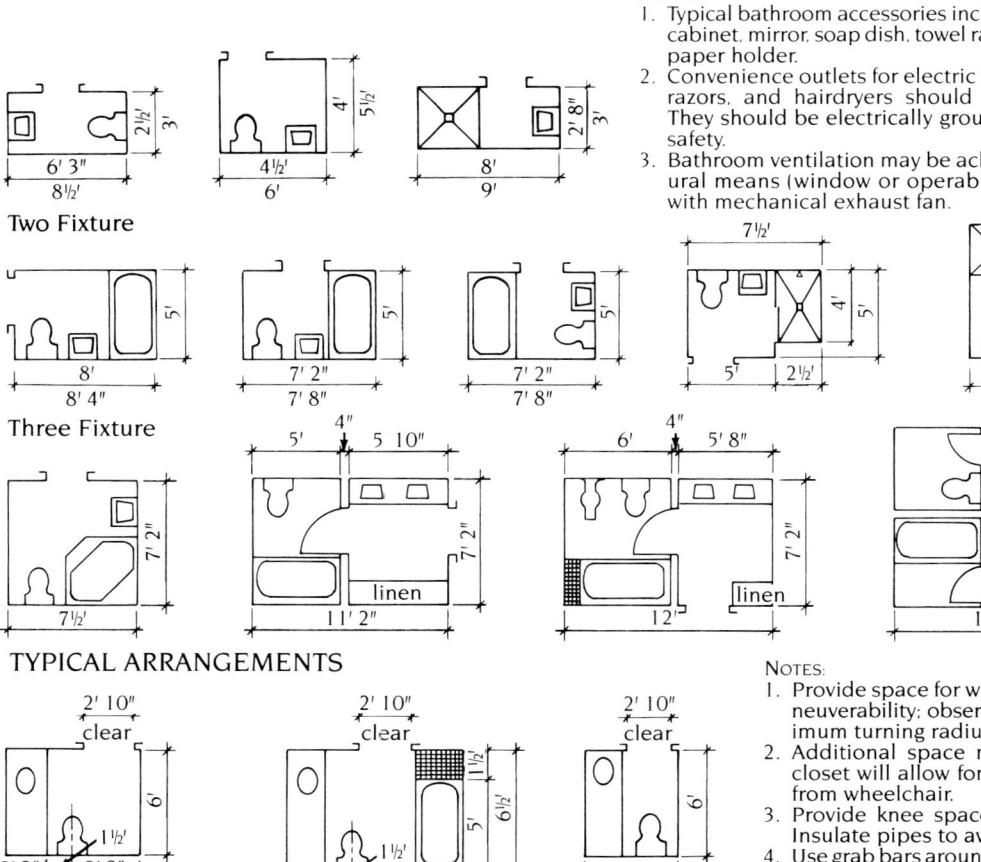

NOTES:
1. Typical bathroom accessories include medicine cabinet, mirror, soap dish, towel rack, and toilet-paper holder.
2. Convenience outlets for electric toothbrushes, razors, and hairdryers should be provided. They should be electrically grounded for user safety.
3. Bathroom ventilation may be achieved by natural means (window or operable skylight) or with mechanical exhaust fan.

NOTES:
1. Provide space for wheelchair maneuverability; observe 5-foot minimum turning radius.
2. Additional space next to water closet will allow for side transfer from wheelchair.
3. Provide knee space under sink. Insulate pipes to avoid scalding.
4. Use grab bars around water closet and tub.
5. Roll-in shower may replace tub and is more convenient for many wheelchair-disabled.
6. Bathroom door to be minimum 32-inch clear opening and to swing outward. Use lever hardware on both sides.

## One Designer's Solutions

Ellen Cheever, CKD, ASID, a practicing bathroom designer, has often faced the challenge of squeezing more bathroom space into a variety of homes. We asked her to share some of her case studies, illustrating solutions to some common problems.

### Bathroom Bumpout

The master bath in this house was cramped and poorly designed. Whoever used the vanity could not help obstructing the passage leading to both the closet and the claustrophobic room housing the toilet and small stall shower.

The only way to maintain the generous proportions of the walk-in closet was to build a 36-inch-deep addition to the house. To minimize the cost, the bumpout was planned so that it would fit beneath the existing roof overhang. The closet was moved, opening up a large area for a new tub, shower, and pedestal lavatory.

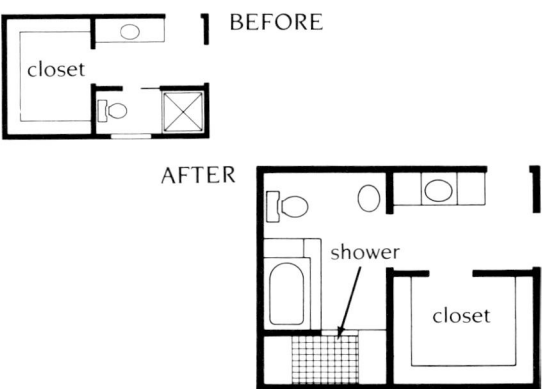

Wanting to keep their large walk-in closet while expanding the cramped master bath, these homeowners made room by adding a small bumpout under the existing roof overhang.

*An Inviting Place for Guests*

The hall bath was adequate for the two children in this family—but the space was not special enough for visitors. The solution: a powder room reserved for guests.

To create two bathrooms where there had been only one, the owners replaced the old tub with a spacious stall shower. They split the vanity into two grooming areas separated by a sliding door. Borrowing some space from the old bathroom, plus a few feet from an adjoining bedroom closet, they added a mirrored powder room with a pedestal lavatory. The closet did not even suffer: By raising the existing pole and adding another one at waist height, they were able to hang the same amount of clothing in the smaller space.

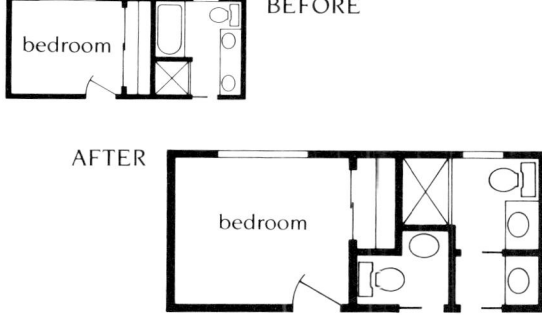

To add a small powder room reserved for visitors, the homeowners borrowed space from the existing family bath and an adjacent bedroom closet. The closet didn't even suffer: By adding a second pole for hanging garments, storage space was not reduced.

*Masterful Minibath*

This small home had only one bath for five family members. The owners had long wanted a master bathroom but did not know where to put it.

The answer involved making the bedroom slightly smaller, changing the proportions of the hall bath and using the existing toilet and tub for the newly created master bath. A small vanity can be closed off from the other fixtures by a sliding door. In the hall bath the old vanity stayed where it was, complemented by a new toilet and stall shower.

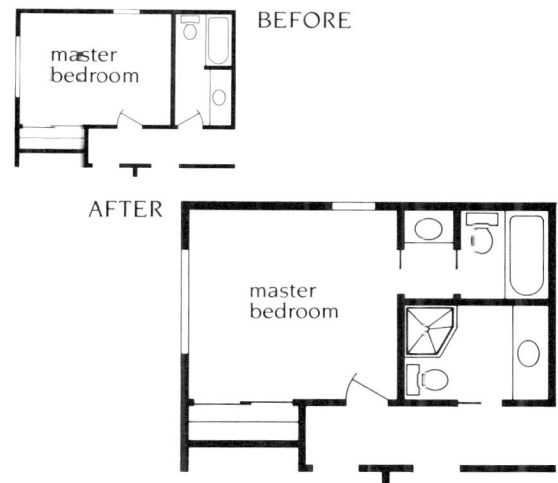

This original hall bath once served an entire family of five. By reshaping the old bath and borrowing floor space from the adjacent bedroom, the owners made room for a small master bath—making life more pleasant for the whole family.

*Rush-Hour Relief*

A busy family of six had one hall bath to serve four children—two girls and two boys. Morning bathroom time was a disaster. By rearranging the floor plan, they created two separate bathing facilities and three grooming stations.

To do it, they moved the closet in the girls' bedroom to the opposite wall. The old tub and toilet remained where they were, but became part of a "new" bathroom, accessible only from the girls' bedroom. The boys' new bathroom, complete with new toilet, single vanity, and stall shower, doubles as a powder room for guests.

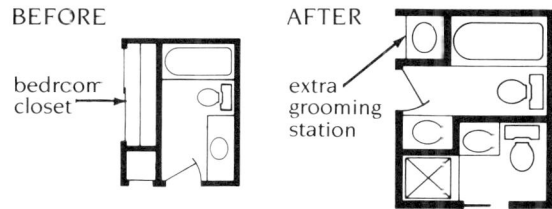

To meet the needs of four busy children, this hall bath was divided into two. The two boys use the reshaped hall bath; the girls use two new grooming stations, now accessible from a bedroom. The displaced closet was moved to another wall.

## Making Your Bathroom Safe

As benign as it might seem, the bathroom can pose some serious hazards—especially in a household with small children or elderly or physically impaired residents. With the right precautions, though, you can greatly reduce the risk of accident or injury in your bath. Here are some thoughts to keep in mind.

In any bathroom, but especially in one used by the elderly or very young children, use nonslip surfaces on floors and in showers and tubs. Save the shiny, slippery tiles for walls and backsplashes, and use a textured surface for floors and showers. Installing grab bars in the tub and shower further reduces the chance of slipping or falling.

Plan for a minimum of sharp corners in your bath. Rounded vanity edges are very popular these days and reduce the risk of injury to a small child. Shower doors also come with rounded edges; some styles are flush-mounted on the tub or floor, eliminating the grooved track that can often cause stubbed toes and stumbling.

If you *must* store medicines and cleaning products in your bathroom, make sure they are clearly labeled and out of the reach of children. (See "Store It Safely" on page 58.) Depending on the circumstances in your home, you may want to install child-proofing devices on cabinets, which allow adults access but keep children out. Remember, too, that cleaning chemicals are often flammable and should be stored in a cool, dry place away from unusually warm surfaces or open flames.

Burns can often occur when a shower is interrupted by a surprise blast of hot water—caused by the turning on of cold water in other areas of the house. To avoid this, consider a thermostatically controlled mixer faucet that will maintain a predetermined temperature throughout your shower. For children's bathrooms, *always* install mixer faucets that move through the cold setting before reaching hot; this will prevent the scalding of little fingers.

The combination of electricity and many water sources makes electrocution the single greatest danger in the bathroom. There are ways, however, to avoid this threat. When planning your bath, don't locate light switches where they might be reached by persons in the tub or shower. Keep battery-powered or electric toys out of the bathroom at all times. Remember to unplug *all* electrical appliances in the bathroom when they are not in use and to keep them out of a child's reach. And *never* use an electrical device—toothbrush, hair dryer, shaver, and so forth—with wet hands, near running water, or while in the tub or shower. Ground-fault circuit interrupters (GFCI) are required by the National Electric Code in all bathroom receptacle circuits. (See "Codes" below.)

## Codes

To many a homeowner, building codes constitute an incomprehensible and mysterious jumble of arcane, arbitrary, and even disagreeable edicts whose sole purpose is to make the owner's life difficult. In reality, the best interests of you, the homeowner, are served not by ignoring or evading the codes but rather by understanding and complying with them. The codes, which cover building, plumbing, and electrical work, are simply sets of rules governing the methods and materials of construction, and their intent is to safeguard the life and property of the citizenry.

These procedures and standards are formulated not by politicians but rather by a committee of experts in associated fields such as engineering, architecture, and contracting. Thus, the codes reflect the currently accepted standards for construction activities. The drafting committee reviews and updates the building codes periodically to incorporate acceptance of new materials and procedures. Once published, these model codes may be adopted by some political jurisdiction such as a city or state as the law in that area. Because there are several competing model codes nationwide, you must ask your local building department which code is applicable to your area.

You should also ask if your locality has made any changes or additions to the published codes. Most localities make some changes to the codes in order to better accommodate local conditions and practices. You often can find code books with addenda pertinent to your locale for sale at legal or technical bookstores. Your building department can advise you of where to purchase the codes or find copies to refer to.

### Benefits of Codes

Although the intent of the codes is to protect the population from shoddy construction, a major benefit is the standardization of building technology. For example, the plumbing code contains a chart showing the proper sizing of all the pipes in the drain-waste-vent (DWV) system, based upon the expected flow rates called "fixture units." Although an individual has the legal right to hire an engineer and perform tests to determine his own pipe sizes, to do so would be pointless because the results would approximate those found in the code. The plumbing and electrical codes contain technical standardization tables and charts for sizing gas pipes, calculating how many wires of what sizes go into a conduit, and so on. Indeed, this sort of information is so valuable that most plumbers and electricians keep copies of the codes near their toolboxes for quick reference. After all, since you must select some size of pipe, you may as well select the right size from the start.

The codes also control the types of materials you must use, and frequently people object to this kind of restriction. The model codes usually acknowledge and permit the use of most materials, but localities may prohibit or restrict the use of some materials. Sometimes this is due to bureaucratic inertia—that is, they just haven't gotten around to adjusting the codes to incorporate new decisions or information—or it may reflect some disagreement regarding the safety or efficacy of a material.

A prime example of such a disagreement is plastic water pipe. Plastic pipe may be allowed in one area while, just a few miles down the road, it is restricted to cold water only; a few miles farther, it may be banned entirely. The reason most often given for restricting or banning the use of plastic pipe is that its safety for carrying drinking water has not been firmly established.

Romex (a type of wiring in which the positive, neutral, and ground wires are in a casing) is another material that is subject to local restriction. Although widely used in America, some localities restrict its use to concealed locations or prohibit it entirely.

Even when these local restrictions seem unreasonable, you should nonetheless comply with the code. The money you might save by not complying rarely equals the consequence of being caught. In plumbing, the most expensive materials controversy revolves around the use of cast iron versus ABS (acrylonitrile-butadiene-styrene) sewer pipe; yet when the in-place costs of each are compared, the difference is only 15 to 20 percent. This is hardly worth the risk of having a plumbing code violation recorded against your property.

Methods and procedures are also governed by the codes, and you should become familiar with them. One area of the code that often gives trouble to do-it-yourself plumbers is pipe transitions. A special fitting is usually required when going from one material to another (for example, copper to galvanized), and some transitions are not allowed at all. (Cast iron to ABS is a prime example.) Changes in direction can be tricky as well. Vertical to horizontal and horizontal to horizontal transitions require fittings of approved sweep or radius. Electricians need to watch the rules for grounding when working with nonmetallic cable and boxes. The locations of switches and fixtures for tubs and spas must conform to the codes. There are requirements for installing ground-fault circuit interrupters (GFCI), which provide shock protection in receptacles for spas or whirlpools, and for any general-purpose outlets in the bathroom. While this list highlights procedures in which the do-it-yourselfer commonly makes mistakes, it is by no means exhaustive, and a more complete understanding of your local codes will be necessary before attempting these types of work.

### Enforcing the Codes

The codes are enforced by inspectors who work for your local building department. Generally, you will need to show them all the work you have done prior to covering it with wallboard or flooring. Usually these people are helpful and cooperative; after all, you both want the same thing: a safe and sanitary installation. You should first meet with your inspector when you apply for your building permit (most locations require a permit prior to doing any work on a building, but especially for any changes to the electrical and plumbing systems); at this time, he can fill you in on any local requirements for doing the work.

Building departments in almost all areas allow you to work on your own single-family dwelling, but you may be required to take a test. These tests, which generally are simple, are administered by your inspector to ensure that you know enough about what you are doing to keep from becoming a hazard to yourself and others. This is very important. Especially with plumbing and electrical work, it is possible to make some very serious mistakes. One example is a man, who will remain nameless, who connected his water line to the gas piping: he had water coming out of his gas range and also destroyed his gas meter.

The best way to ensure a good relationship with your inspector is to consult with him early and often—let him know what you intend to do and how you are going to do it. While none of us likes to have others pass judgment on our efforts, it is easier to accept suggestions and modify plans before the fact rather than have to tear out some unacceptable work and do it all over again.

The code book and inspector can be valuable resources for you to use in building your new bathroom, or they can be terrible obstacles. The choice is yours.

## Making the Right Connections

More than any other room, the bathroom is a collection of connections. With unseen inlets and outlets for water and air, power supplies for heat, lights, and ventilation, a bathroom could be dominated by hookups. But bathrooms only operate by their connections; they succeed by their design, their amenities, and certainly their location. And nowhere is that success more important than when it comes to adding a new bathroom.

It's a simple truth that Americans want more bathrooms. They add convenience and increase privacy; they sell homes; they are in demand. So when you plan a new bathroom or powder room, your first priorities should be with putting it in the optimum location and with arranging fixtures and other elements to best serve the space, the design, and your needs. The plumbing, electrical, and ventilation connections may be tricky—and trickier can be costlier—but they're never (99.9 percent never) impossible. This section will show you some common and not-so-common ways to run pipes, wires, and vents that should eliminate "the connection factor" as an obstacle to achieving the best bathroom design and location. Whether or not there's a wall, there's a way.

### Water Ins and Outs

Since plumbing connections are the most numerous of all bathroom hookups, they usually need the most careful planning and sometimes the most creative routing to keep them concealed. In the plumbing trade the two main connections are the hot and cold water supply and the drain-waste-vent system (DWV). The latter includes the drains, the traps, and the vents, all of which keep your system sanitary and trouble-free. The DWV system also uses the biggest pipes (1½- to 4-inch diameter) and are usually considered first in planning the plumbing.

Drains, of course, lead to the sewer or septic system. Vents do two things: They provide an exhaust route for noxious sewer gases, and they provide air to the drains to ensure unimpeded drainage. Traps are connected to the tub, shower stall, and lavatory and are always filled with water. The water is there to stop sewer gases from flowing into the bathroom through these drains. The water that's always standing in toilets serves the same purpose. And without vents the traps could be siphoned of their water, or gases could literally bubble their way through the traps.

When you're adding a bathroom close to another, you may have the option of connecting new drains with existing ones

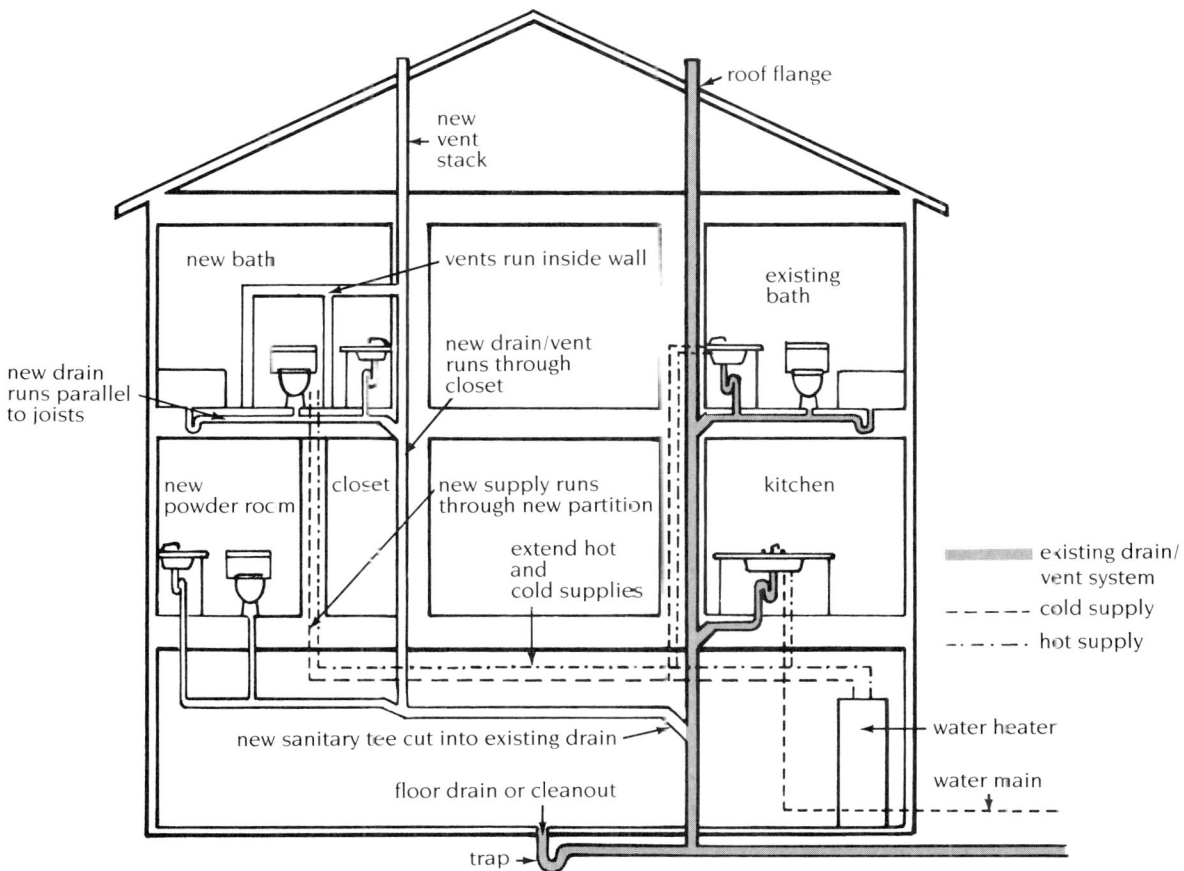

When adding new bathrooms, you can always consider the option of connecting them to existing drains, as in this example. In this case a new vent stack was required. The new supply line runs through the new partition, and the new drain/vent runs through the closet.

and tying new vents into the main vent stack (depending on what local codes allow). But when a new bathroom is rooms away from an existing one, you may have to start fresh. First-floor bathrooms located over unfinished basements usually present the least problem for drains, since new lines can be run across or along joists as needed. If the house is built over a crawl space, there's still no problem as long as there's room to crawl around and hang a 3- to 4-inch drain line from the joists.

For houses built on slabs there can be a bit more difficulty. Holes and channels must be cut through the slab to accept interconnecting drains from all the fixtures. Then a horizontal hole must be dug or drilled underground through the perimeter foundation to make way for the soil pipe. Fur-

ther trenching would be needed to connect this pipe to the main house waste line, allowing for a slope of ⅛ to ¼ inch for every foot of horizontal run. (This is the requirement for any drain line.)

If you're adding a bathroom to a finished basement and the house drain is below the basement floor, draining the toilet and other fixtures will also require chopping holes and channels in the slab to bury drain lines. If that drain is higher and you really want a bathroom down there, you'll need a *sewage lift* pumping system to push waste from a small, sealed holding tank up to the house drain.

Once the route for the toilet drain is established, you can assume that the lavatory and tub or shower will tie right in with T and Y fittings designed for these purposes.

In the same collection of fittings are those that allow connections for vent pipes. Bathroom layout and code requirements will determine the exact way the fixtures must be vented, but ultimately the other end will have to pass up through the roof, away from windows, operable skylights, and any other opening that might take in what the vent pipe lets out.

It is common to run the vent pipe through any convenient frame wall, including exterior walls, since the line doesn't carry any water. If the required size is too large for the existing cavity, it's possible to run two smaller-diameter lines through the wall, to be rejoined before going through the roof. In regions with even occasional snowfall, the pipe should extend at least 14 to 18 inches above the roof plane, or whatever is enough to keep it above the deepest accumulations.

Providing the water supply for a bathroom over a basement should be no more trouble than routing the drain line. The hot and cold water lines need only be ½ inch (inside diameter) for all fixtures. On long runs over 30 feet, the hot water line should be run through insulation sleeves. For bathrooms over crawl spaces, supply pipes should be run through interior walls, except in the most southern climates. Even then it may be best to keep pipes out of exterior walls, because as recent winters have shown, hard frosts don't conform to climate maps. One option is to route them up from a utility room into an unfinished attic, traveling *under* a blanket of insulation and down through a partition into the bathroom.

### Ground-Fault Circuit

To power lights, a fan vent, and the plugged-in load of a hair dryer, the bathroom should have its own 15-amp ground-fault circuit, the wire for which must come directly from the circuit breaker panel or subpanel. A fan vent can be wall mounted (away from a window), or a 3- or 4-inch duct can be run for a more remote outlet. Electricians use rigid and flexible ducting, with the latter often being easier to pull up through existing walls. And in any bathroom there's got to be an air *inlet* to replace fan-vented air. Usually just having a crack between the door and the threshold will allow a sufficient supply of make-up air.

### Heating the Bath

How do you heat a new bathroom? It may or may not be economical to extend the supply and return lines of an existing hot water heating system or a duct from a hot air system. A small powder room, for example, will have relatively minimal heating needs due to size and intermittent use. This is where a short (24-inch maximum) run of electric baseboard can be the most economical heat source, compared to the higher installation cost of hot water or hot air heat. Another electric option is a ceiling-mounted radiant heater, which can provide comfortable heat on demand and with constant thermostatic control.

In a master or family bathroom, on the other hand, it can ultimately be cheaper to extend an existing gas- or oil-fired system, since such heat will be one- to two-thirds cheaper than electric heat. Sometimes the outlet of a hot air duct is concealed in the toe-kick space of the vanity cabinet, where toes get the royal treatment. One way of providing some hot water heat can only be described as fun: You can buy a serpentine towel rack formed from brass- or chrome-plated pipe that you connect to the supply and return lines. It will warm your towels and at least part of the bathroom.

### Upper-Floor Bathrooms

Supplying utilities to upper-floor bathrooms can bring out the most creative routes for pipeline concealment. After all, concealment is the name of the game, and while the options for it are limited, they should provide solutions to almost any routing and concealment problem.

As with a new first-floor bathroom, backing a new bathroom up to an existing one makes it possible to tie in with the existing drains and water supplies. (Any new bathroom should have its own electrical circuit.) But like all routing options, this one is very site-specific. Your plumber might tell you that it would be cheaper to bring in new drain and water lines all the way from the first floor or basement, rather than tear into the wall and floor to get at the old plumbing. But if you do make a direct connection, be sure to provide separate shutoff valves for the new bathroom. That will at least allow for the servicing of the new bath without shutting down the original bathroom (although the reverse would not be true). When you tap into an existing line, the ideal, of course, is to put valves on both sides so that either bath can be shut down individually.

The next play in this routing game is to run the drain line through an existing wall; the main difficulty here would be that the wall cavity may not be deep enough for even 3-inch pipe and fittings. In that case the wall can be opened up and deepened with furring strips, then closed in with a new wall finish after the pipe is in place.

If the new bathroom is horizontally offset from this wall, the drain can be run through the space created by the floor joists. Luck will be with you if the joists run in the same direction as the drain route, but if they don't, a few inches of flooring or first-floor ceiling will have to be taken out to expose the crossing joists for drilling or notching. It will be best to plan for a minimum of joist crossing, but where it can't be avoided, the size of the hole or notch should be no more than one-fourth the width of the joist. A 2 × 8, for example, can have a 2-inch hole or notch without creating a structural risk. That rule of thumb works for water lines (½ or ¾ inch), shower drains (2 inches) and sink drains (1½ inches), but not the toilet drain (3 or 4 inches), to which all other drains usually connect. Joist cuts for that size pipe will have to be reinforced with added lumber and/or steel straps (which will require removal of an even wider strip of flooring or ceiling material).

Faced with that kind of work or expense, you might want to look harder for routing alternatives. If the exterior walls are solid masonry, a *chase* could be boxed out or built into a corner, big enough to carry drain and water supply lines, as well as a possible wire or two. Pipe and wall insulation would be important for protecting the hot *and* cold water lines even though they are on the interior. (According to Murphy's Law, some

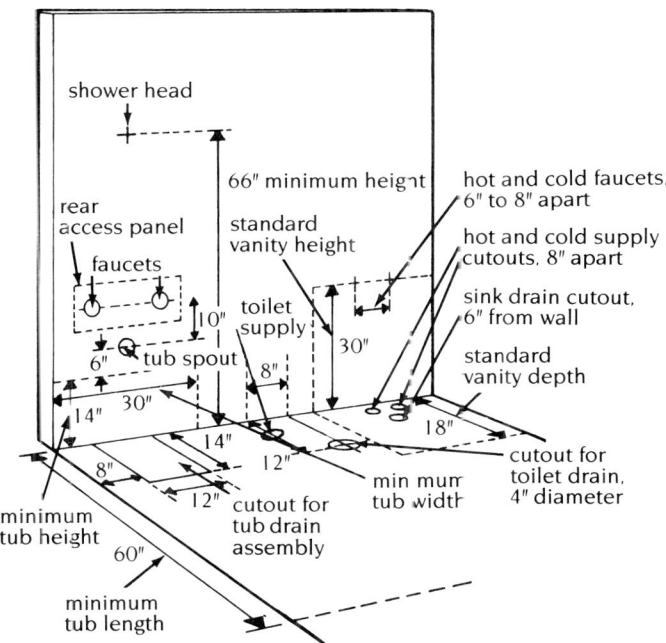

Part of the routing game involves roughing in the dimensions for fixtures, cabinets, drains, and supply lines. Shown here are dimensions for a typical installation.

once-in-a-lifetime combination of super-low winter temperatures and a heating system failure *will* conspire to freeze and burst those lines.)

There may already be a ready-made, easy-access chase available in the form of a closet or a floor-to-ceiling cabinet where the pipes will be only semiexposed. And if you're really strapped for a horizontal route, it's not uncommon for plumbers to run large and small pipes through the soffit above kitchen cupboards and thence up into the new bathroom, or down through a cabinet or wall. Other details of drain installation include providing a cleanout and an access panel behind the tub faucet. The cleanout is a port of entry for a snake in case of clogging, and the access panel allows for possible servicing of the faucet.

Again, a route established for the drain will also be a likely path for the water supply lines, perhaps even power lines although their small size makes it easier to run them through thinner walls that won't accept a drain. If the vent line can run straight up through the roof, all the better, but if bends must be made, it is recommended that they be no sharper than 45 degrees. If the air vent is easily run, the exhaust line for the fan vent should also be easy. An alternative to exhausting the fan vent through yet another appurtenance on the roof is to run it over to a grille in the roof soffit. One less roof vent is one less source for possible leaks.

Armed with these sorts of options, you should be able to have your bath where you want it, equipped with all the right connections, the kinds that you make once and forget about forever.

## Installing Ventilating Fans

The installation of bathroom ventilating fans is pretty much a straightforward job for construction contractors, but a few fine points and suggestions are worth mentioning. One problem, especially in cold climates, is having the moisture condense out of the humid flow of air where the duct runs through cold attic spaces. This liquid moisture runs back into the fan housing causing wet ceilings, dripping, and rusted fan components.

A solution to the problem is to vent the duct pipe through a gable wall in the attic (not through the roof), and to insulate the duct with R-11 fiberglass. The horizontal pipe run in the attic can also be sloped to cause any condensate to run downstream toward the vent. (Never terminate the duct in an open attic space!)

Another problem is caused by the *stack effect*—the natural updraft of warm air that can cause a constant draft, especially through a cheap or poor fitting backdraft damper at the outside vent. One design scheme solves this and the previous problem. The ventilating fan duct can be run inside the bathroom wall *down* to the basement or crawl space and to the outside through a band joist or foundation wall. This eliminates the stack-effect drafts and prevents any condensation from falling back into the fan. Don't forget to put a screen over the grade-level exhaust vent to keep little critters out. Also, no matter what the duct design, ensure free airflow into the bathroom by undercutting the door an inch or installing a low-mounted grille.

## How Long Will It Take, and How Much Will It Cost?

As you plan your new bath, you will have to consider the construction steps involved, how much time they will take, and how much each will cost. You should be as precise as possible when estimating these costs; you don't want to run out of money before your bathroom is finished! Estimating construction requirements for your bath will also help you decide how much of the project you can do on your own, and how much should be contracted to professionals.

To help you plan better—and perhaps save some money in the process—we have included some information from the *Means Home Improvement Cost Guide*.[1] This is one of the most authoritative reference guides for home builders and remodelers, and the information in the following tables and illustrations will give you a general idea of the materials, labor, and costs required for each of four types of baths: half bath, full bath, master bath, and deluxe bath.

The estimates provided in the tables are based on the requirements for baths composed of deluxe materials. If you plan to use standard materials and white fixtures in your bath project, you can deduct 25 to 30 percent from the total contractor's fee for each type of bath. Additional costs may be incurred if fixtures must be relocated. Note also that these figures are national averages; prices for labor and materials may vary slightly from state to state.

## Half Bath, Deluxe

Often a half bath is located in an area of your home where more decorative and deluxe features are desired—perhaps off a

---

1. The information on pp. 134-39 ("Half Bath, Deluxe" through "Deluxe Bath") is copyrighted by R. S. Means, Inc. It is reprinted from *Means Home Improvement Cost Guide* with permission.

recreation room or a room where you do most of your entertaining. A deluxe half bath may also be in order simply because you want to upgrade the facility, in keeping with other improvements throughout your dwelling.

*Level of Difficulty.* The deluxe half bath is a fairly demanding project for even experienced do-it-yourselfers. The two most difficult tasks involved in the renovation are the plumbing procedures and the floor and wall ceramic tile installations. Both of these jobs require specialized skills and a considerable degree of expertise. Beginners can handle the ceramic work, but only if they are given ample instruction beforehand and guidance during the installation. If you have not done any plumbing work in the past, you should leave the fixture installations to professionals, even if you are an accomplished do-it-yourselfer. Handymen and experts should be able to complete a great deal of this project, including tile instal-

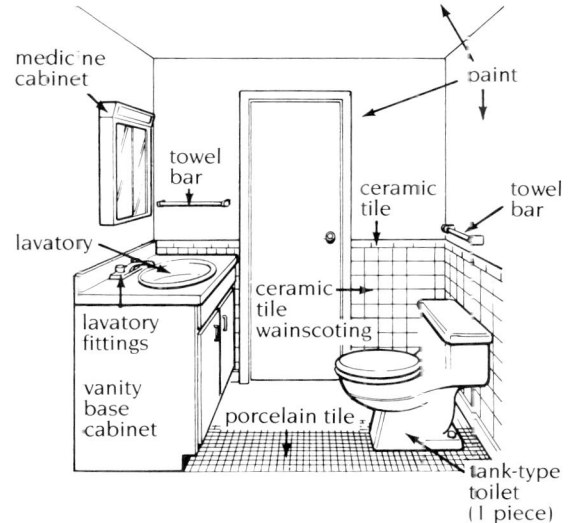

lation, but they will need to obtain the specialized tools for ceramic work and seek some instruction at the start. In using the professional man-hour estimates, add 100 percent to the time if you are a beginner, 50 percent if you are an experienced handyman, and 20 percent if you are an expert.

## Half Bath, Deluxe
### Project Size 4' × 5'

| Description | Quantity | Man-hours | Cost of Materials |
|---|---|---|---|
| Rough in frame for medicine cabinet, using 2" × 4" stock | 8 lin ft | 0.5 | $ 2.25 |
| Painting, ceiling, walls, and door, primer and 1 coat | 142 sq ft | 1.5 | 15.45 |
| Medicine cabinet, with mirror, stock, 16" × 22", lighted | 1 each | 1.5 | 100.00 |
| Vanity base cabinet, deluxe, 2 door, 30" wide | 1 each | 2.0 | 135.00 |
| Vanity top, plastic laminated, maximum | 1 each | 1.0 | 42.00 |
| Lavatory, with trim, porcelain enamel on cast iron, 18" round, in color | 1 each | 2.5 | 145.00 |
| Fittings for lavatory | 1 set | 8.5 | 66.00 |
| Towel bars, stainless steel, 18" long | 2 each | 1.0 | 41.00 |
| Toilet-paper holder, surface mounted, stainless steel | 1 each | 0.5 | 21.00 |
| Walls, ceramic-tile wainscoting, thin set, 4¼" × 4¼" tiles | 20 sq ft | 2.0 | 31.00 |
| Flooring, porcelain tile, 1 color, 1' × 1" tiles | 20 sq ft | 2.0 | 46.00 |
| Toilet, tank type, vitreous china, floor mounted, 1 piece, in color | 1 each | 3.0 | 565.00 |
| Fittings for toilet | 1 set | 8.5 | 100.00 |
| Totals | | 34.5 | $1,359.70 |

**Contractor's Fee, Including Materials:** **$2,910**

## Full Bath, Deluxe

The deluxe full bath includes the amenities and upgraded fixtures to provide an attractive and durable addition to any home. For the additional expense of deluxe features like a one-piece toilet, a sliding shower door, and ceramic tile, this bath offers first-quality materials for a relatively modest investment, especially if you opt to do most of the work on your own.

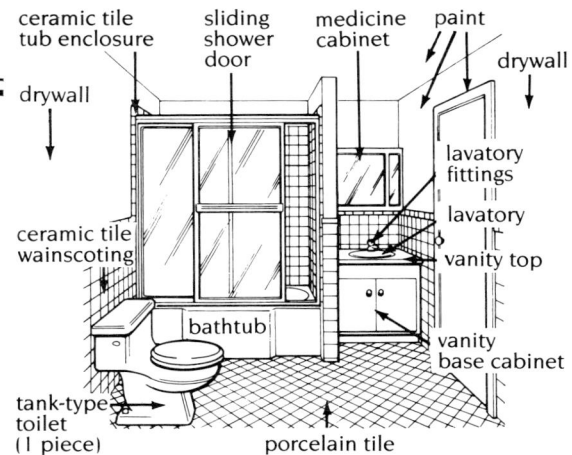

*Level of Difficulty.* The deluxe full bath project poses certain challenges, and expediency is a prime consideration, especially if your home has just one bathroom facility. For all but the expert level of do-it-yourselfers, a plumber should be hired to do the fixture installations. Beginners should also hire someone to do the tile work for this project. In time, a poor tiling job will cost you many times over the installer's fee in leakage and water problems around the tub and shower. Beginners can figure on 150 percent added to the man-hours estimate on other parts of the project. They are advised to seek professional assistance along the way. Handymen should contract the plumbing and add 70 percent to the man-hours estimate for all other operations involved in the renovation. Experts who can handle the plumbing should be able to complete the entire project with about 30 percent added to the professional estimate.

### Full Bath, Deluxe
**Project Size 7' × 8'**

| Description | Quantity | Man-hours | Cost of Materials |
|---|---|---|---|
| Partition wall between vanity and tub, 2" × 4" plates and studs, 16" O.C., 8' high | 64 lin ft | 1.0 | $ 17.80 |
| Rough-in frame for medicine cabinet, using 2" × 4" stock | 10 lin ft | 0.5 | 2.80 |
| Drywall, ½" thick, on walls, water-resistant, taped and finished, 4' × 8' sheets | 2 sheets | 1.5 | 26.00 |
| Painting, ceiling, walls, and door, primer and 1 coat | 230 sq ft | 2.0 | 25.00 |
| Vanity base cabinet, deluxe, 2 door, 30" wide | 1 each | 2.0 | 185.00 |
| Vanity top, Formica covered | 1 each | 1.0 | 41.00 |
| Lavatory, with trim, porcelain enamel on cast iron, 18" round, in color | 1 each | 2.5 | 145.00 |
| Fittings for lavatory | 1 set | 8.5 | 66.00 |
| Bathtub, recessed, porcelain enamel on cast iron, with trim, mat bottom, 5' long, in color | 1 each | 4.0 | 370.00 |
| Fittings for bathtub and shower | 1 set | 9.5 | 83.00 |
| Sliding shower door, deluxe, tempered glass | 1 each | 2.0 | 320.00 |
| Medicine cabinet, sliding mirror doors, 34" × 21", lighted | 1 each | 2.0 | 165.00 |
| Walls, ceramic tile, shower enclosure and wainscoting, thin set, 4¼" × 4¼" tiles | 140 sq ft | 12.5 | 220.00 |
| Flooring, porcelain tile, 1 color, 1" × 1" tiles | 36 sq ft | 3.5 | 82.00 |
| Toilet, tank type, vitreous china, floor mounted, 1 piece, in color | 1 each | 3.0 | 435.00 |
| Fittings for toilet | 1 set | 8.5 | 100.00 |
| Toilet-paper holder, surface mounted, stainless steel | 1 each | 0.5 | 21.00 |
| Towel bar, stainless steel, 30" long | 1 each | 0.5 | 23.00 |
| Totals | | 65.0 | $2,327.60 |

**Contractor's Fee, Including Materials: $5,160**

## Master Bath, Deluxe

The accessories and amenities offered in this deluxe master bath reflect the quality of larger, more expensive homes. The four-fixture project offered in this plan involves a considerable commitment of money and time. If you plan to accomplish some or all of this renovation on your own, seek the assistance of knowledgeable people. Good advice can save you money and prevent damage to fixtures and materials.

*Level of Difficulty.* Installing this bathroom is a major job for even the accomplished remodeler. The extensive tile work and complexity of the plumbing fixtures dictate that even the most experienced worker will need some advice from a professional. In this case we suggest that the expert add 25 percent to the man-hours given. The home handyman should have the plumbing contracted and get assistance on the tile work. Jobs like constructing the partition at the

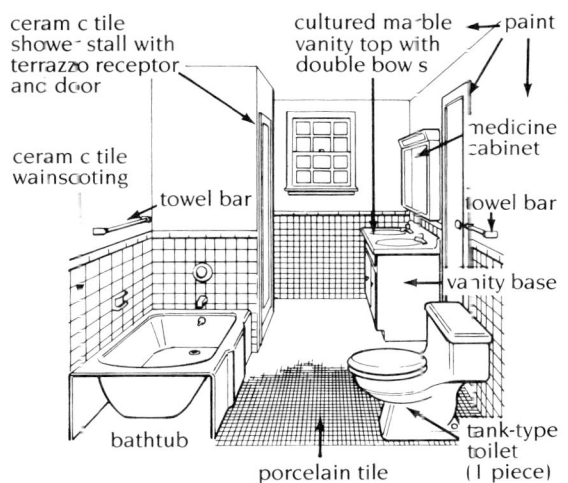

head of the tub and drywalling and finishing the shower stall are well within the realm of most experienced do-it-yourselfers. Handymen should add 60 percent to the man-hours for these and the other remaining tasks. Beginners could attempt the medicine cabinet, towel bars, and toilet accessories installation and could also save on labor costs by painting the walls, ceiling, door, and trim. They should add 100 percent to the man-hours for these items and leave the rest of the work to professional contractors.

### Master Bath, Deluxe
### Project Size 8' × 10'

| Description | Quantity | Man-hours | Cost of Materials |
|---|---|---|---|
| Partition wall for shower stall, 2" × 4" plates and studs, 16" O.C., 8' high | 152 lin ft | 2.5 | $ 42.00 |
| Rough-in frame for medicine cabinet, using 2" × 4" stock | 16 lin ft | 0.5 | 4.45 |
| Drywall, ½" thick, on shower-stall walls, water-resistant, taped and finished, 4' × 8' sheets | 5 sheets | 3.0 | 64.00 |
| Painting, ceiling, walls, and door, primer and 1 coat | 330 sq ft | 3.0 | 56.00 |
| Vanity base cabinet, deluxe, 2 door, 72" wide | 1 each | 4.0 | 500.00 |
| Vanity top, cultured marble, 73" × 22", double bowl | 1 each | 5.0 | 250.00 |
| Fittings for lavatory | 2 sets | 16.5 | 150.00 |
| Shower stall, terrazzo receptor, 36" × 36" | 1 each | 8.0 | 545.00 |
| Shower door, tempered glass, deluxe | 1 each | 2.0 | 320.00 |
| Bathtub, recessed, porcelain enamel on cast iron, with trim, mat bottom, 5' long, in color | 1 each | 4.0 | 370.00 |
| Fittings for bathtub and shower | 1 set | 19.0 | 130.00 |
| Medicine cabinet, center mirror, 2 end cabinets, 72" long, lighted | 1 each | 4.5 | 340.00 |
| Walls, ceramic tile, shower stall and wainscoting, thin set, 4¼" × 4¼" tiles | 170 sq ft | 15.5 | 265.00 |
| Flooring, porcelain tile, 1 color, 1" × 1" tiles | 40 sq ft | 3.5 | 91.00 |
| Toilet, tank type, vitreous china, floor mounted, 1 piece, in color | 1 each | 3.0 | 565.00 |
| Fittings for toilet | 1 set | 8.5 | 100.00 |
| Towel bars, stainless steel, 30" long | 2 each | 1.0 | 46.00 |
| Toilet-paper holder, surface mounted, stainless steel | 1 each | 0.5 | 21.00 |
| Totals | | 102.0 | $3,799.45 |

**Contractor's Fee, Including Materials: $8,290**

## Deluxe Bath

If your home has the space to accommodate a deluxe bath, or if you are building an addition large enough for such a room, this remodeling plan will help you in selecting materials and designing the facility. The project is a costly one, as only top-of-the-line fixtures and materials are recommended to complement the size and intended comfort and luxury of this room. Many different layouts are possible in the design of a five-fixture deluxe bathroom, as long as the available floor area allows for them and for the various amenities and accessories. If your house or addition is not large enough to accommodate the facility or if you do not have the minimum 12-by-18-foot area recommended for a deluxe bath, then you might reconsider doing the project or arrange, at added expense, to alter the floor plan in the area where the facility is to be located. A deluxe bath requires adequate floor space, and cramming the fixtures into too small an area or reducing the bath's open space will only detract from its intended

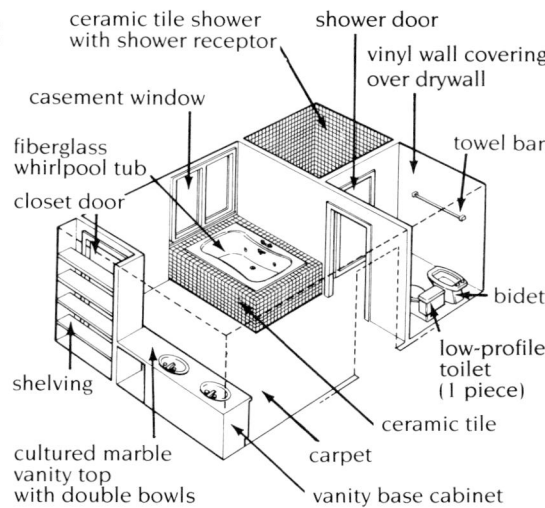

### Deluxe Bath
Project Size 12' × 18'

| Description | Quantity | Man-hours | Cost of Materials |
|---|---|---|---|
| Partition walls, 2" × 4" plates and studs, 16" O.C., 8' high | 400 lin ft | 6.0 | $ 110.00 |
| Framing around bathtub, 2" × 4" stock | 80 lin ft | 3.0 | 22.00 |
| Drywall, ½" thick on walls and ceilings, water-resistant, taped and finished, 4' × 8' sheets | 32 sheets | 18.5 | 410.00 |
| Subflooring, underlayment-grade plywood, ½" thick, 4' × 8' sheets | 6 sheets | 2.5 | 100.00 |
| Vanity base cabinet, deluxe, 4 door, 21" × 76" | 1 each | 4.0 | 500.00 |
| Vanity top, including basins, cultured marble | 1 each | 5.0 | 230.00 |
| Fittings for lavatory | 2 sets | 16.5 | 130.00 |
| Bathtub, whirlpool, molded fiberglass, 56" × 46" | 1 each | 16.0 | 2,600.00 |
| Fittings for bathtub | 1 set | 9.5 | 83.00 |
| Shower receptor and fittings | 1 each | 11.0 | 215.00 |
| Shower door, tempered glass, deluxe | 1 each | 2.0 | 320.00 |
| Window, 4' × 4' 6", plastic clad, casement type | 1 each | 2.0 | 385.00 |
| Doors, 6-panel pine doors, 2' 6" wide × 6' 8" high | 2 each | 2.0 | 220.00 |
| Trim for doors, window, and baseboard, $^9/_{16}$" × 3½" wide | 180 lin ft | 6.0 | 125.00 |
| Painting, ceiling and trim, primer and 1 coat | 800 sq ft | 6.5 | 87.00 |
| Tile, ceramic, shower and bathtub, 4¼" × 4¼" tiles | 210 sq ft | 19.0 | 330.00 |
| Wallpaper, vinyl, fabric backed, medium weight | 560 sq ft | 9.5 | 425.00 |
| Shelving, 10" wide, prefinished, 4' long | 4 each | 2.0 | 110.00 |
| Toilet, one piece, low profile | 1 each | 3.0 | 755.00 |
| Fittings for toilet | 1 set | 8.5 | 100.00 |
| Bidet, vitreous china, white trim | 1 each | 3.5 | 605.00 |
| Fittings for bidet | 1 set | 9.0 | 68.00 |
| Carpet, wool, including pad | 24 sq yd | 3.5 | 650.00 |
| Mirror over vanity, plate glass, 6' × 4' | 1 each | 2.5 | 145.00 |
| Totals | | 169.0 | $8,725.00 |

**Contractor's Fee, Including Materials: $18,600**

luxury. Because of the magnitude of the project and the high cost of the fixtures and materials, do-it-yourselfers are advised to take a realistic look at the renovation and seriously consider hiring a contractor to install the facility.

**Level of Difficulty.** If the expensive plumbing fixtures and other costly building materials in this luxurious bath are within your budget and you have a home large enough to accommodate them, you might find it most expedient to hire a contractor to do the installations. Tasks like the painting and wallpapering can be completed by the homeowner to cut some of the cost, and beginners can accomplish these jobs without much difficulty. Handymen and expert do-it-yourselfers who want to have a hand in constructing the facility should leave the plumbing, ceramic, and carpeting installations to the professionals, but they should be able to complete most of the other jobs involved in the project. Experts should add about 30 percent to the professional time estimates for those tasks which they intend to do; handymen, about 70 percent.

## Making Choices and a Budget

As you plan your new bath, use the spaces below to record the various components of the room as you select them. Using this checklist will help you make decisions about what to include in your new bathroom as well as serve as a record of those decisions. You'll need a description of each item you plan to include in your bath (i.e., a synthetic marble countertop with built-in sink; a drop-in, enameled cast-iron sink; a fiberglass whirlpool tub; and so forth) and its brand name. You'll need to get even more specific when you complete the budget worksheet.

### Accessories

Shower faucets _____ (description); brand name _____
Shower head(s) _____ (description); brand name _____
Sink faucets _____ (description); brand name _____
Tub faucets _____ (description); brand name _____

Soap dish _____ (description); brand name _____
Toilet-paper holder _____ (description); brand name _____
Towel bars _____ (description); brand name _____
Towel warmer _____ (description); brand name _____

Washer/dryer _____ (description); brand name _____
Water heater _____ (description); brand name _____
Ventilation system _____ (description); brand name _____

Stereo/radio _____ (description); brand name _____
Telephone _____ (description); brand name _____
Television _____ (description); brand name _____

### Cabinets and Closets

Vanity cabinet(s) of _____ (laminate, wood, combination, other)
Brand name or cabinetmaker _____
Other cabinets, closets or shelving _____
_____ (description)

*continued*

### Cabinets and Closets (continued)

Items you plan to store in your bath (consider the kind, amount, and size of the space you need to store each item):

- \_\_\_\_ bath oils, salts
- \_\_\_\_ compact mirrors
- \_\_\_\_ drinking cups
- \_\_\_\_ hair-care items
- \_\_\_\_ medicines
- \_\_\_\_ shoes
- \_\_\_\_ toys and games
- \_\_\_\_ cleaning supplies
- \_\_\_\_ dental-care items
- \_\_\_\_ electric shaver
- \_\_\_\_ hair dryer
- \_\_\_\_ nail-care items
- \_\_\_\_ soap
- \_\_\_\_ towels
- \_\_\_\_ clothing
- \_\_\_\_ distilled water
- \_\_\_\_ grooming aids
- \_\_\_\_ makeup
- \_\_\_\_ linens
- \_\_\_\_ tissues
- \_\_\_\_ other

### Countertops

Countertop(s) of _____ (material)
Brand name _____

### Fixtures

Bidet _____ (description); brand name _____
Toilet _____ (description); brand name _____
Urinal _____ (description); brand name _____

Shower stall _____ (description); brand name _____
Sink(s) _____ (description); brand name _____
Tub(s) _____ (description); brand name _____

Hot tub _____ (description); brand name _____
Sauna _____ (description); brand name _____
Spa _____ (description); brand name _____
Steam room _____ (description); brand name _____
Whirlpool _____ (description); brand name _____

### Lighting

Accent lighting _____ (description); brand name _____
_____ (description); brand name _____
Overhead lighting _____ (description); brand name _____
_____ (description); brand name _____
Task lighting _____ (description); brand name _____
_____ (description); brand name _____
Skylight(s) _____ (description); brand name _____
Window(s) _____ (description); brand name _____

### Walls, Floors, and Ceilings

Ceiling _____ (description); brand name _____
Floor covering _____ (description); brand name _____
Tub surround _____ (description); brand name _____
Shower surround _____ (description); brand name _____
Wall covering _____ (description); brand name _____
_____ (description); brand name _____

## Bath Budget Worksheet

**Permits** $
- Building _____
- Electric _____
- Plumbing _____
- Mechanical _____

**Removal of construction trash**
- Dumpster _____
- Dump fee _____
- Trash hauling _____

**Labor**
- Demolition _____
- Carpentry
  - Rough _____
  - Finish _____
  - Installation of vanity _____
- Wiring
  - Rough _____
  - Finish _____
- Plumbing
  - Rough _____
  - Finish _____
- Drywalling
  - Hanging _____
  - Taping and sealing _____
- Countertop(s) _____
- Floors _____
- Finish Work
  - Painting _____
  - Tiling _____
  - Wallpapering _____

**Materials**
- Cabinetry _____
- Closet(s) _____
- Countertop(s) _____
- Door(s) _____
- Faucet(s) _____
- Fixtures
  - Bidet _____
  - Hot Tub _____
  - Sauna _____
  - Sink(s) _____
  - Shower stall _____
  - Spa _____
  - Steam room _____
  - Toilet _____
  - Tub _____
  - Urinal _____
  - Whirlpool _____
- Mirror(s) _____

**Materials** *(continued)* $
  - Skylight(s) _____
  - Window(s) _____
  - Other _____

**Miscellaneous items**
- Carpentry
  - 2 × 4s _____
  - Headers _____
  - Miscellaneous lumber _____
  - Nails _____
  - Insulation _____
- Electric supplies
  - Wire _____
  - Boxes _____
  - Connectors _____
  - Plugs, switches, and dimmers _____
  - Ground-fault circuit interrupters _____
  - Miscellaneous supplies _____
- Lighting fixtures
  - Recessed _____
  - Surface-mounted _____
- Plumbing
  - Pipe _____
  - Connectors and fittings _____
- Drywall
  - Tape, joint compound, and corner fittings _____
- Finishing materials
  - Moldings _____
  - Paint _____
  - Wallpaper _____
  - Window treatment(s) _____

**Design fee** _____

## Keep Your Bath Bright

| Surface | Preventive Care | Heavy-duty Maintenance | Special Considerations |
|---|---|---|---|
| Carpeting | Daily vacuuming and the occasional application of a deodorizing compound will prevent odor buildup and mold growth | Have the carpet professionally cleaned at least once a year. Treat with an aerosol rug cleaner periodically. To remove stains, blot—don't rub. Use a stain and spot remover | Carpeting not tacked down will be easier to maintain. Avoid excess water |
| Corian (Du Pont) 2000X (Formica) | For vanities and countertops, wipe daily with a damp cloth to remove water stains | Occasional use of a Scotch-Brite pad or scouring powder renews these surfaces. For deeper scratches and stains, use fine sandpaper (320-400 grit) and buff with a Scotch-Brite pad | Wipe up chemical spills immediately; consult manufacturers for care instructions |
| Cultured marble | Wipe down regularly with warm water; a little mild soap in the solution will prevent water marks | Impossible to repair subsurface scratches | Caustic substances such as drain cleaners can damage this surface. Do not use abrasive cleansers to remove stains |
| Fiberglass | Towel off after each use to prevent water spotting and soap-scum buildup. Liquid or paste automotive wax restores shine and helps to resist stains and scratches | Remove heavy stains with a nonabrasive bathroom cleaner. Tough stains might be coaxed out with white automotive compound | Abrasive cleansers will scratch fiberglass |
| Glass | Wipe mirrors, shower enclosures, and windows regularly with a soft cloth; this prevents filming | Use conventional glass cleaners or ammonia to remove water spots, dirt, and soap scum | Abrasive cleansers will scratch glass |
| Laminate | Wipe around sink and tub areas with a damp cloth. A thin film of furniture polish or wax provides added protection against stains and scars | Remove mildew and tough stains with a nonabrasive cleaner | Do not use bleaches, abrasive cleansers, or scouring pads, since they will scratch |
| Marble | Wipe countertops with a slightly damp cloth; dust floors regularly with a dustcloth or dry mop. A nonyellowing floor wax will help to seal and protect marble from water and stains | Clean floors periodically with a solution of diluted ammonia or hydrogen peroxide. Stains can be removed with poultices. Use untreated flour or white tissue as a base; the liquid will vary depending on the type of stain: acetone for oil stains; rust | Marble is sensitive to acids and oils. Don't place cosmetics or other substances containing oils directly on a marble surface. Wipe up spills immediately; don't let water sit |

| Surface | Preventive Care | Heavy-duty Maintenance | Special Considerations |
|---|---|---|---|
| Marble (*continued*) | — | remover for rust stains; hydrogen peroxide for organic stains | — |
| Metal | Wipe off faucets each day with a soft cloth. Disinfect every so often | Use a nonabrasive cleaner to remove heavy soap scum and dirt. For rust and tarnish, use an automotive chrome cleaner | — |
| Tile | Toweling off tile surfaces—especially in the shower area—will help to prevent mildew and grime buildup. Seal grout with three coats of lemon oil or grout sealer; grout will resist staining better | An all-purpose cleaner or a solution of vinegar and water works well on walls and floors. For areas that have heavy mildew buildup, scrub with ammonia or bleach mixed with water—*do not mix ammonia and bleach!* Tough stains or grout can be tackled with a grout cleaner like X-14 and a stiff toothbrush. For very stained tile *only*, use a scouring-powder paste | Do not use steel-wool pads on tile surfaces as they can contribute to rust stains. Do not use harsh cleansers; avoid abrasives |
| Vinyl floors | Sweep regularly. Applying a floor wax every so often will make vinyl shiny and easier to clean | Wash periodically with a general-purpose household detergent, diluted with water; always rinse well | — |
| Vinyl wall coverings, paint | Wipe down regularly with a damp sponge or soft-bristle brush | Remove stains on painted walls with commercial degreasers or cleaners. Clean wallpaper with a solution of water and 2-3 tablespoons of household bleach | Test cleaners on a small portion of painted or papered surfaces before treating the whole wall. Walls should be clean and smooth before papering; this prevents buckling and peeling |
| Vitreous china | Wipe with a damp sponge | Use a nonabrasive bathroom cleaner or ammonia and water for heavy-duty cleaning. Remove tough stains with a cream of tartar paste; apply, let dry, and remove with a damp cloth | Although vitreous china can tolerate them, abrasives will eventually etch its surface |
| Wood | Sweep or vacuum floors regularly with a brush attachment. The application of a polyurethane finish will ease a wood floor's maintenance needs. Seal walls to protect them from moisture | For woods with a polyurethane finish: Remove stains with a sponge mop and a solution of warm water, mild detergent, and clear, distilled vinegar. For unfinished floors: Wax every three months, using a wax that contains a cleaning solution for stains, heel marks, and so forth | Sunlight will discolor wood and necessitate sanding. Do not *wax* a floor with a polyurethane finish. Don't let water stand on wood floors |

# Helpful Addresses

## Organizations

American Home Lighting Institute
230 N. Michigan Ave.
Chicago, IL 60601

American Institute of Architects (AIA)
1735 New York Ave. NW
Washington, DC 20006

American Society of Heating,
Refrigerating and Air-Conditioning
Engineers (ASHRAE)
1791 Tullie Circle NE
Atlanta, GA 30329

American Society of Interior Designers
1430 Broadway
New York, NY 10018

California Redwood Association
591 Redwood Hwy.
Suite 3100
Mill Valley, CA 94941

Cultured Marble Institute
435 N. Michigan Ave.
Suite 1717
Chicago, IL 60611

Home Ventilating Institute
30 W. University Dr.
Arlington Heights, IL 60004-1893

Illuminating Engineering Society
345 E. 47th St.
New York, NY 10017

National Center for Appropriate
Technology (NCAT)
P. O. Box 3838
Butte, MT 59702

National Kitchen and Bath Association
124 Main St.
Hackettstown, NJ 07840

National Kitchen and Bath Association
Ontario Chapter
c/o Duncan McKerracher, CKD
Chatelaine Kitchen Design Limited
3323 B. Mainway Dr.
Burlington, Ontario L7N 1A6

National Spa & Pool Institute
2111 Eisenhower Ave.
Alexandria, VA 22314

## Manufacturers
### Air-to-Air Heat Exchangers

Des Champs Laboratories
P. O. Box 440
East Hanover, NJ 07936

NuTone Inc.
Madison and Red Bank Rds.
Cincinnati, OH 45227

## Cabinet Hardware and Other Accessories

Baldwin Hardware Corp.
841 Wyomissing Blvd.
Reading, PA 19603

Barclay Products Ltd.
424 N. Oakley Blvd.
Chicago, IL 60612

Franklin Brass Manufacturing Co.
5353 Grosvenor Blvd.
Los Angeles, CA 90066

Germain Manufacturing
1368 Fontenay Crescent
Ottawa, Ontario K1V 7K6

Grass America, Inc.
P. O. Box 1019
1377 S. Park Dr.
Kernersville, NC 27284

Grass Canada
7290 Torbram Rd., Unit 19
Mississauga, Ontario L4T 3Y8

Häfele America
203 Feld Ave.
P. O. Box 1590
High Point, NC 27261

Häfele Canada
6345 Netherhart Rd.
Mississauga, Ontario L5T 1B8

LaVona's Hand-Crafted Ceramics
19007 Stateline
Belton, MO 64012

Mepla, Inc.
P. O. Box 1469
High Point, NC 27261

Omnia Industries, Inc.
49 Park St.
P. O. Box 263
Montclair, NJ 07042

## Cabinets

Allmilmö Corp.
P. O. Box 629
70 Clinton Rd.
Fairfield, NJ 07006

Aristokraft, Inc.
P. O. Box 420
Jasper, IN 47546

Canac Kitchens Ltd.
360 John St.
Thornhill, Ontario L3T 3M9

Diamond Cabinets
A Tappan Division
P. O. Box 547
Hillsboro, OR 97123

Excel Wood Products Co., Inc.
One Excel Plaza
Lakewood, NJ 08701

Gerber Plumbing Fixtures
4656 W. Touhy Ave.
Chicago, IL 60646

Heritage Custom Kitchens, Inc.
215 Diller Ave.
New Holland, PA 17557

Home-Crest Corp.
P. O. Box 595
Goshen, IN 46526

International Cabinet Co.
Facelifters Division
200 Liberty Ave.
Brooklyn, NY 11207

Kemper
Division of Tappan Co.
P. O. Box 1567
Richmond, IN 47375

Kitchens from Germany, Ltd.
6900 Peachtree Industrial Blvd.
Suite F
Norcross, GA 30071

Les-Care Kitchens, Inc.
One Les-Care Dr.
Waterbury, CT 06705

Merillat Industries, Inc.
5353 W. U.S. 223
Adrian, MI 49221

Perma-Bilt Industries
19308 S. Normandie Ave.
Torrance, CA 90502

Poggenpohl USA Corp.
6 Pearl Ct.
Allendale, NJ 07401

Quakermaid
Rte. 61
Leesport, PA 19533

H. J. Scheirich Co.
250 Ottawa Ave.
P. O. Box 37120
Louisville, KY 40233

Triangle Pacific Corp.
16803 Dallas Pkwy.
P. O. Box 660100
Dallas, TX 75248

Universal-Rundle Corp.
P. O. Box 960
New Castle, PA 16103

Wood-Mode Cabinetry
Snyder Co.
Kreamer, PA 17833

Yorktowne Cabinets
P. O. Box 231
Red Lion, PA 17356

## Composting Toilets

Clivus Multrum USA, Inc.
14-A Eliot St.
Cambridge, MA 02138

## Faucets

Alsons Corp.
525 E. Edna Pl.
Covina, CA 91723

American-Standard
555 River Rd.
Piscataway, NJ 08854

American-Standard
80 Ward St.
Toronto, Ontario M6H 4A7

Artistic Brass
Division of Norris Industries, Inc.
3136 E. 11th St.
Los Angeles, CA 90023

The Chicago Faucet Co.
2100 S. Nuclear Dr.
Des Plaines, IL 60018-5999

Danfoss Inc.
16 McKee Dr.
Box 606
Mahwah, NJ 07430

Delta Faucet Co.
A Division of Masco Corp. of Indiana
55 E. 11th St.
P. O. Box 40980
Indianapolis, IN 46280

Delta Faucet of Canada Ltd.
250 Baseline East
Bowmanville, Ontario L1C 1A4

Eljer Plumbingware
Three Gateway Center
Pittsburgh, PA 15222

Elkay Manufacturing Co.
2222 Camden Ct.
Oak Brook, IL 60521

Epic
8630 E. 33rd St.
Indianapolis, IN 46226

Franklin Brass Manufacturing Co.
5353 Grosvenor Blvd.
Los Angeles, CA 90066

Grohe America, Inc.
2677 Coyle Ave.
Elk Grove Village, IL 60007

Harden Industries, Inc.
P. O. Box 59911
13813 S. Main St.
Los Angeles, CA 90059

Jado Bathroom and Hardware
Manufacturing Corp.
P. O. Box 1759
670 Garcia Ave.
Pittsburg, CA 94565

Kallista, Inc.
200 Kansas St.
San Francisco, CA 94103

Kinkead Co.
101 S. Wacker Dr.
Chicago, IL 60606

Kohler Co.
444 Highland Dr.
Kohler, WI 53044

Kohler Ltd.
195 The West Mall
Suite 314
Etobicoke, Ontario M9C 5K1

Kolson, Inc.
(distributor of Dornbracht)
653 Middle Neck Rd.
Great Neck, NY 11023

KWC/Western State Manufacturing Corp.
2610 S. Yale St.
Santa Ana, CA 92704

Moen Group
Stanadyne, Inc.
377 Woodland Ave.
P. O. Box 4007
Elyria, OH 44036

Paul Associates
155 E. 55th St.
New York, NY 10022

Peerless Faucet Co.
55 E. 111 St.
Indianapolis, IN 46280

Phylrich International
1000 N. Orange Ave.
Los Angeles, CA 90038

Price Pfister, Inc.
13500 Paxton St.
P. O. Box 637
Pacoima, CA 91331-0637

Santile International Corp.
W. Loop Business Park
1201 W. Loop North, Suite 170
Houston, TX 77055

Sherle Wagner International, Inc.
60 E. 57th St.
New York, NY 10022

Speakman Co.
P. O. Box 191
Wilmington, DE 19899

Sterling Faucet Co.
P. O. Box 798
Morgantown, WV 26505

## Fixtures

Acriform Engineering Inc.
395 Mulock Dr.
P. O. Box 327
Newmarket, Ontario L3Y 4X7

American-Standard
555 River Rd.
Piscataway, NJ 08854

American-Standard
80 Ward St.
Toronto, Ontario M6H 4A7

The Broadway Collection
Division of Broadway Industries, Inc.
250 N. Troost
Olathe, KS 66061

Eljer Plumbingware
Three Gateway Center
Pittsburgh, PA 15222

Elkay Manufacturing Co.
2222 Camden Ct.
Oak Brook, IL 60521

Ginger's Bathrooms
945 Eglinton Ave. E.
Toronto, Ontario M4G 4B5

IFO Water Management Products
(Colton-Wartsila)
2882 Love Creek Rd.
Box 349
Avery, CA 95224

Kohler Co.
444 Highland Dr.
Kohler, WI 53044

Kohler Ltd.
195 The West Mall
Suite 314
Etobicoke, Ontario M9C 5K1

Mansfield Plumbing Products
150 First St.
Perrysville, OH 44864

Microphor, Inc.
452 East Hill Rd.
P. O. Box 490
Willits, CA 95490

Owens Corning Fiberglas Corp.
Fiberglas Tower
Toledo, OH 43659

Poggenpohl USA Corp.
6 Pearl Ct.
Allendale, NJ 07401

Pogi Designs, Inc.
International Business Center
11 Empire Blvd.
South Hackensack, NJ 07606

Porcelite International, Inc.
14560 Southlawn La.
Rockville, MD 20850

Porcher, Inc.
612 N. Michigan Ave.
Chicago, IL 60611

Ruddy
(distributor of Eljer products)
1300 Eglinton Ave. E.
Mississauga, Ontario L4W 1K8

Sherle Wagner International, Inc.
60 E. 57th St.
New York, NY 10022

Thetford Corp.
P. O. Box 1285
Ann Arbor, MI 48106

Villeroy & Boch
Ceratec Inc.
100 Rossdean Dr.
Weston, Ontario M9L 2S1

## Baths

### Fixtures (continued)

Villeroy & Boch (USA) Inc.
P. O. Box 103
Interstate 80 at New Maple Ave.
Pinebrook, NJ 07058

### Floor Coverings (see also "Tile" below)

Armstrong World Industries, Inc.
P. O. Box 3001
Lancaster, PA 17604

Azrock Industries, Inc.
Azrock Floor Products Division
P. O. Box 34030
San Antonio, TX 78265

Country Floors, Inc.
300 E. 61st St.
New York, NY 10021

Einstein Moomjy
526 Rte. 17
Paramus, NJ 07652

Galaxy Carpet Mills, Inc.
850 Arthur Dr.
Elk Grove Village, IL 60007

Hartco, Inc.
P. O. Box 1001
Oneida, TN 37841

Karastan Rug Mills
Division of Fieldcrest Mills
919 Third Ave.
New York, NY 10022

Mannington Mills, Inc.
P. O. Box 30
Salem, NJ 08079

C. H. Masland & Sons
Carlisle Springs Rd.
Carlisle Springs, PA 17013

Memphis Hardwood Flooring Co.
P. O. Box 7523
1551 Thomas St.
Memphis, TN 38107

Missouri Hardwood Flooring Co.
P. O. Box 117
Birch Tree, MO 65438

Monsanto Textiles Co.
1460 Broadway
New York, NY 10036

National Oak Flooring Manufacturers Association
8 N. Third St.
Suite 810, Sterick Bldg.
Memphis, TN 38103

Natural Vinyl Floor Co., Inc.
P. O. Box 1302
Florence, AL 35631

Sears, Roebuck & Co.
Sears Tower
Chicago, IL 60684

J. P. Stevens & Co., Inc.
Aberdeen, NC 28315

### The "itty bitty" GroLite

Zelco Industries, Inc.
630 S. Columbus Ave.
Mt. Vernon, NY 10550

### Laminates

Consoweld Corp.
700 Durabeauty La.
Wisconsin Rapids, WI 54494

Formica Canada Inc.
2255 Sheppard Ave. E.
Willowdale, Ontario M2J 4Y5

Formica Corp.
Wayne Interchange Plaza II
155 Rte. 46 W.
Wayne, NJ 07470

Laminart, Inc.
1330 Mark St.
Elk Grove, IL 60007

Micarta Division
Westinghouse Electric Corp.
Hampton, SC 29924

Nevamar Corp.
8339 Telegraph Rd.
Odenton, MD 21113

Pioneer Plastics
Division of LOF Plastics, Inc.
Pionite Rd.
Auburn, ME 04210

Suba Manufacturing, Inc.
Bldg. 116
Benicia Industrial Park
Benicia, CA 94510

Suncraft Moldings, Inc.
650 SE Ninth St.
Bend, OR 97702

Wilsonart Information Center
Ralph Wilson Plastics Co.
600 General Bruce Dr.
Temple, TX 76501

### Lighting

Aladdin Industries, Inc.
P. O. Box 100255
Nashville, TN 37210

Capri Swivelier Co.
33 Rte. 304
Nanuet, NY 10954

Duro-Test Corp.
2321 Kennedy Blvd.
North Bergen, NJ 07047

Dynascan Corp.
6460 W. Cortland St.
Chicago, IL 60635

Forecast Lighting Co.
500 N. Oak St.
Inglewood, CA 90302

General Electric Co.
Campus Center, Suite 106
120 Gibraltar Rd.
Horsham, PA 19044

GTE Products Corp.
Sylvania Lighting Center
100 Endicott Dr.
Danvers, MA 01923

Halo Lighting
Cooper Industries
400 Busse Rd.
Elk Grove Village, IL 60007

Lightolier Genlyte, Inc.
346 Claremont Ave.
Jersey City, NJ 07305

Lutron Electronics Co., Inc.
Suter Rd.
Coopersburg, PA 18036

Moore Lambert Industries, Inc.
2237 Colby Ave.
P. O. Box 64428
Los Angeles, CA 90064

Nessen Lamps, Inc.
621 E. 216th St.
New York, NY 10467

North American Philips Lighting Corp.
One Westinghouse Plaza
Bloomfield, NJ 07003

Peerless Electric Co.
747 Bancroft Wy.
Berkeley, CA 94710

Progress Lighting
Subsidiary of Walter Kidde and Co., Inc.
G St. and Erie Ave.
Philadelphia, PA 19134

R E C Specialties, Inc.
530 Constitution Ave.
Camarillo, CA 93010

Sears, Roebuck & Co.
Sears Tower
Chicago, IL 60684

Task Lighting Corp.
3423 Second Ave.
P. O. Box 1094
Kearney, NE 68847

Thomas Industries, Inc.
207 E. Broadway
Louisville, KY 40232

### Marble, Cultured Marble, and Synthetic Marble

E. I. Du Pont de Nemours & Co.
(synthetic marble)
1007 Marketing St.
Wilmington, DE 19898

Du Pont of Canada Ltd. (synthetic marble)
Toronto Dominion Tower,
Box 26
Toronto, Ontario M5H 1B6

Elite Marble (cultured marble)
Division of Kestom Industries Inc.
751 Farewell St.
Oshawa, Ontario L1H 6N2

Formica Canada Inc. (synthetic marble)
2255 Sheppard Ave. E.
Willowdale, Ontario M2J 4Y5

Formica Corp. (synthetic marble)
Wayne Interchange Plaza II
155 Rte. 46 W.
Wayne, NJ 07470

Phillipsburg Marble Co., Inc. (marble)
River Rd.
Phillipsburg, NJ 08865

Romarco Corp. (cultured marble)
P. O. Box 2218
Morganton, NC 28655

### Renovating and Resurfacing

The Renovator's Supply, Inc.
744 Northfield Rd.
Millers Falls, MA 01349

The Sink Factory
2140 San Pablo Ave.
Berkeley, CA 94702

### Saunas and Steam Machines

Amerec Corp.
P. O. Box 3825
Bellevue, WA 98009

Automatic Steam Products Corp.
4320 34th St.
Long Island City, NY 11101

Finnleo Sauna of the West
9475 SW Oak St.
Portland, OR 97223

General Recreation of Atlanta, Inc.
3120 Maple Dr.
Atlanta, GA 30305

Helo, Inc.
28 Fahey St.
Stamford, CT 06907

Steamist Co. Inc.
One Altman Dr.
Rutherford, NJ 07070

ThermaSol Ltd.
100 Leyland Dr.
Leonia, NJ 07605

Viking Leisure Products Co.
P. O. Box 9157
Marietta, GA 30065

### Specialty Tubs, Hot Tubs, Spas

Acriform Engineering Inc.
395 Mulock Drive
P. O. Box 329
Newmarket, Ontario L3Y 4X7

Almost Heaven Hot Tubs Ltd.
Rte. 219
Renick, WV 24966

Artistcraft Limited
1892 Mattawa Ave.
Mississauga, Ontario L4X 1K1

Bruce Manufacturing, Inc.
1826 N. Military Dr.
Bruce Crossing, MI 49912

California Cooperage, Inc.
P. O. Box 3
San Luis Obispo, CA 93406

California Redwood Spa Co.
7751 Alabama Ave.
Canoga Park, CA 91304

Florida Hot Tub Co.
4634 State Rd. 84
Fort Lauderdale, FL 33313

HessCo Industries
160 E. Foundation Ave.
La Habra, CA 90631

Hydro-Spa, Inc.
3741 Telegraph Rd.
Piru, CA 93040

International Spa and Tub Institute
P. O. Box 19531
Irvine, CA 92713

Jacuzzi Canada Ltd.
330 Humberline Dr.
Rexdale, Ontario M9W 1R5

Jacuzzi Whirlpool Bath, Inc.
298 N. Wiget La.
P. O. Drawer J
Walnut Creek, CA 94596

Kohler Co.
444 Highland Dr.
Kohler, WI 53044

Novi American, Inc.
3245 Berkeley Lake Rd.
Duluth, GA 31036

Pearl Baths, Inc.
9224 73rd Ave. N.
Minneapolis, MN 55428

The Soft Bathtub Co.
P. O. Box 81125
Seattle, WA 98108

Universal-Rundle Corp.
P. O. Box 29
New Castle, PA 16103

Viking Leisure Products Co.
P. O. Box 9157
Marietta, GA 30065

Water Jet Corp.
8431 Canoga Ave.
Canoga Park, CA 91304

### Tankless, Point-of-Use Water Heaters

Chronomite Laboratories
21011 S. Figueroa St.
Carson, CA 90745

Thermar Corp.
Melrose Square
Greenwich, CT 06830

### Tile

American Olean Tile Co.
1000 Cannon Ave.
P. O. Box 271
Lansdale, PA 19446-0271

W. R. Bonsal Co.
P. O. Box 241148
Charlotte, NC 28224

The Briare Co. Inc.
51 Tec St.
Hicksville, NY 11801

Endicott Clay Products
Endicott, NE 68350

Florida Tile
Division of Sikes Corp.
P. O. Box 447
Lakeland, FL 33802

Hastings Tile & Il Bagno Collection
201 E. 57 St.
New York, NY 10022

International Collection
1288 S. La Brea Ave.
Los Angeles, CA 90019

Italian Tile Center
499 Park Ave.
New York, NY 10022

Mid-State Tile Manufacturing, Inc.
P. O. Box 1777
Lexington, NC 27292

Monarch Manufacturing, Inc.
1 E. Twohit St.
P. O. Box 2041
San Angelo, TX 76902

Olympia Floor and Wall Tile Co.
1000 Lawrence Ave. W.
Toronto, Ontario M6B 4A8

Ramca Ltd.
1185 Caledonia Rd.
Toronto, Ontario M6A 2X2

Summitville Tiles, Inc
Summitville, OH 43962

U.S. Ceramic Tile Co.
Division of Spartek, Inc.
1275 Raff Rd. SW
Canton, OH 44711

Villeroy & Boch
Ceratec Inc.
100 Rossdean Dr.
Weston, Ontario M9L 2S1

Villeroy & Boch (USA) Inc.
P. O. Box 103
Interstate 80 at New Maple Ave.
Pinebrook, NJ 07058

Walker and Zanger
(West Coast Ltd.)
1832 S. Brand Blvd.
Glendale, CA 91204

Washington Mills Ceramics Corp.
31 Airport Rd.
P. O. Box 112
Lake Wales, FL 33853

Wenczel Tile Co.
200 Enterprise Ave.
P. O. Box 5308
Trenton, NJ 08638

### Tub/Shower Enclosures

Abitibi-Price Corp.
Building Products Group
Troy, MI 48084

**Tub/Shower Enclosures** (continued)

Acriform Engineering Inc.
395 Mulock Drive
P. O. Box 329
Newmarket, Ontario L3Y 4X7

Alumax/Magnolia Division
P. O. Box 40
Magnolia, AR 71753

American Shower Door Co.
P. O. Box 2119
Santa Monica, CA 90406

Aqua Glass, Inc.
P. O. Box 412
Industrial Park
Adamsville, TN 38310

F. E. Bieze Import Canada Ltd.
(distributor of Huppe)
466 Trafalgar Rd.
Oakville, Ontario L6J 3H9

Monarch Manufacturing, Inc.
1 E. Twohit St.
P. O. Box 2041
San Angelo, TX 76902

Philips Industries Inc.
Lasco Division
3255 E. Miraloma
Anaheim, CA 92806

Plaskolite, Inc.
P. O. Box 1497
Columbus, OH 43216

The Shower Door Company of America
One Permalume Pl. NW
P. O. Box 20202
Atlanta, GA 30325

Showerlux Canada Ltd.
1380 Birchmount Rd.
Scarborough, Ontario M1P 2E6

Sterline Manufacturing Corp.
410 N. Oakley Blvd.
Chicago, IL 60612

Swan Corp.
408 Olive St.
St. Louis, MO 63102

Tub-Master Corp.
413 Virginia Dr.
Orlando, FL 32803

**Vintage Bath Fixtures and Accessories**

A*Ball Plumbing Supply
1703 W. Burnside
Portland, OR 97209

Barclay Products, Ltd.
424 N. Oakley Blvd.
Chicago, IL 60612

Bath Queen Refinishing
119 Raymeville Dr.
Markham, Ontario L3P 4M7

Bathtub King Refinishing Ltd.
4615 Burgoyne St.
Mississauga, Ontario L4W 1G3

Crème de la Crème Vintage Plumbing
342 Queen St. E.
Toronto, Ontario M5A 1S8

Cumberland General Store
Rte. 3
Crossville, TN 38555

DeWeese Woodworking Co.
P. O. Box 576
Philadelphia, MS 39350

P. E. Guerin, Inc.
23 Jane St.
New York, NY 10014

Rejuvenation House Parts Co.
901-C N. Skidmore
Portland, OR 97217

Sunrise Specialty Co.
2210 San Pablo Ave.
Berkeley, CA 94702

Surrey Shoppe Interiors
665 Centre St.
Brockton, MA 02402

Tennessee Tub, Inc. & Tub Liner Co.
6682 Charlotte Pike
Hillwood Village
Nashville, TN 37209

The Walker Mercantile Co.
P. O. Box 129
Bellevue, TN 37221

W. T. Weaver & Sons, Inc.
1208 Wisconsin Ave.
Washington, DC 20007

# CREDITS

### Notes
### A New Version of the Bath

By Catherine M. Cassidy except for the following: "Questions to Answer before You Begin," "Renew," "Replace," "Redesign," and "Making Room for the Bath" by Ellen Cheever.

### The Working Parts

By Catherine M. Cassidy except for the following: "An Efficient Flush," "Faucets: Plain and Fancy," and "Tub and Shower Faucets" by Ellen Cheever. "Sinks," "The Basic Bathtub," and "Shower Stalls" by Catherine M. Cassidy and Ellen Cheever. "Whirlpools, Hot Tubs, and Spas," "Steam Adds Sizzle," "Finish with a Sauna," and "Heat Lamps" by Patrick J. Galvin. "What about Sunlamps?" by Marguerite Smolen.

### Storage in the Bath

By Marguerite Smolen.

### The Finishing Touches

By Catherine M. Cassidy except for the following: "On the Walls" and "The Floor" by Ellen Cheever. "Ventilation" by David Sellers. "Plants in Your Bath" and the table "Great Plants for the Bath" by Suzanne Nelson.

### Gallery: A Tour of Fine Baths

By Catherine M. Cassidy.

### Workbook: The Basics of Bath Design

"Drawing a Floor Plan," "Making Your Bathroom Safe," and "Making Choices and a Budget" by Catherine M. Cassidy. "One Designer's Solutions" by Ellen Cheever. "Codes" by Michael Hammran. "Making the Right Connections" by Joe

Carter. "Installing Ventilating Fans" by David Sellers. "How Long Will It Take, and How Much Will It Cost?" reprinted, with permission, from *Means Home Improvement Cost Guide*.

## Photography Credits

Below are the credits for each photograph. The first name is that of the photographer, followed by the names of the designer, craftsman, or photo stylist, when applicable.

**Title page:** Mitchell T. Mandel; design, Rhoda Schuman Interiors; photo styling, J. C. Vera. **Page vi:** courtesy of Kohler Company; design, Marilynn W. Schall, ASID. **Page 1:** © 1986 by Mary Fote; design, Karen Nelson and Joan Silver.

"A New Version of the Bath": **Page 3:** Mitchell T. Mandel; design, Joe Bracchitta, CKD, Tarrytown, N.Y. **Page 4:** courtesy of Alumax/Magnolia Division. **Page 5:** Mitchell T. Mandel; design, Harry Teague, AIA, Aspen Colo. **Page 6:** courtesy of Armstrong World Industries, Inc. **Page 7:** Mitchell T. Mandel; design, Richard M. Sibly, AIA, Atlanta. **Page 8:** Mitchell T. Mandel; design, Angela Smallwood and Steve Smith, Atlanta; photo styling, Lucretia Arpad. **Page 9:** J. Michael Kanouff; design, Peter Hardell and Karl Oppen, Sonoma County, Calif. **Page 10:** J. Michael Kanouff; design, Ellen Cheever, CKD, ASID, Sacramento, Calif. **Page 11:** courtesy of Wilsonart Decorative Laminates. **Page 12 (upper):** courtesy of Kaufman Meeks, Inc., Houston, Tex., photo by Rob Muir; design, Kaufman Meeks, Inc. **Page 12 (lower):** courtesy of Kohler Company; design, William M. Manly, FASID. **Page 13 (upper):** courtesy of Columbus Coated Fabrics. **Page 13 (lower):** Robert Perron; design, Robert Gelormino. **Pages 14-15:** J. Michael Kanouff; design, Fred Karren, San Francisco. **Page 19:** Mitchell T. Mandel; design, Allison Moreland, Allentown, Pa.

"The Working Parts": **Page 21:** courtesy of American-Standard. **Page 22:** courtesy of Water Conservation Systems, Concord, Mass. **Page 25:** courtesy of Paul Associates, New York, N.Y. **Page 26 (clockwise from top right):** courtesy of Phylrich International; courtesy of Hastings Tile & Il Bagno Collection; photo by J. Michael Kanouff, design by Peter Hardell; courtesy of Eljer Plumbingware; photo by Mitchell T. Mandel, design by Thomas Caswell, photo styling by Lucretia Arpad. **Page 27 (clockwise from top right):** courtesy of Porcher, Inc.; courtesy of Sherle Wagner International, Inc.; courtesy of Eljer Plumbingware; courtesy of Sunrise Specialty Company; courtesy of Kohler Company. **Page 30:** Ken Paul; design, Rick Cowlishaw, Passive Solar Architects, Monument, Colo. **Page 31 (upper):** Mitchell T. Mandel design, Steve Myrwang, Myrwang Associates Architects, Seattle, Wash.; **Page 31 (lower):** courtesy of American-Standard. **Page 33:** courtesy of Plaskolite. **Page 34 (clockwise from top):** courtesy of Eljer Plumbingware; photo by J. Michael Kanouff, design by Roberta and James Godbe, Carmel, Calif.; courtesy of Soft Bathtub Company. **Page 35 (clockwise from upper right):** photo by J. Michael Kanouff, design by Anthony Cutri, San Francisco; Rodale Press Photo Dept.; courtesy of Porcher, Inc.; courtesy of Jacuzzi Whirlpool Bath. **Pages 36-37 (left to right):** Mitchell T. Mandel; photo styling, Michael Koenig. **Pages 39 and 43:** Mitchell T. Mandel; design, Linda Ziegenfuss; photo styling, J. C. Vera. **Page 41:** © 1985 by Mary Fote for *The Renovation Handbook*; design, Volgesi & Propst Architects, Toronto, Canada.

"Storage in the Bath": **Page 45:** © 1985 by Mary Fote for *The Renovation Handbook*; design, Andrew Volgyesi, Volgyesi & Propst Architects, Toronto, Canada. **Page 48:** Mitchell T. Mandel; design, David J. Shaw, AIA, John's Island, S.C. **Page 50:** J. Michael Kanouff; design, Karl Oppen, Sonoma County, Calif. **Page 51:** courtesy of American Olean Tile Company; design, Joy Wulke. **Page 53:** Mitchell T. Mandel; design, Richard M. Sibly, AIA, Atlanta; photo styling, Lucretia Arpad. **Page 56 (clockwise from top right):** courtesy of Wilsonart Decorative Laminates. Mitchell T. Mandel; design Richard M. Sibly, AIA, Atlanta; photo styling, Lucretia Arpad. Courtesy of Poggenpohl USA Corp. Courtesy of T + L Royal Inc., Charlotte, N.C. Courtesy of Wilsonart Decorative Laminates. **Page 57 (top left):** courtesy of Poggenpohl USA Corp. **Page 57 (others):** Mitchell T. Mandel; design, Steven Johnson of Interior Concepts, Atlanta, and Michael Cantin, St. Charles Cabinets of Atlanta; photo styling, Lucretia Arpad.

"The Finishing Touches": **Page 61:** Robb Miller, courtesy of Kaufman Meeks, Inc., Houston, Texas; design, Kaufman Meeks, Inc. **Page 62:** Mitchell T. Mandel; design, Richard M. Sibly, AIA, Atlanta; photo styling, Lucretia Arpad. **Page 64:** courtesy of California Redwood Association; design, Robert J. Hendle, Sr. **Page 65:** photo by Elliot Fine, courtesy of Italian Tile Center; design, André Putman. **Page 66:** courtesy of Owens-Corning Fiberglas Corp.; design, Beverly Truop with Mark I. Kaufman. **Page 68:** photo by Eric Figge, courtesy of Brion S. Jeannette & Associates, Newport Beach, Calif.; design, Brion S. Jeannette, AIA. **Page 73:** Mitchell T. Mandel; photo styling, J. C. Vera and Michael Koenig. Products shown are available from Kohler Direct Marketing, Inc., P. O. Box 998, Ridgely, MD 21660. **Page 74:** photo by Michael Peck, reprinted with permission from *Colorado Homes & Lifestyles*.

"Gallery: A Tour of Fine Baths": **Page 78:** Carl Doney; photo styling, Kay Lichthardt. **Page 79:** Robert Reck. **Pages 80-81:** J. Michael Kanouff. **Pages 82-83:** Mitchell T. Mandel. **Pages 84-85:** Mitchell T. Mandel; photo styling, J. C. Vera. **Pages 86-87:** photo by Greg Hursley, courtesy of Alan Y. Tariguchi Architects and Associates. **Pages 88-89:** Mitchell T. Mandel; photo styling, J. C. Vera. **Pages 90-91:** Mitchell T. Mandel; photo styling, Lucretia Arpad. **Pages 92-93:** Photo by Vic Tomasyan, courtesy of Brion S. Jeannette & Associates. **Pages 94-95:** David Kenik. **Pages 95-97:** Mitchell T. Mandel; photo styling Lucretia Arpad. **Pages 98-99:** Mitchell T. Mandel; photo styling, J. C. Vera. **Pages 100-101:** © 1986 by Mary Fote. **Pages 102-3:** Mitchell T. Mandel; photo styling J. C. Vera. **Pages 104-5:** courtesy of the Italian Trade Commission. **Pages 106-9:** Mitchell T. Mandel; photo styling, Lucretia Arpad. **Pages 110-11:** Carl Doney; photo styling, Kay Lichthardt. **Pages 112-13:** Mitchell T. Mandel. **Pages 114-15:** Robert Reck. **Pages 116-17:** Mitchell T. Mandel. **Page 118:** Robert Perron. **Page 119 (left):** J. Michael Kanouff. **Page 119 (right):** Mitchell T. Mandel; photo styling, J. C. Vera. **Pages 120-21 (upper):** © 1986 by Mary Fote. **Page 121 (lower):** Carol Besler for *Bath & Kitchen Marketer*. **Page 122:** Mitchell T. Mandel; design, David J. Shaw, AIA, St. John's Island. **Page 123:** Mitchell T. Mandel; design, Ryland W. Koets, AIA, Atlanta.

## Credits for "Gallery: A Tour of Fine Baths"

"Windows on Their World" (pp. 80-81): **house and bath design** by Sears Barrett, Equinox Design Group, 6000 S. Ulster Ave., Suite 206, Englewood, CO 80111; **construction** by Norman Nadolsky, Custom Concepts Inc., 6000 S. Ulster St., No. 206, Englewood, CO 80111; **cabinet hardware** by Baldwin Hardware Corp.; **cabinetry** in white laminate custom-built by C & G Woodworking, Parker Colo.; **countertop** is Formica with bullnose trim by Imagini from C & G Woodworking; **lighting** by Lightolier Genlyte; **mirrors and shower stall enclosure** by Monarch Manufacturing, Denver, Colo.; **shower and sink faucets, sink, toilet, and tub** by Kohler (tub is Birthday Bath); **tile floor covering and tub surround** is Cerdissa from C & G Woodworking; **windows and skylights** by Pozzi Window Co., Denver, Colo.

"An Unplanned Oriental Bath" (pp. 82-83): **house and bath design** by Joseph Boggs Studio/Architects, 1333 H St. NW, Washington, DC 20005; **cabinetry** by

149

Heritage Custom Kitchens; **countertop, shower stall, and tub surround** are tile by American Olean; **floor covering** is tile by Santerno Italian Tile Co.; **hot tub** of cypress by California Cooperage; **lighting** (except paper globe over hot tub) by Lightolier Genlyte; **shower and sink faucets, sink, and toilet** by Kohler; **windows**: window by hot tub is custom-designed Plexiglas, bent at 90° angle to accommodate corner; other windows by Weather Shield; **window blinds** are vertical and miniblinds by Levolor Lorentzen, Lyndhurst, N.J.

"A Bath in the Woods" (pp. 84-85): **house and bath design** by Harrison Fraker (formerly of the Princeton Energy Group), School of Architecture, 110 Architecture Bldg., 89 Church St. SE, Minneapolis, MN 55403; **additional design** by Kyle Van Dyke and Larry Lindsey, Princeton Energy Group, 575 Ewing St., Princeton, NJ 08540; **accessories** by Baldwin Hardware Corp.; **bidet; shower, sink, and tub faucets; and toilet** by Kohler; **countertop and built-in sink** are Corian by Du Pont; **floor covering** is ceramic tile by American Olean; **glass block** by Pittsburgh Corning Corp.; **lighting** by Lightolier Genlyte; **perfume sculptures** by Charles Kumnick, Hopewell, N.J.; **shower stall** by Lasco; **whirlpool tub** by Water Jet Corp.; **windows** by Andersen; **window blinds** by Verosol USA, Pittsburgh, Pa.

"A Tranquil Retreat" (pp. 86-87): **house and bath design** by Alan Y. Taniguchi, F.A.I.A., Alan Y. Taniguchi Architects and Associates, 1609 W. Sixth St., Austin, TX 78703; **construction** by Jackson/King Builders, 9601 W. Beebe Cave Rd., Austin, TX 78745; **cabinetry** of pine custom-built by Jackson/King; **countertop** is laminate by Wilsonart; **floor covering** is laminated yellow pine; **lighting** by Lightolier Genlyte (overhead lights), Nessen Lamps (lights on headboard), and Progress Lighting (steplights); **refrigerator** by Sub-Zero Freezer Co., Inc., P. O. Box 4130, Madison, WI 53711; **shower and sink faucets, sinks, toilet, and whirlpool bath** by Kohler.

"A Bath of Soft, Soothing Colors" (pp. 88-89): **bath design** by Rhoda Schuman Interiors, 27 Millbrook Rd. W., Stamford, CT 06902; **construction** by Bruce Bentzig, Bentzig Builders, 23 Trautwein Crescent, Closter, NJ 07624; **bidet, sink faucets, and toilet** by American-Standard; **cabinetry** by Boos Custom Woodworking Co., Inc., Plainview, N.Y.; **countertop and built-in sink** are Corian by Du Pont; **floor covering** is tile by American Olean; **shower faucet** by Moen Group/Stanadyne; **shower stall** custom-designed of tile by American Olean; **steam machine** is Mr. Steam by Automatic Steam Products Corp.; **tub faucets** by Grohe America; **wall covering** by First Editions Wallpaper and Fabrics, Inc.; **whirlpool tub** by Jacuzzi Whirlpool Bath; **windows and skylights** by Andersen as well as custom designs.

"A Bath of Color" (pp. 90-91): **bath design** by Cassandra and Michael Caton; **design consultant** was T. Duffy and Associates Interior Design, 6900 Roswell Rd., Suite K-2, Atlanta, GA 30328; **additional bath design** by Michael Cantin, St. Charles Cabinets of Atlanta, Inc., 3487 Northside Pkwy. NW, Atlanta, GA 30327; **house design** by Deck House Inc., Acton, Ma.; **cabinetry** by St. Charles Fashion Kitchens; **countertop and built-in sink** are Corian by Du Pont; **lighting** by Forecast Lighting Co., Atlanta, Ga. (above vanity and in toilet compartment), Lightolier Genlyte (above tub area), and Nessen Lamps (swing-arm lamps near closet); **mirrors** custom-designed by North Fulton Glass and Mirror Co., Roswell, Ga.; **shower faucets** by the Broadway Collection; **shower stall** custom-designed with brass by North Fulton Glass and Mirror Co.; **sink faucets** by Artistic Brass; **steam machine** by Steamist; **tile** by Villeroy & Boch; **toilet** by Kohler; **wall covering** in toilet compartment is wallpaper by Groundworks, Inc., New York, N.Y.; **whirlpool tub** by Jacuzzi Whirlpool Bath.

"A Garden Bath" (pp. 92-93): **bath design** by Brion S. Jeannette, A.I.A., Brion S. Jeannette & Associates, 470 Old Newport Blvd., Newport Beach, CA 92663; **project manager** was Michael Beam of Brion S. Jeannette & Associates; **bidet, sink, and toilet** by Kohler; **cabinetry** is custom-built of oak; **countertop** is tile by Latco Tile Products Co., Los Angeles, Ca.; **floor covering** is carpet and tile by Latco Tile Products Co.; **lighting** by Halo Lighting; **shower, sink, and tub faucets, and decorative accessories** by Artistic Brass; **shower stall** is custom-built of tile with enclosure by Century Windows; **tub and tub surround** built from imported Italian tile.

"An Octagonal Bath" (pp. 94-95): **bath design** by Philippe Favet, Interior Designer, P. O. Box 4672, Portsmouth, NH 03801; **cabinetry** custom-designed of mahogany and maple by Favet; **ceiling** constructed of mahogany and pine; **lighting** by Progress Lighting; **mirrors** by New Hampshire Glass Co., Portsmouth, N.H.; **stained-glass window** in cupola custom-designed by John Whalen, York Beach, Maine.

"A Bath of Simply Stated Luxury" (pp. 96-97): **house and bath design** by Karel Pruner, A.I.A., Karel Pruner & Associates—Architects, 2110 Powers Ferry Rd., Suite 470, Atlanta, GA 30339; **construction** by Clarkcraft, Inc., 6720 Powers Ferry Rd., Suite 100, Atlanta, GA 30339; **cabinet hardware** by Forms & Surfaces, Inc.; **cabinetry** custom-built by Clarkcraft; **countertop** is laminate by Wilsonart; **floor covering** is ceramic tile by Florida Tile; **shower and steam unit closure** by Shower Door Company of America; **sink and shower faucets** by Grohe America; **sinks** by Kohler; **steam machine** by Viking Leisure Products; **toilet** by American-Standard; **tub, tub surround, and wall covering** are Italian ceramic tile by Zumpano Enterprises, Atlanta, Ga.; **whirlpool tub** by Viking Leisure Products; **window** is custom-designed with wood casements by Rolscreen/Pella.

"The Best of Both Worlds" (pp. 98-99): **house and bath design** by Barbara and David Bollinger; **cabinetry** custom-built of cherry wood by Brader's Woodcraft Laury's Station, Pa.; **countertop and built-in sinks** are Corian by Du Pont; **floor covering and tub surround** are imported marble; **lighting** by Lightolier Genlyte; **mirrors** custom-designed by S & H Mirror, Slatington, Pa.; **shower, sink, and tub faucets** by Harden; **shower stall** custom-designed of imported marble; **toilet** by Kohler; **whirlpool tub** by Aqua Glass; **windows** by Marvin Window.

"A Bath of European Elegance" (pp. 100-101): **bath design** by Barbara Munn, Yorkville Design Centre, 70 Yorkville Ave., Toronto, Ontario M5R 1B9; **interior design** by Ginger's Bathrooms, 945 Eglinton Ave. E., Toronto, Ontario M4G 4B5; **bidet, sinks, and toilet** by Cesame S.P.A. of Italy, imported by Ginger's Bathrooms; **cabinetry** by Yorkville Design Centre; **countertop, floor and wall covering, and shower stall** are genuine marble; **lighting** by Residential Lighting Co., Toronto, Ontario; **mirrors** by Mirror L'Image, Toronto, Ontario; **shower and sink faucets** by VIP S.A.S. of Italy, imported by Ginger's Bathrooms; **whirlpool tub** by Metaliberica S.A. of Spain, imported by Ginger's Bathrooms; **windows** by Rolscreen/Pella.

"A Split-Level Country Bath" (pp. 102-3): **bath design** by Robin and Sam Landis; **cabinetry** by Elmer Bachman; **custom railing** by Jost Iron Works, Allentown, Pa.; **lighting** by Lighting Fixture and Supply Co., Allentown, Pa.; **sink and shower faucets** by Moen Group/Stanadyne; **toilet and whirlpool tub** by Universal-Rundle Corp.; **windows** by Andersen.

"A Body and Soul Room" (pp. 104-5): **bath design** by Eric Bernard Designs, 177 E. 94th St., New York, NY 10028; **audio and remote-control systems** by Audio Command Systems, Inc., Rockville Centre, N.Y.; **chaise lounge** designed by Frank A. Hall & Sons, Inc., New York, N.Y.; **closet** contains automatic garment checking device by Railex Corp., New

York, N.Y.; **computer** by Radio Shack, Fort Worth, Tex.; **decorative accessories** by Muriel Karasik Galleries, New York, N.Y.; **doors for bath and closet** by Wyatt Co., New York, N.Y.; **fabric** on chaise lounge custom-woven by Jeffrey Aronoff, New York, N.Y.; **gym equipment** by Marcy Fitness Products, Alhambra, Calif.; **lighting** by Bridget Beier of Kliegel Brothers, Long Island, N.Y. (programmed lighting projections), Novitas, Inc., Santa Monica, Calif. (motion detector), Roberto Tamez of Progress Lighting, (track lighting); **lighting concept** by James Nuckolls, I.A.L.D., with Stephen Roche of Incorporated Consultants Limited, New York, N.Y.; **steam machine** by Steamist; **swivel stool** by Dakota Jackson, Long Island City, N.Y.; **tile** by Marazzi USA, Dallas, Tex.; **whirlpool tub** by Jacuzzi Whirlpool Bath.

"A Terrarium Bath" (pp. 106-7): **bath design** by Steven Johnston, Interior Concepts, 3838 Peachtree Dunwoody Rd., Atlanta, GA 30342; **additional bath design** by Michael Cantin, St. Charles Cabinets of Atlanta, Inc., 3487 Northside Pkwy. NW, Atlanta, GA 30327; **cabinetry** by St. Charles Fashion Kitchens; **countertop and built-in sink** are Corian by Du Pont; **floor covering** is carpeting; **furniture** in the bath by Directional, Inc., New York, N.Y.; **shower, sink, and tub faucets and toilet** by Kohler; **shower stall** custom-designed with imported Italian ceramic tile and cultured marble; **whirlpool tub** by Jacuzzi Whirlpool Bath; **window treatments** by Peachtree Window and Door Co., Atlanta, Ga.

"A Bath of Wide Open Spaces" (pp. 108-9): **bath design** by Thomas A. Caswell, Designer, St. Charles Cabinets of Atlanta, Inc., 3487 Northside Pkwy., Atlanta, GA 30327; **cabinetry** by St. Charles Fashion Kitchens; **countertop, floor covering, shower stall, and tub surround** are ceramic tile from Associated Products, Division of Sandsy, Inc., Atlanta, Ga.; **sink and shower faucets** by Kohler; **spa** by Jacuzzi Whirlpool Bath; **steam bath** by Steamist; **toilet and tub** by Kohler.

"City Sophistication" (pp. 110-11): **bath design** by Heidi Kleinman, 107 Demarest Ave., Bloomingdale, NJ 07403 (Architect for Morpurgo Architects, Saddle River, N.J.); **cabinetry** by J. Berger Custom Cabinetry, Hackensack, N.J.; **countertop** is Corian by Du Pont; **glass block** by Pittsburgh Corning Corp.; **floor covering** is Italian white marble, imported by Continental Creative Co., Lodi, N.J.; **shower faucets** by Grohe America; **shower stall** custom-designed of ceramic tile and white marble; **sink and sink faucets** by Kroin Architectural Complements, Cambridge, Mass.; **toilet** by American-Standard.

"A Victorian Bath" (pp. 112-13): **bath design** by Spurgeon Smith; **decorating** by Joyce Smith; **floor covering** by Armstrong; **toilet** by Kohler; **tub and brass fixtures** by Barclay Products.

"A Spa with a View of Pikes Peak" (pp. 114-15): **house design and construction** by Dominique Gettliffe, Architect D.P.L.G. (licensed by France), Zenith Concepts, Star Rte. 1153, Woodland Park, CO 80863 and Lee Cerioni, builder, of Terra-Sol, Inc., P. O. Box 3009, Colorado Springs, CO 80934; **automated curtains** (insulating curtain wall system) by Huntington Ead Inc., Broomfield, Colo.; **floor covering** of redwood deck, continuous to outside; **lighting** of built-in ceiling spots by Halo; **mirrors** on waterfall by Accent Glass Co., Colorado Springs, Colo.; **spa** by Pacific Spas, Marquis Corp., Independence, Oreg.; **windows** by Rocky Mountain Solar Glass, Boulder, Colo.

"An Atrium Spa—Underground" (pp. 116-17): **house and atrium design** by Joe Hylton & Associates, Earth Shelter and Solar Design Architects, 313 E. Boyd St., Norman, OK 73069; **ceiling** is made of hand-pressed tin; **countertops** are Formica; **floor covering** is ceramic tile by John Paschal Tile Co., Oklahoma City, Okla.; **lighting** by Halo Lighting; **wall covering** is pine car siding; **windows** by Rolscreen/Pella.

"Small Baths": "His and Hers" (p. 118): **design of baths** by Janine J. Newlin, CKD, ISID, J. J. Newlin Interiors, 42 Whippoorwill Rd., Chappaqua, NY 10514; **construction** by Skip Gorenfo, Box 95, Rte. 22, Bedford, NY 10506.

"His": **blinds** by Levolor Lorentzen, Lyndhurst, N.J.; **countertop** with integral bowl is Corian by Du Pont; **fan/light** by NuTone; **floor covering** is Marazzi 8 × 8 white tile from Marazzi USA, Inc., Dallas, Tex.; **shower stall** with Corian interior, and tile floor by American Olean; **sink and shower faucets and body sprays** by Grohe America; **toilet** by Kohler; **vanity** is Formica ColorCore made by Westchester Design House, Armonk, N.Y.; **walls** are Gabbinelli 5 × 10 mirrored tile from House of Ceramics, Portchester, N.Y.

"Hers": **countertop** is Formica ColorCore; **fan/light** by NuTone; **floor covering** is Shell by American Olean; **lighting** by NuTone; **mirror/medicine cabinet** by Allibert, Inc., Edison, N.J.; **sink and faucet** by Kohler; **steeping tub** by Kohler with **tub faucets** by Grohe America; **tub surround** of Shell by American Olean; **vanity** is Formica ColorCore with design by Janine and made by Westchester Design House; **wall covering** is overglazed design onto American Olean Shell with design by Phyllis Traynor, Phyllis Traynor Designs, P. O. Box 355, Scotts Corners, Pound Ridge, NY 10576.

"Fitting It All In" (p. 119): **house and bath design** by Richard R. Heinemeyer, Architect, 180 Cook St., Denver, CO 80206; **cabinetry** is custom-built of Nevamar laminate; **countertop** also of Nevamar laminate; **floor covering** is tongue and groove oak; **lighting** by Lightolier Genlyte; **shower and sink faucets, sink, and toilet** by American-Standard; **tile** imported from Japan; **whirlpool tub** by Kohler.

"Victorian Charm" (p. 119): **bath design** by Peter I. Ripsom., A.I.A., 1024 Chew St., Allentown, PA 18 02; **decorative accessories** by Renovator's Supply; **floor covering** is hexagonal ceramic tile, imported by Tile Distributors of Allentown, Pa.; **lighting** by Hinkley Lighting Co., Cleveland, Ohio (wall fixtures), NuTone (heat light/vent fixture); **shower and sink faucets and shower curtain rod** by Sunrise Specialty Co.; **sink** by Phylrich International; **toilet** is salvaged antique; **tub** is salvaged antique with new polyurethane finish by Bathtub Refinishing Co., Wescosville, Pa.; **vanity** is antique oak washstand converted to lavatory; **wall covering** is pine wainscoting.

"Pretty and Feminine" (p. 120): **bath design** by Karen Nelson of Ginger's Bathrooms, 945 Eglinton Ave. E., Toronto, Ontario M4G 4B5, and Joan Silver; **fixtures** from Ginger's Bathrooms (vanity basin by Porcher, faucet by Zarri, tub by Dafne); **countertop** is marble.

"A Bath in a Closet" (p. 120): **bath design** by Barbara Munn, Yorkville Design Centre, 70 Yorkville Ave., Toronto, Ontario M5R 1B9; **additional design** by Ginger's Bathrooms, 945 Eglinton Ave. E., Toronto, Ontario M4G 4B5; **faucet** by the Broadway Collection; **floor and wall covering** is marble from Caledonia Marble, Toronto; **lighting** by Residential Lighting, Toronto; **mirror** by Mirror L'Image, Toronto; **sink** by Sintisa of Italy, imported by Ginger's Bathrooms; **toilet** by Cesame S.P.A. of Italy, imported by Ginger's Bathrooms.

"Making Bath Time Playtime" (p. 121): **bath design** by Ann Louise of the Children's Design Centre, Inc., 549 Eglinton Ave. W., Toronto, Ontario M5N 1B5; **countertop** is Formica; **sink, toilet, and tub** by American-Standard; **vanity** by Canac Kitchens Ltd.

"Mirror, Mirror on the Wall" (p. 121): **bath design** by Karen Nelson of Ginger's Bathrooms, 945 Eglinton Ave. E., Toronto, Ontario M4G 4B5 and Joan Silver; **floor covering** is imported marble; **sink** by Valdarez, imported by Ginger's Bathrooms; **toilet** by Kohler.

# INDEX

Page numbers in **boldface** indicate entries for tables, graphs, and illustrations.

## A

Accessories, 54-55, 72-73, **73**
Addresses, list of, 144-48
Air Movement and Control Association, 71
Air-to-air heat exchangers, 72
American Olean Tile Company
    Cerámica Companions by, 21, 25, **27**
    Whisper Colors and Patterns by, 21
American Society of Heating, Refrigerating and Air-Conditioning Engineers (ASHRAE), 71
American-Standard
    bidets by, 24
    Ellisse by, **36**
    faucets by, 36
    Sensorium whirlpool by, 31, **31**
    Whisper Colors and Patterns by, 21
Artistic Brass
    Dual-Finish Lever Handles by, **36**
    Onyx-460 series by, **37**
    Wedgwood by, **37**
Atriums, 116-17
Automatic dispensers, 5

## B

Backsplashes, 54
Barrett, Sears, 80
Basements, baths in, 131, 132
Bathon, Heidi and Gregory, 118
Bathtubs. *See* Tubs
BathWomb, 31
Bernard, Eric, 104-5
Bidets, 4, 23-24
Birthday Bath, **81**
Bodyrooms, 6-7, **6, 87, 104, 105**
Boggs, Joseph, 83
Bollinger, Barbara and David, 98-99
Broadway Collection
    La Coquille Petite by, **36**
Budget worksheet, 141
Bumpouts, use of, 126, **126**
Butler, Diane and Robert, 106-7

## C

Cabinetry
    American-style, 49
    colors for, 51
    custom-built, 49
    European-style, 49, **56**
    factory-built, 49
    knock-down, 50
    laminate, 50, 51, **51, 58-59**
    mirrored, 55, **56**
    particle-board, 50
    stock, 49
    vanities, 48-49, **48, 50**
    wood, 49, **59**
Carpeting, 9, 65-66, **142**
Cast-iron
    sinks, 25
    tubs, 28
Caswell, Tommy, 108-9
Caton, Cassie and Michael, 90-91
Ceilings, 60-61, 64
    luminescent, 67
Cerámica Companions, 21, 25, **27**
Ceramic tile
    for countertops, 52-53, **58**
    for floors, 64
    maintenance of, **143**
    for tubs, 29, **35**
    use of, 4, **4,** 6, 18
    for walls, 62-63, **62**
Cerioni, Lee, 114
Cheever, Ellen, 126
Children's baths, 7-8, **7,** 60, 68, 121, **121,** 128
Children's Design Centre, 121
China, vitreous
    maintenance of, **143**
    sinks of, 25, **25**
Cleaning of bathrooms, 73, **142-43**
Clivus Multrum
    composting toilets by, 23
Codes
    benefits of, 129
    enforcing the, 129-30
    purpose of, 128-29
Color Coordinates program, 21
Colorcore, 63, 111
Colors, **65**
    for cabinets, 51
    for children's bath, 7, **7**
    dark, 61
    for fixtures, 4, 20
    to spruce up a bath, 18
Colton Wartsila
    Ifö Cascade unit by, **22,** 23
Compartmentalizing, 7, **14**
Composting toilets, 23
Computers, 4, 105
*Consumer Reports,* 41
Corian, 25, 29, 52, 53, **58**
    maintenance of, **142**
Costs of
    deluxe bath, **138**
    full bath, deluxe, **136**
    half bath, deluxe, **135**
    master bath, deluxe, **137**
    redesigning, 14-15, **14, 15**
    renewing, 13, **13**
    replacing, 13, **13**
Countertops, 51
    ceramic tile, 52-53, **58**
    Corian, 53, **58**
    laminate, 52, **58-59**
    marble, 53, **53, 58**
    materials for, 52
    2000X, 53
Cultured Marble Institute, 25

## D

Delta Faucet Company, 36
    Award Collection by, **37**
Deluxe bath, 138-39, **138**
Des Champs Laboratories, 72
Designing baths
    budget worksheet, 141
    codes, 128-30
    cost of, 134
    heating requirements, 132
    installing ventilating fans, 134
    keeping records of your choices, 139-40
    length of time needed, 134
    problems, how to deal with, 126-27
    safety and, 128
    upper-floor baths, 132-34
    water connections, 130-32
Dimmers, 68
Doors, pocket versus swinging, 17
Double sinks, 7, 83
Drain-waste-vent-system (DWV), 130-32
Dressing areas, 5
Dressing room inserts, 55, 58
Du Pont de Nemours & Company, E. I.
    Corian by, 25, 29, 52, 53, **59,** 142

## E

Electrical outlets, **57,** 68
Electric heaters, 41
Eljer Plumbingware
    bidets by, 24
    Blended Hues by, **34**
    Cerámica Companions by, 21, 25, **27**
    sinks by, **26**
    tubs by, **34**
Energy-saving innovations, 4, 37
    shower heads, 38
    toilets, 22-23, **22,** 37
Eric Bernard Designs, 104
European design, 4, 36, 49, **56, 65**
Evanson, Stephanie and Jack, 86-87
Exercise equipment, 4, 6-7, **6, 87**

## F

Family baths, 7, 17
Fan-assisted ceiling heaters, 41
Faucets
    chrome versus brass, 36
    foreign-made, 37
    how to select, 36
    mixer, 128
    shower and tub, 37-38
    sink, 36-37
    styles, **36, 37**

## Index

Favet, Philippe, 94
Fiberglass
    maintenance of, **142**
    shower stalls, 32
    sinks, 24-25
    spas, 31
    tubs, 28
Fireplaces, 4
Fisher, Anna and Art, 80-81
Fixtures
    antique, 38-39
    colors for, 4, 20
    selecting, 12, **12**
Fixture sizes and clearances
    for bidets and lavatories, **124**
    for showers, **125**
    for toilets, **125**
    for tubs, **125**
Flexwatt Corporation, 41
Floor plans
    drawing of, 125, **126**
Floors, 60
    carpeting for, 65-66
    ceramic tile for, 64
    marble for, 64
    vinyl, 64-65
    wood, 65
Formed-steel tubs, 28
Formica Corporation
    2000X by, 25, 29, 52, 53, **58**, **142**
Fraker, Harrison, 84
Full bath, deluxe, 136, **136**
Furniture, 72

### G
Gas heaters, 40
Gelormino, Robert, **13**
Gettliffe, Dominique, 114
Ginger's Bathrooms, 120, 121
Glass
    maintenance of, **142**
    use of, 4, 18, **62**, **69**
Glass block, 70, **84**
"Greek, The," tub, 17
Greer, Marsha and Scott, 116-17
Grohe America
    faucets by, 36
GroLite, 75
Ground-fault circuit interrupters, 68, 128, 129, 132
Gym-baths, 6-7, **6**

### H
Hahne, Linda and Wally, 92-93
Hair dryers, in-wall, 4
Half bath, deluxe, 134-35, **135**
Handicapped, baths for the, 9, **39**, **126**
Hastings Tile & Il Bagno Collection
    sinks by, **26**
Haviland Vanity, **25**
Heated towel bars, 5, 55
Heaters, types of, 40-41
Heating systems
    improving, 40-41
    options for, 41, 132
Heat lamps, 42
Heinemeyer, Diana and Richard, 119
Home Ventilating Institute (HVI), 71
Hot tubs, 8, **8**, 9, 29, 30-31, **30**, **82**

Huppe
    shower enclosures by, 33
Hylton, Joe, 116

### I
Ifö Cascade unit, **22**, 23

### J
Jarek, Claire and Ted, 94-95
Jeannette, Brion S., 92

### K
Karlin, Edward, 96-97
Karren, Fred, **14**
Kleinman, Heidi, 110
Knock-down cabinets, 50
Kohler Company
    Antique Series by, **37**
    bidets by, 24
    Birthday Bath by, **81**
    Color Coordinates program of, 21
    Environment Masterbath by, 31
    faucets by, 36
    "Greek, The," tub by, 17
    sinks by, **26**, **27**
    toilets by, 121

### L
Laidman, Cecily, 84-85
Laminates, 29
    for cabinets, 50, 51, **51**, **58-59**
    for countertops, 52, **58-59**
    maintenance of, **142**
    tamboured, 51-52
    for walls, 63
Landis, Robin and Sam, 102-3
Larry, Fern and Mitchell, 121
Laundry facilities, 7, 42-43, **43**
"Lift" sink, 25
Lighting, 66
    diffused overhead, 67
    electric, 66-68, **67**
    incandescent versus fluorescent, 68
    luminescent ceiling and, 67
    natural, **68**, 69-70
    night-lights, 68
    recessed, 67, **67**
    space and, 18
    theatrical, 67, **95**
    underwater, 30
Louise, Ann, 121
Luminescent ceiling, 67

### M
Mansfield Plumbing Products
    Quantum by, 23
    urinals by, 23
Marble
    cultured, 53, **53**, **58** 142
    for floors, 64
    maintenance of, **142**, **143**
    use of, 4, 9, 25, **59**
    for walls, 62
Master bath, deluxe, 137, **137**
Master baths, 5, 17-18
Means *Home Improvement Cost Guide*, 134
Metal
    maintenance of, **143**
Mirrors
    on cabinets, 55, **56**, **86**

    on ceilings, 64
    floor-to-ceiling, 6
    to increase space, 4, **14**, 18, **90**, **100**, **101**, **108**, **121**
    maintenance of, **142**
    triptych, 85, **85**
    for walls, 63
Mr. Steam, **40**, 89
Moen Group/Stanadyne
    gooseneck faucet by, 36
    Moen Widespread by, **36**
Mudrooms, 8
Munn, Barbara, 100, 120

### N
National Spa & Pool Institute, 32
Nelson, Karen, 120, 121
Newlin, Janine, 118
Night-lights, 68
NuTone, 72

### O
Onyx, cultured, 25

### P
Paint
    for ceilings, 64
    spray, 38
    for walls, 63
Particle-board cabinets, 50
Paul Associates
    Haviland Vanity by, **25**
Pedestal sinks, 4, 24
Phylrich
    sinks by, **26**
Plants
    lists of, **76-77**
    use of, 4, 73-75, **74**, 106, **106**, **107**
Plaskolite
    Bath Wraps by, 32-33
Plastic piping, 129
Platforms
    for tubs, 29
Plumbing
    connections, 130-32
    materials, 129
Porcher
    fixtures by, **27**
Powder rooms, 7, 16-17
Pruner, Karel, 96

### Q
Quantum, 23

### R
Radiant heating systems, 41, **88**, 132
Railex automatic garment organizer, 105
Recessed lighting, 67, **67**
Refrigerators, small, 5
Remodeling
    cost to redesign, 14-15, **14**, **15**
    cost to renew, 13, **13**
    cost to replace 13, **13**
    questions to ask, 10-12
    ways to spruce up a bath, 18-19
Resurfacing, 38-39
Romex wiring, 129
Routing of pipes, 133, **133**
Rubber floors, 6

## Index

**S**
Safety in bathrooms, 58, 128
Saunas, 5, 40, **40, 41**
Schuman, Rhoda, 88
Scott, Heather and Allen, 100-101, 120
*Sensible Way to Enjoy Your Spa or Hot Tub: An Essential Safety Guide, The*, 32
Sensorium whirlpool, 31, **31**
Sewage lift pumping system, 131
Sherle Wagner International
   sinks by, 25, **27**
Shower curtains, 33
Shower heads, 38
Shower stalls
   ceramic tile for, **35**
   corner, **35**
   curtains for, 33
   doors for, 33
   faucets for, 37-38
   fiberglass, 32
   space for, 17
   with tubs, 32, **33**
Silver, Joan, 120, 121
Sinks, 24-25, **26-27**
   cast-iron, 25
   double, 7, 83
   faucets for, 36-37
   fiberglass, 24-25
   integral countertop, 25
   pedestal, 4, 24
   separate, 24-25
   vanity-top, 24
   vitreous-china, 25, **25**
   wall-hung, 24
Skylights, 4, 9, **15**, 18, 70
Small baths, 7-8, **7, 118-21**
Smith, Joyce and Spurgeon, 112-13
Soft Bathtub Company
   soft tubs by, 29
Solicor, 63
Space
   around tubs, **15**
   creating, 15-16
   lighting and, 18
   mirrors to increase, 4, **14**, 18, **90, 100, 101, 108, 121**
   for powder rooms, 16-17
   skylights to increase, 4, 9, **15**, 18, 70
   for tubs or shower stalls, 17
Space-stretchers, 4
Spas, 8, 9, **9**, 29, 30-31, **30, 114**
   fiberglass, 31
   outdoor, **31**
   portable, 31
   questions to ask before buying, 32
Stack effect, 134
Steam machines, 39, **40**
Steam rooms, 5
Stereo equipment, 4, 9

Stone
   use of, 29
Storage space, 11, **11, 13**, 18-19, **19, 56-57**. *See also* Cabinetry
   above toilets, 47
   accessories and, 54-55
   around windows, 47
   for clothes, 55, 58
   planning of, 44-45, **46**
   selection of storage devices, 46-47
   types of, 47
Strachan, Joan and Michael, 82-83
Sunken tubs, 29
   soft tubs, 29, **34**
Sunlamps, 42
Sunrise Specialty Company
   sinks by, **27**
Sunspaces, 5, 8, 70
Superinse, 23
Sussman, Lila and Richard, 88-89
Swan Corporation
   Shower Shell by, 33

**T**
Taniguchi, Alan, 87
Tankless heaters, 40-41
Telephones, 4
Television sets, 4
Texas A&M University, Texas Engineering Experiment Station of, 70-71
Theatrical lighting, 67, **95**
Thetford Corporation
   Superinse by, 23
Thorpe, Phil, 84-85
Toilets, 22-23, **22**
   composting, 23
   storage space above, 47
Towel bars, **56**
Tub rooms, 8-9, **8**
Tubs, **34**. *See also* Hot tubs; Spas; Whirlpool tubs
   basic, 28
   cast-iron, 28
   ceramic tile, 29, **35**
   faucets for, 37-38
   fiberglass, 28
   formed-steel, 28
   oversized, 28-29
   platforms for, 29
   soft, 29, **34**
   space and, **15**, 17
   sunken, 29
Tucker, Susan and Tom, 114-15
2000X, 25, 29, 52, 53, **58**
   maintenance of, **142**

**U**
Underwater illumination, 30
Underwriters Laboratories, 30, 68

U.S. Dept. of Housing and Urban Development (HUD), 71
Upper-floor baths, 132-34
Urinals, 23

**V**
Vanities, 48-49, **48, 50**
Ventilating fans
   installing, 134
   use of, 70-72, **71**
Ventilation, 70-72
Villeroy & Boch, 90
   "Lift" sink by, 25
Vinyl floors
   maintenance of, **143**
Vinyl tiles, 64-65
Vinyl wall coverings
   maintenance of, **143**

**W**
Wall heaters, 41
Wall-hung sinks, 24
Wallpaper, 18, 63, 64
Walls, 60, 61
   ceramic tile for, 62-63, **62**
   decorative laminates for, 63
   marble for, 62
   mirrors for, 63
   paint for, 63
   wallpaper for, 63
   wood for, 63-64, **64**
Water connections, 130-32
Water experience rooms, 8-9
Waterfall, indoor, 114-15
Water heaters, 40
Water Jet Corporation
   BathWomb by, 31
Weaver, Susan, 119
Wet bars, 4, 9
Whirlpool tubs
   Sensorium whirlpool, 31, **31**
   use of, 4, 5, 29-30, **29, 31, 35, 84, 94, 97, 98, 106, 107**
Windows
   storage space around, 47
   treatment of, 18, 69
   use of, **80**
Witt, Juanita and Frank, 110-11
Wonderboard, 62-63
Wood
   cabinets, 49, **59**
   for ceilings, 64
   for floors, 65
   maintenance of, **143**
   use of, 4, **4**, 9, 18, 29
   for walls, 63-64, **64**

**Z**
Ziegenfuss, David, **39**